THE HISTORY AND CONQUEST OF

common diseases

the history and conquest of

Donald C. Balfour	M.D., LL.D., D.Sc., F.R.C.S. Eng.
E. M. Brockbank	M.B.E., M.D., F.R.C.P.
William Brockbank	M.A., M.D., F.R.C.P.
Harold Burrows	C.B.E., Ph.D., F.R.C.S. Eng.
Douglas J. Campbell	T.D., F.R.C.P., D.P.H.
A. P. Cawadias	O.B.E., M.D., F.R.C.P.
W. S. C. Copeman	O.B.E., M.D., F.R.C.P.
Terence East	M.A., D.M., F.R.C.P.
A. White Franklin	M.B., B.Ch., F.R.C.P.
Edward F. Hartung	M.D.
William G. Lennox	M.D.
Ralph H. Major	M.D.
Lewis J. Moorman	M.D., B.S., F.A.C.P.
Edward L. Murphy	M.D., M.R.C.P.
George Rosen	M.D., Ph.D.
R. Scott Stevenson	M.D., F.R.C.S. Ed.
C. H. Stuart-Harris	M.D., F.R.C.P.

common

diseases

EDITED BY

WALTER R. BETT

M.R.C.S., L.R.C.P., F.R.S.L., F.S.A. Scot.

norman : university of oklahoma press

By WALTER R. BETT

Editor and contributor, *The History and Conquest of Common Diseases* (Norman, 1954)

The Preparation and Writing of Medical Papers for Publication (London, 1953)

The Infirmities of Genius (London and New York, 1952)

Osler: The Man and the Legend (London, 1951)

The Short-lived Spring: Poems (London, 1934)

Editor and contributor, *A Short History of Some Common Diseases* (London, 1934)

Library of Congress Catalog Card Number: 54–10060

Copyright 1954 by the University of Oklahoma Press, Publishing Division of the University. Composed and printed at Norman, Oklahoma, U.S.A., by the University of Oklahoma Press. First edition.

To the Library Staff
of the Royal Society of Medicine
with admiration, affection, and gratitude

"Would—would that there were

A book on that shelf

To teach an old man

To teach himself!—"

—Walter de la Mare: *In a Library*

preface

THE forerunner of this book, *A Short History of Some Common Diseases,* was published in 1934 by the Oxford University Press in London. Intended "mainly for students and practitioners of medicine, and possibly also for patients," it has long been out of print, and the majority of the original contributors have since died. The present volume is virtually a new book. It is intended mainly for patients, but also for the medical profession. The editor is grateful to his distinguished colleagues who have lavished their time, their learning, and their wit upon its production; and to his secretaries, Miss Sylvia J. Caveley and Mr. T. H. Bishop, for their untiring and cheerful help. The book is dedicated as a reward and as a tribute of affection and gratitude to the library staff of the Royal Society of Medicine for reasons which it is hoped will be obvious to them, but not to others.

WALTER R. BETT

London
August, 1954

contents

THE HISTORY AND CONQUEST OF

common diseases

BY GEORGE ROSEN
M. D., Ph. D.*

chapter 1 / acute communicable diseases

(DIPHTHERIA, SCARLET FEVER,
MEASLES, GERMAN MEASLES,
SMALLPOX, CHICKEN POX,
MUMPS, AND WHOOPING COUGH)

THE HISTORY of disease is fundamental for an understanding of the development of medicine and of the history of civilization. Sickness is a constant phenomenon in human life, and man everywhere endeavors to deal with it as best he can. Studies in paleopathology have shown not only the antiquity of disease, but also that it has always occurred in the same basic forms, such as infection, inflammation, disturbances of development and metabolism, traumatism, and tumors. But while these basic types have not changed, the incidence and prevalence of illness have varied from time to time and from place to place. Knowledge of such changes in the occurrence of disease is essential for an understanding of the health problems faced by communities in the course of human history, and of the thoughts and actions of those who dealt with them.

Faced with problems of endemic or epidemic disease, communities and individuals have acted in terms of some prevailing concept of the nature of illness. On the primitive level of knowledge this is gen-

* Director of preventive services, Health Insurance Plan of Greater New York, and professor of public health education, School of Public Health, Columbia University, New York. He has written several books and papers on medical history, and has been editor of the *Journal of the History of Medicine*.

erally couched in supernatural terms. Modern medicine, on the other hand, seeks to understand and manage illness by studying normal and morbid structures and processes in the body. Modern medicine identifies and differentiates many distinct diseases, defining the picture of a disease as clearly as possible in terms of its symptoms, location, and cause. This concept of distinct disease entities is, however, of comparatively recent origin.

Ancient and medieval physicians did not generally distinguish different diseases as such, but were concerned rather with various groups of symptoms exhibited by sick people. Such evidences of disordered health were explained by theories about the abnormal mixture of the body fluids (humoralism), or by the constricted and relaxed states in the solid parts of the body (solidism). As long as such conceptions of diseases prevailed, physicians could not, in the nature of the case, concentrate attention on specific seats of disease. But as soon as illness in many instances was found to be associated with local lesions in organs or in tissues of these organs, and the existence of organ pathology could be correlated with groups of signs and symptoms observed at the bedside, there emerged a concept of distinct diseases, such as diphtheria, pneumonia, and typhoid fever.

Certain difficulties must, therefore, be faced in studying the history of disease. If the very concept of disease has changed so much in the course of time, how can we decide which modern disease was meant in a document created centuries or millennia before our time? Furthermore, how shall we establish the incidence and prevalence of disease in earlier periods and in various parts of the world? After all, reasonably adequate statistical data on health and disease exist only in economically advanced countries, and even in these for only the past 100 or 150 years. Yet, despite these limitations and difficulties, it is possible to trace the history of numerous diseases—in some cases from antiquity, in others from more recent periods to the present.

The transmissibility of certain diseases was noted long before the causes of contagion were known, and communicable diseases have been recognized for many centuries. There is no doubt that the ancient world was repeatedly visited by epidemics. The possible existence of smallpox in Egypt around 1100 B.C. was suggested by M. A. Ruffer. He examined a mummy of the Twentieth Dynasty, in which the skin was "the seat of a peculiar vesicular or bulbous eruption which in

4

form and general distribution bore a striking resemblance to that of smallpox."[1]

However, the first distinct references to acute communicable diseases occur in the literature of Greco-Roman antiquity. Thucydides has a vivid account of the epidemic which broke out at Athens in the second year of the Peloponnesian War.[2] Curiously enough, there is an apparent absence of most communicable diseases in the writings of the Hippocratic collection. There is no mention of smallpox or measles, nor is there any certain reference to diphtheria, chicken pox, or scarlet fever. The great plague of Athens does not appear in the Hippocratic writings. Yet there is an unmistakable clinical description of mumps in the book known as *Epidemics I*.[3] Attention is centered chiefly on endemic disease in the Hippocratic works; included are such conditions as colds, pneumonia, malarial fevers, inflammations of the eyes, as well as various unidentified illnesses.[4]

Despite these limitations, classical antiquity provides a useful point of departure for a survey of the history of some acute communicable diseases. This chapter will present the history of diphtheria, scarlet fever, measles, German measles, smallpox, chicken pox, mumps, and whooping cough. The evolution of our knowledge of these diseases falls into three major periods, each marked by a characteristic mode of approach to the problems raised by these ailments. The first period, extending from antiquity to the end of the eighteenth century, was characterized by the use of observation. Clinical cases were recorded, and epidemic outbreaks were described. During the second period, beginning in the later eighteenth century, attention was concentrated on establishing more exact knowledge of essential pathological changes through the study of gross and microscopic morbid anatomy. The development of the microscope and of the doctrine of cellular pathology provided the major investigative tools for this period. The third period, extending from the latter part of the nineteenth century to the present, has been marked by an endeavor to establish a specific, microbiologic etiology for each communicable disease, to study the immunologic reactions of the body to infection, and to apply this knowledge for prevention, diagnosis, and treatment. This knowledge was developed through the brilliant use of the laboratory experiment and applied with dramatic success through organized public health measures. The phenomenal results achieved in the control of acute communicable diseases, particularly the reduction in mortality during infancy, childhood, and young adulthood, have brought a fundamental change in the problems of public health, especially in economically advanced countries.

§ DIPHTHERIA

Classical medical literature contains numerous references to severe sore throats, often ending in death. However, owing to the ambiguity of the terms employed by Greek and Roman writers, it is difficult to recognize diphtheria with any degree of certainty in these early accounts of ulcerous sore throat. The Greek word *kynanchē* (cynanche) was applied to various forms of acute inflammatory disease of the throat and larynx, characterized by difficulty in swallowing and in breathing to the point of suffocation. The equivalent term in Latin was *angina*.[5] While we are certainly unable to draw any firm conclusion from the symptoms described, it is probable that diphtheria was included under these comprehensive clinical concepts.

Several Hippocratic treatises contain tantalizing statements suggestive of diphtheria and its sequelae. In *Epidemics II* the writer mentions certain complications of cynanche, among them a nasal voice, difficulty in swallowing, escape of fluid through the nostrils when drinking, and inability to stand upright. Similarly, in the aphoristic collection *On dentition,* two statements seem to suggest diphtheria. The one states that "In cases of ulcerated tonsils, the formation of a membrane like a spider's web is not a good sign" (XXIV). According to the other, "Ulcers on the tonsils that spread over the uvula alter the voice of those who recover" (XXXI).[6] These comments may refer to diphtheria and the nasal voice of diphtheritic paralysis.

While there is a justifiable doubt whether the Hippocratic writings deal with diphtheria, the clinical picture of the Egyptian or Syriac ulcer described by Aretaeus the Cappadocian in the second century A.D. may be identified as diphtheria with greater certainty. He gives a clear description of a severe inflammatory disease of the throat, attacking children particularly, and accompanied by the formation of a whitish or discolored membrane covering the throat, which might extend into the mouth or descend into the windpipe, causing difficulty in breathing or suffocation. In the chapter of his

6

treatise *On the causes and symptoms of acute diseases,* where he discusses ulcerations about the tonsils, Aretaeus says:

> Ulcers occur on the tonsils; some, indeed, of an ordinary nature, mild and innocuous; but others of an unusual kind, pestilential, and fatal. Such as are clean, small, superficial, without inflammation and without pain, are mild; but such as are broad, hollow, foul, and are covered with a white, livid, or black concretion, are pestilential. Aphtha is the name given to those ulcers. But if the concretion has depth, it is an Eschar and is so called: but around the eschar there is formed a great redness, inflammation, and pain of the veins, as in carbuncle; and small pustules form, at first few in number, but others coming out, they coalesce, and a broad ulcer is produced. And if the disease spread outwardly to the mouth, and reach the columella (*uvula*) and divide it asunder, and if it extend to the tongue, the gums, and the alveoli, the teeth become loosened and black; and the inflammation seizes the neck; and these die within a few days from the inflammation, fever, foetid smell, and want of food. But if it spread to the thorax by the windpipe, it occasions death by suffocation within the space of a day.[7]

Aretaeus goes on to say that the disease was engendered in Egypt and Syria, particularly in Coelesyria, hence the name Egyptian and Syrian ulcer. He also noted that in extremely severe cases of the disease before death occurred, food and drink were regurgitated through the nostrils, hoarseness and loss of speech supervened, and there was great difficulty in breathing. Finally, such patients were released from their agony by death.

Aëtius of Amida, a writer who flourished in the sixth century A.D., described a similar disease. He noted that it occurred "most frequently in children, but also in adults and most of all in those who being in a bad state of health are particularly liable to seasonal disease." Aëtius mentions also that "In some cases the uvula is eaten up and when the sores have prevailed a long time and deepened, a cicatrix forms over them and the patient's speech becomes rather husky and, in drinking, liquid is diverted upward to the nostrils. I have known a girl die even after forty days when already on the way to recovery."[8]

There would seem to be small doubt that these authors had observed cases of diphtheria and had noted various postdiphtheritic sequelae. Furthermore, from an epidemiological viewpoint, the disease appears to have been endemic in the Mediterranean area, occurring in Italy, Greece, Syria, and Egypt, and may have been especially prevalent around the eastern and southeastern shores of the Mediterranean. That there were recurrent epidemic outbreaks may, perhaps, be inferred from a statement by Macrobius. He speaks of an epidemic at Rome in A.D. 380, during which sacrifices were offered to a certain goddess for the liberation of the Roman people from a disease called angina.[9] Aëtius' remark on the seasonal occurrence of the disease which he described strengthens this inference.

From the sixth century to the sixteenth century the occurrence of diphtheria is shrouded in darkness, only fitfully illuminated by scanty and incomplete reports of epidemics of sore throat.[10] According to the Chronicle of St. Denis in A.D. 580, a great flood was followed by a "plague" called *Esquinancie* (*Squinancia*). For the year A.D. 856 Baronius recorded the occurrence of an epidemic of sore throat (*pestilentia faucium*) at Rome. Cedrenus noted an epidemic sickness known as cynanche, which was prevalent in 1004 in some provinces of the Byzantine Empire and was very fatal. A similar epidemic is also mentioned by Baronius for the year 1039 at Rome. Gilbertus Anglicus wrote in the twelfth to thirteenth century of a *squinantia* which sometimes caused death by suffocation. In the fourteenth century John of Arderne seems to have observed similar cases in England, which he called *sqwynancy*.[11] A fatal epidemic of sore throat occurred in 1337 in Holland.[12] A plague fatal to many children prevailed in 1382 in a number of European countries, among them England, Germany, and France.[13]

No doubt some of the epidemics recorded during the Middle Ages were diphtheria. However, in view of the difficulty in written reports of differentiating diphtheria from the anginal forms of scarlet fever, it is impossible to be certain of the precise biological nature of individual epidemics, even when specified as "throat" epidemics. This is true as well of clinical and epidemiological reports during the sixteenth, seventeenth, and eighteenth centuries. Even with these qualifications, however, it is clear that during the sixteenth century diphtheria emerged in Europe as a serious epidemic disease, first in the Low Countries, along the Rhine and in France, later in the western Mediterranean area, in the Iberian Peninsula, and Italy. Hecker in his account of the sweating sickness in England in 1517 described a ful-

8

minating, inflammatory disease of the throat that was often fatal in a day, the victims dying of suffocation.[14] The tongue and pharynx were covered with a tough whitish membrane, which in many cases was removed every two hours. The disease appeared first in Holland and later the same year at Basel, where within eight months it killed two thousand people. The chronicle of Frank von Word described a similar outbreak for the Rhine district, in which "men's tongues and throats were covered as with a fungus and turned white."[15] Other outbreaks occurred in 1544 and 1545 in lower Germany and along the Rhine, in 1557 in France and Germany, in 1564 along the lower Rhine, in Belgium, in Alsace, Switzerland, and, perhaps, also in Denmark, and again in 1576 along the Rhine.[16]

Clinical observations by contemporary physicians indicate that diphtheria was involved in these epidemics. In 1560 Joost van Lom (1500–63) published his *Observationum medicinalum* at Antwerp. He discussed cases of sore throat in which breathing is difficult and swallowing impeded, so that liquids drunk are regurgitated through the nostrils. He wrote:

The mouth is open wide, gasps for cool air and discharges a frothy saliva. The tongue hangs out and it frequently agitated like that of over-ridden horses. The liquor drunk returns through the nostrils, the lips become livid, and the neck is rendered rigid and contracted. Sight and hearing are dull, and on account of the violence of the suffocation, the patient neither knows what he hears or says or does, till at last being seized with a syncope he dies.[17]

Why such patients suffocated was indicated by Guillaume de Baillou (1538–1616), a French physician, who has left us striking descriptions of the plague, rheumatic fever, diphtheria, and whooping cough. In describing the epidemic constitution of 1576 at Paris, he relates that people died after taking ill with a sore throat. They developed a swelling of the pharynx, a growling hoarseness, and difficulty in breathing. Baillou reports the case of a boy who died of this disease and whose body was examined after death. "The surgeon said he sectioned the body of the boy with this difficult breathing, & with the disease (as I said) of unknown cause; sluggish resisting phlegm, was found which covered the trachea like a membrane and the entry & exit of air to the exterior was not free: thus sudden suffocation."[18] In discussing

9

a similar epidemic in 1576, Baillou suggested the opening of the throat to prevent suffocation. Although tracheotomy had been mentioned in antiquity and the Middle Ages, it was first practiced extensively by Marco Aurelio Severino (1580–1656), an Italian anatomist and surgeon, in 1610 during an epidemic of diphtheria at Naples.

A series of deadly epidemics that swept the Spanish and Italian peninsulas from the end of the sixteenth century made possible the next important contributions to the developing knowledge of diphtheria.[19] From 1583 to 1618 Spain and Portugal were ravaged. The disease flared up anew in 1630, once again in 1666, and in 1690 was still considered prevalent in Spain and Portugal. From Spain the disease spread to Italy, first breaking out in 1618 at Naples and then spreading all over southern Italy and Sicily between 1618 and 1620. In 1642 and 1650 diphtheria was again epidemic in Italy in a highly malignant form. In Spain the disease was known popularly as *garrotillo,* because the suffocation which ended the patient's life resembled that brought about by garroting, the Spanish method of executing criminals. The year 1613, when a murderous epidemic ravaged Spain, became known as *anno de los garrotillos.* The colloquial designation in Italy was *male in canna,* gullet disease. Physicians gave it various Latin names: *morbus suffocans, morbus strangulatorius,* and *angina ulcerosa.*

These epidemics called forth a large number of excellent studies by Spanish and Italian physicians. Full, lucid accounts were given by the following:

Villa-Real, J. de (1611): *De signis, causis, essentia, prognostico et curatione morbi suffocantis.* Alonso y de los Ruyzes de Fontecha, J. (1611): *Disputationes medicae super ea quae Hippocrates, Galenus, Avicenna, necnon at alii Graeci, Arabes, et Latini de anginarum naturis, speciebus, causis, et curationibus scripsere diversis in locis; et circa affectionem hisce temporibus vocatan Garrotillo* . . . . Perez de Herrera, C. (1615): *Brevis tractatus de essentia, causis, notis, praesagio, curatione et praecautione faucium et gutturis anginosorum ulcerum, morbi suffocantis Garrotillo Hispane appellati.* Perez Cascales, F. (1611): *Liber de affectionibus puerorum, una cum tractatu de morbo illo vulgariter garrotillo appellato* . . . . Sgambatus, J. A. (1620): *De pestilente faucium affectu Neapoli saeviente opusculum.* Carnevalis, J. B. (1620): *De epidemico strangulatorio affectu*

Acute Communicable Diseases

.... Cletus, A. (1620): *De morbo strangulatorio opus*. Nola, F. (1620): *De epidemio phlegmone anginoso grassante Neapoli.*

Almost without exception, these writers, as well as others who have not been mentioned, accepted the communicable character of the disease. In discussing the problem of communicability an Italian author, Cortesius of Messina, who published a book on the disease in 1625, relates the following case: A warden of St. Francis, who had been taken ill with an inflammation of the tonsils and uvula, complained of bad breath. To make sure that his breath was foul, he asked a particular friend of his to smell it. In the presence of Cortesius the man did what the warden requested; a few hours later he took to his bed with a sore throat and died of suffocation four days later. "From this instance," says Cortesius, "I have come to the conclusion that the disease is more or less contagious."[20]

Various authors indicated that the diagnostic signs of the disease were not always the same. Nevertheless, all agreed on certain common features, such as the appearance of the diphtheritic membrane, the septic character of the disease, and the difficulty in breathing. Villa Real described the membrane as elastic like wet leather or parchment, having observed this fact when patients coughed up the membrane, or in the course of post-mortem examinations. He also mentioned the high mortality of the hemorrhagic form of the disease. Herrera described cutaneous diphtheria, and Sgambati pointed out that the formation of the membrane was not always accompanied by ulceration.

Treatment consisted in the application of leeches at the beginning of the illness. Later in the disease scarification was employed as well as topical application of acids, alum, copper, arsenic, and other cauterizing substances. As previously indicated, tracheotomy was frequently performed in Italy.

Interest in these epidemics was not limited to Spain and Italy. In 1646 a small book entitled *De angina puerorum, campaniae siciliaeque epidemica* was published at Paris by Thomas Bartholin (1616–80), known for his work in anatomy.[21] This was a careful clinical study in which Bartholin expressed the view that the disease is contagious. Furthermore, he was impressed by the involvement of the nervous system. "It has the insidious character," he says, "of a toxic disease, in which air contaminated with the virus is inhaled through the nos-

11

trils and works its way surreptitiously through the cribriform plate to the brain within." As evidence of its relationship to the nervous system, Bartholin described the occurrence of weakness and squint in a child following recovery. His book also contained a short discourse on tracheotomy by Moreau, professor of medicine at Paris. The discourse was a reply to a request by Bartholin for an opinion on the value and safety of this operation for preventing suffocation of children suffering from diphtheria. Moreau reported that he had performed it twice in adults, with recovery in both cases. He saw no reason why the operation could not be performed with equal success in children.

Slowly but surely the differentiation of epidemic sore throat of a malignant type as a specific disease was being made. Toward the end of the seventeenth century, however, the violence of the disease appears to have abated, and the interest of physicians in it declined. This is not to say that the disease was completely absent. As the eighteenth century advanced, diphtheria again became increasingly prevalent in Europe and broke out as well in Great Britain and America, although nowhere with such virulence as in the Spanish and Italian epidemics of the preceding century. The French botanist Joseph-Pitton de Tournefort (1656–1708) reported an epidemic of malignant sore throat among children on the Ionian Islands, particularly in Milos, in 1701. In the same year outbreaks occurred anew in certain Spanish provinces.[22]

The American colonies, however, suffered the first major attack of the eighteenth century. Between 1735 and 1740 a deadly epidemic, commonly known as the throat distemper, broke over New England.[23] From the various descriptions and discussions of the disease it seems clear that the term "throat distemper" covered both diphtheria and scarlet fever. The first large-scale outbreak began at Kingston, New Hampshire, early in 1735. "The general description of [the disease]," wrote a contemporary historian, "is a swelled throat, with white or ash-colored specks, an efflorescence on the skin, great debility of the whole system, and a strong tendency to putridity." In 1736 William Douglass described it as "a new epidemical eruptive military fever with an *angina ulcusculosa.*"

Actually, outbreaks of throat distemper had been reported in the American colonies in the seventeenth century.[24] Cotton Mather noted that "in December, 1659, the (until then unknown) Malady of Bladders in the Windpipe, invaded and removed many children; by Opening of one of them the Malady and Remedy (too late for very many) were discovered." In succeeding years sporadic outbreaks of contagious throat infections were recorded: New England, 1673; Virginia, 1686; Connecticut, 1689; and South Carolina, 1724. From accounts of such outbreaks it seems quite clear that diphtheria and scarlet fever had been prevalent in the colonies before the murderous storm broke at Kingston.

Beginning in 1735 the epidemic wave involved all New England, spreading out from two foci, one at Kingston, the other in Connecticut. The relationship between these foci is unknown; most probably they represent spontaneous outbreaks. By 1740 most of the New England area had been affected by the throat distemper, and epidemics were breaking out in other sections. Early in 1736 the disorder spread to Rhode Island, Connecticut, and New Jersey; and by 1740 New York had been involved. Gradually the disease moved south, reaching Pennsylvania in 1746 and South Carolina in 1750–51.

The throat distemper continued to flare up in various parts of the colonies during the later eighteenth century. From 1750 to 1755 it was constantly present in New England and New York. Philadelphia experienced a major outbreak in 1763, and New York was attacked in 1769. Based upon his experience in this epidemic, Samuel Bard (1742–1821), professor of medicine at King's College, in 1771 published a monograph entitled *An enquiry into the nature, cause and cure of the angina suffocativa, or sore throat distemper, as it is commonly called by the inhabitants of this city and colony.* It contains a classic description of diphtheria, including an account of the findings in three autopsies performed by Bard. In each instance he was able to demonstrate the diphtheritic membrane in the windpipe.[25] He also pointed out that the disease was confined to children under the age of ten, for the most part, and that it was communicable, being transmitted from person to person. An epidemic that occurred in South Carolina in 1770 was described by Lionel Chalmers in *An account of the weather and diseases of South Carolina,* which appeared in 1776. He noted that the disease was limited to children under fifteen. Those attacked suffered from an inflammation of the entire throat, which eventually became ulcerated. In some cases this morbid process was accompanied by hoarseness and a fetid breath. Patients died when the infection spread down the windpipe and obstructed breathing.[26]

Beginning around the middle of the eighteenth century, epidemics of malignant sore throat were observed in France, Italy, Holland, Switzerland, Germany, and Sweden.[27] During the period 1745–50 there were outbreaks at Paris, Versailles, Orléans, Lille, Rouen, Amiens, Châlons-sur-Marne, Montpellier, and other places in France. The malady recurred at Paris in 1758, 1759, and 1762; a number of towns in Normandy were attacked in 1774; and there was an outbreak at Poitiers in 1787. A severe epidemic occurred in Italy at Cremona and in its vicinity in 1747; other outbreaks were observed at Ponte Lungo in 1759 and in Istria in 1786. In the Low Countries epidemics were reported in 1745–46, later at Utrecht in 1750 and 1769–70, and at Rotterdam and Dordrecht in 1754. Epidemics were reported in Germany in 1754–55 and 1790. From 1755 to 1762 there was an epidemic in Sweden which attacked a number of towns, among them Stockholm and Uppsala.

Concurrently, outbreaks of malignant, ulcerative sore throat also began to be noted in the British Isles. Devon and Cornwall were visited during 1734 and the following years, and then in 1739 cases of "putrid" sore throat were observed in London. A Dr. Joseph Letherland identified this condition as the *garrotillo* of the earlier Spanish writers. A severe epidemic in Cornwall in 1748 was described by John Starr, a physician of Liskeard. He termed the disease *morbus strangulatorius* and drew attention to a false membrane in the trachea as the main lesion. Nevertheless, he also noted many other signs and symptoms, including a skin rash. Epidemic occurrence of similar cases was noted by other writers, among whom two of the more prominent were John Fothergill (1712–80) and John Huxham (1692–1768). Fothergill encountered an epidemic of ulcerous sore throat in and about London in 1746 and several years thereafter. On the basis of this experience in 1748 he published *An account of the sore throat attended with ulcers*. Essentially, he described an acute febrile disease, characterized by a severe ulcerative inflammation of the throat, associated in most cases with a generalized scarlet rash on the body. From a close reading of his work it is clear that Fothergill was really describing scarlet fever in most of his cases, although there probably were a few instances of diphtheria among them. In 1757 Huxham wrote *A dissertation on the*

14

malignant, ulcerous sore-throat, derived from his experience with the Cornish epidemic first described by Starr. While the emphasis in his account is on a disease of the throat and the trachea, so many other symptoms are enumerated, including a red eruption on the body, it is evident that Huxham had encountered both diphtheria and scarlet fever and had failed to differentiate them.

This confusion of diphtheria with scarlet fever is characteristic of the eighteenth century. To be sure, it had been noted in Boston in 1736 that the throat distemper acted differently in different places, almost as if it were two distinct diseases, but this view did not prevail.[28] Furthermore, the existing confusion was intensified still further through the publication in 1765 of Francis Home's *An enquiry into the nature, cause, and cure of the croup.* Home laid great stress on the laryngeal and tracheal involvement in diphtheria. While giving a graphic account of the membranous inflammation of the larynx and trachea, he did not realize that this was simply one aspect of a broader disease entity which had been described by other physicians as *garrotillo, angina maligna,* and *morbus strangulatorius.* In fact, Home proposed that a new name, *suffocatio stridula,* be given to the condition, because "the sharp stridulous voice which I can resemble to nothing more nearly than the crowing of a cock . . . is the true diagnostic sign of the disease."[29] Finally, not only did he make a symptom pathognomonic of a distinct morbid entity, but he gave it a popular name, the "croup," which was vague in its meaning.

The confusion which centered round the conditions known as throat distemper, *angina maligna,* croup, and scarlatina, prevailed throughout the remainder of the eighteenth century and during the early decades of the nineteenth. The situation is well illustrated by a remark of Thomas Bateman in 1819. Commenting on the occurrence of measles, scarlet fever, and chicken pox in London in 1812, he wrote:

Little has occurred that is worthy of particular remark, in the progress of the diseases above enumerated, except a singular extension of the inflammation of the throat, in a case of scarlatina, to the internal membrane of the trachea, producing a true *croup.* It may possibly be doubted, whether the croup did not actually supervene, incidentally, at the time when the scarlatina was present; but, as it occurred just when the angina was at its acme, and the eruption disappearing, it seems more probable that it was a mere extension of the original inflammation. The patient, however, coughed up a cylindrical tube of coagulated lymph, of nearly four inches in length; but from this she experienced only temporary relief, and died two days afterwards.[30]

Nevertheless, it was during this period that the method was created which was to put diphtheria and other communicable diseases on a sound clinical foundation, thus making possible their further investigation. In the seventeenth century a new and important approach to the problem of the nature of illness was made by Thomas Sydenham, an Englishman. He was not primarily concerned with the ultimate nature of disease, his interest being directed rather to the phenomena observed at the bedside. Furthermore, he thought in terms of diseases rather than of disease as a general condition, and was firmly convinced that it was possible to draw up a complete picture of each disease, much as one described a plant or animal. By abstracting the pathological symptoms which he saw repeatedly in individual sick people, and co-ordinating them into separate groups, Sydenham arrived at a conception of a disease as an entity, an objective thing in itself. This idea of disease descriptions was taken up and developed further during the eighteenth century. These efforts to describe and classify morbid conditions had great shortcomings. Symptoms furnished the only basis upon which diseases could be distinguished, with the result that symptoms exhibiting a superficial similarity but differing widely in significance and pathogenesis were often grouped together. There was as yet no clear-cut idea of the intimate relationship between organ pathology and clinical observation. This situation is reflected in the status of knowledge concerning diphtheria in the eighteenth century.

This clinical trend was paralleled by an anatomical approach to the study of disease. Anatomical investigation had been sedulously cultivated for centuries, and in the course of innumerable dissections and autopsies, a mass of pathological observations was collected. Gradually the view gained ground that the reactions observed in human beings under the stress of disease are related to the lesions found after death. This idea was first given effective expression by Giovanni Battista Morgagni (1682–1771) in his work *De sedibus et causis morborum* (On the seats and causes of disease), which appeared in 1761 at Venice. In this famous book, Morgagni showed conclusively that disease has a definite seat in the organs and that pathological changes in organs are responsible for most symptoms. By firmly linking the symptoms which constitute the clinical picture of a disease to an anatomical base which explained them, Morgagni opened up the possibility of observing the mechanism of disease and indicated the path to be followed by future research in medicine.

The fusion of the clinical and anatomical trends and their systematic application was the great contribution of the Paris school of clinical pathologists from 1800 to 1850. In their work there emerged from the confusion of the eighteenth century a relatively clear and critical picture of diseases based upon the idea that there was a definite connection between the clinical findings at the bedside and the anatomical lesions observed in various organs at autopsy.

Application of this method to the problem of *angina maligna* produced a fundamental advance toward an understanding of diphtheria and gave the disease its present name. Down to about 1860 *angina maligna* prevailed widely in only one part of Europe, namely France, and it was there that this advance was made by Pierre-Fidèle Bretonneau (1778–1862), chief physician to the Hospice Général at Tours. In 1818 an epidemic designated as "scorbutic gangrene" of the mouth and throat appeared among soldiers in garrison at Tours. Shortly thereafter the civilian population near the barracks was attacked by *angina maligna*. Bretonneau studied the epidemic with scrupulous care, maintaining accurate records of his clinical observations and post-mortem studies. The epidemic prevailed from 1818 to 1820. During this period, Bretonneau performed sixty autopsies and endeavored to establish the character of the disease. In 1821 his observations and conclusions were presented to the Academy of Medicine at Paris. He undertook to prove that scorbutic gangrene of the gums, croup, and malignant angina were all forms of a specific disease. These observations, augmented by a great deal of additional material, were then published in 1826 under the title *Des inflammations spéciales du tissu muqueux, et en particulier de la diphthérite, ou inflammation pelliculaire*. This classic work swept away the concepts of croup and malignant angina, establishing in their place the doctrine of *diphthérite* as a specific disease.[31] Bretonneau coined the term *diphthérite*

from the Greek word *diphthera* (a piece of leather, a prepared hide);
in 1855, in his final memoir on the subject, he dropped it for the term
diphthérie (diphtheria) which we use today.

Bretonneau had a clear concept that communicable diseases are
specific and that this specificity is determined in large measure by the
nature of the disease cause. Based on his investigations, he concluded
that diphtheria was a specific disease (*enfin une affection morbide sui
generis*), where the characteristic anatomical feature, the false membrane, resulted from some unknown special agent acting on the body.
He knew that in man diphtheria was communicable, having traced
the disease from family to family in several deadly epidemics. According to Bretonneau, then, the diagnosis of diphtheria depended on its
epidemic occurrence and the exclusion of other diseases in which
false membranes were produced as a result of inflammation.

Bretonneau's doctrine was generally accepted in France, where it
was popularized especially by Armand Trousseau, one of his students
and long a leading French clinician. Medical opinion in Britain and
in other European countries was more divided. Although Bretonneau's concept was remarkably clear and accurate, the problem of
differentiating diphtheria from other clinically similar conditions was
still not completely solved. Nor could it be until the postulated
causative agent was discovered and its etiologic relationship to the disease demonstrated. Bretonneau did not attempt to relate the communicable principle of *diphthérite* to microscopic organisms which were
already known and were being discussed in his time. Indeed, it was
not until the close of the nineteenth century that this essential aim in
the investigation of diphtheria was finally achieved.

While Bretonneau's concept of diphtheria was a fundamental
contribution toward an understanding of the disease, it still left a
number of problems to be resolved. What was the anatomical character of the diphtheritic membrane? What other tissue changes occurred during the disease and how were they produced? Could the
disease be produced experimentally? Was the disease communicable?
If the disease was transmissible, was this due to a specific microorganism? What was the most effective way to treat and to prevent diphtheria? These problems were approached from three directions. A
number of investigators, particularly in Germany, under the influence
of Virchow's cellular pathology, undertook to study the pathological

tissue changes in diphtheria. A second direction of original research was the experimental approach to diphtheria. Efforts were made to produce false membranes by chemical and physical agents in the throat or trachea of animals, in order to ascertain the mechanism by which such products developed. Other investigations were undertaken to establish experimentally whether or not diphtheria was communicable. Research of this type was carried out on animals and humans. Related to this approach was the third area of investigation, the elucidation of the specific etiology of the disease.

An important factor in furthering these researches was the pandemic of diphtheria which broke out at various points in Europe and North America between 1856 and 1858 and soon spread to almost every part of the globe.[32] During the earlier part of the nineteenth century France, Norway, and Denmark had been the only countries severely affected by epidemics of diphtheria, but after the fifth decade of the century the disease was to be found in all civilized communities of the temperate zone. While the incidence and severity of diphtheria varied widely during this period, it was overwhelmingly a disease of childhood, not of adult life. A second epidemic wave appeared in Europe around 1890, which then declined steadily over the next thirty years.

While the spread of diphtheria gave great impetus to research, the results were generally confusing. Apart from the work of Friedrich Trendelenburg and Max Joseph Oertel, pathological anatomists and experimental investigators contributed little to establish Bretonneau's concept on a firmer foundation. Trendelenburg in 1869 reported the successful inoculation of diphtheritic material in animals; and his results were confirmed and extended by Oertel in 1871 in an elaborate investigation.[33] The solution of the problem was to come, however, from another direction—from those studies intended to elucidate the etiology of disease in terms of specific microorganisms.

As soon as the conceptual and technical bases of bacteriology were laid by Louis Pasteur and Robert Koch, attempts were made to see whether diphtheria was caused by a pathogenic microbe. After more than a decade of research, which produced more confusion than certainty, a positive contribution was made by Edwin Klebs (1834–1913) in 1883. At the Congress for Internal Medicine held at Wiesbaden that year, he claimed that diphtheria was caused by rod-shaped bacteria, some exhibiting a clubbed form. They appeared to be limited to the diphtheritic membrane, none having been found in the blood or organs of patients who had died of the disease.[34]

The following year, 1884, this finding was confirmed and extended in the exhaustive study published by Friedrich Loeffler (1852–1915), an assistant to Koch at the *Kaiserliche Gesundheitsamt,* Berlin.[35] The difficulties of earlier workers had arisen because they had operated with impure cultures of microorganisms. A simple method for the pure cultivation of bacteria was devised by Robert Koch in 1881, and within a few years had disclosed definitely the causes of numerous communicable diseases. This method was applied by Loeffler in his classic investigation; the causative agent of diphtheria was identified as a non-motile, rod-shaped bacterium, of which one or both ends frequently presented a swollen appearance, and exhibiting considerable variations in length. This is the organism now known as *Corynebacterium diphtheriae.* Loeffler found the bacteria in thirteen cases of clinical diphtheria. Cultures of the organisms were highly pathogenic for guinea pigs and small birds, and when inoculated into the trachea of rabbits, pigeons, and fowl, yielded typical false membranes. He also confirmed Klebs's finding that while the bacteria were associated with the diphtheritic membrane, especially in its deeper layers, they were not present in the internal organs. Finally, Loeffler found typical virulent bacilli in a healthy child, indicating the existence of problems still to be investigated.

The specific agent postulated by Bretonneau was now known, and attention could be turned to the questions: How was the disease produced? How was it transmitted? What were the most effective means for diagnosing, treating, and preventing diphtheria? These have been the lines of research that have occupied investigators of diphtheria during the past seventy years and with such success that today any community that wishes to do so, can within a relatively short time almost completely prevent the occurrence of diphtheria.

The first important line of investigation on these problems was initiated in a series of three papers published between 1888 and 1890 by Émile Roux (1853–1933) and Alexandre Yersin (1863–1943), two French bacteriologists.[36] On the basis of his finding that diphtheria bacilli were present at the site of the membrane but could not be recovered from internal organs, Loeffler had suggested that the disease was due to a poison elaborated by the microbe. Roux and Yersin proved that the bacillus produces such a poison, which can be separated from the bacterial cells themselves and when inoculated into animals is capable of producing the symptoms and type of death characteristic of infection with the diphtheria bacillus. Finally, stressing the importance of demonstrating the diphtheria organism in the diagnosis of the disease, they developed a technique which essentially has been employed by all subsequent investigators.

The work of Roux and Yersin was fundamental not only in clarifying the mechanism of the disease and in developing a suitable diagnostic technique, but equally in providing a point of departure for investigations which led eventually to effective methods for treatment and control. Their investigations aroused intense interest, and efforts were undertaken to create an artificial immunity to diphtheria. On December 3, 1890, Karl Fraenkel (1861–1915) published in the *Berliner Klinische Wochenschrift* the results of his studies showing that it was possible to establish an artificial immunity in guinea pigs by injecting them with attenuated cultures of diphtheria bacilli.[37] The following day Emil von Behring (1854–1917) and his Japanese coworker, Shibasaburo Kitasato (1852–1931), published in the *Deutsche Medizinische Wochenscrift* an account of immunity to tetanus.[38] In this brief but fundamental paper they pointed out that the immunity of rabbits and mice which had been treated with tetanus cultures depends on the capacity of the cell-free blood serum to render innocuous the toxic substances elaborated by the tetanus bacillus. This capacity was so durable that it still exhibited its activity when the immune serum was injected into the bodies of other animals. A week later (December 11, 1890) Behring alone published a paper on immunization against diphtheria, in which the essential facts reported in the earlier communication were confirmed as well for this disease. Thus the foundation was laid for the specific serum therapy and prophylaxis of diphtheria as well as of other communicable diseases. A year later, on Christmas night, 1891, a child in von Bergmann's clinic in Berlin became the first person to be treated with diphtheria antitoxin. It was not, however, until after Roux, on September 4, 1894, read his classic paper at the Eighth International Congress of Hygiene and Demography at Budapest that diphtheria antitoxin began to be employed generally.

These brilliant discoveries must, however, also be seen in a larger frame of reference. They are products of a long period of research in which the bactericidal and immunological properties of the blood have been thoroughly studied. Since the discovery of diphtheria anti-toxin, continued investigation of the blood has yielded other effective substances for the prevention and treatment of disease. These will be discussed in relation to some of the other acute communicable diseases.

While bacteriology was revolutionizing the diagnosis and treatment of diphtheria, an important method for the relief of respiratory difficulty in laryngeal diphtheria was published in 1885 by Joseph O'Dwyer (1841–98), a New York physician.[39] Intubation, the method proposed by O'Dwyer, was not actually new, having been mentioned and discussed in medical literature at various times from Hippocrates onward. Pierre Joseph Desault had used it in the eighteenth century, and it had again been revived in 1858 by Loiseau and Bouchut. The operation of tracheotomy, already practiced in Italy in the sixteenth century, had been brought into favor by Bretonneau and Trousseau, and could not be supplanted by the practice of intubation. In 1881 Sir William Macewen of Glasgow reported several cases in which tubes ten to fourteen inches long had been passed into the larynx to relieve obstruction of breathing. O'Dwyer's work, however, revived the practice and successfully introduced it into the operative treatment of laryngeal diphtheria.

New York City was the scene of other important contributions. It was here that the new knowledge of bacteriology was first really applied in public health practice. In 1892, as a result of the cholera epidemic in Hamburg, New York City established a bacteriological laboratory in the Health Department; this was the first municipally operated public health laboratory in the United States.[40] After the cholera scare was over, the laboratory, instead of being discontinued, began to employ bacteriological procedures for the control of diphtheria. In 1893 a young physician, William Hallock Park (1863–1939), was placed in charge of this work as bacteriological diagnostician and inspector of diphtheria. In the same year, Park and Alfred L. Beebe, his assistant, carried out a series of investigations in which they definitely established the concept of the carrier in diphtheria and demonstrated the value of routine bacteriological examination in the diagnosis of the disease. In 1895 a report of this work was issued as

22

Scientific Bulletin No. 1 of the New York City Health Department.[41] Loeffler and others had noted virulent bacilli in the throats of well individuals, as well as the persistence of infecting organisms during convalescence. It was in connection with the cholera epidemic of 1892–93, however, that the significance of the human carrier as a source of infection was generally realized. In 1893 Koch emphasized the importance of the convalescent carrier, but while he recognized the role of the well carrier, he did not regard such individuals as important. Park and Beebe examined forty-eight well family contacts to diphtheria cases and demonstrated the bacillus in twenty-four cases. They concluded "that the members of a household in which a case of diphtheria exists should be regarded as sources of danger unless cultures from their throats show the absence of diphtheria bacilli." The last important piece of knowledge was thus provided for an understanding of the process by which the disease was transmitted within a community.

Diphtheria could now be diagnosed and treated with a high degree of effectiveness. The next important advance was to be made in its prevention and control. This was achieved eventually by active mass immunization, a method developed logically from earlier knowledge on the use of diphtheria antitoxin as a passive immunizing agent as well as a therapeutic agent. In 1902 Dzierzgowsky showed that immunization in a human being could be achieved by increasing doses of diluted toxin.[42] The use of toxin neutralized by antitoxin was then suggested by Theobald Smith in 1909.[43] Von Behring in 1913 substituted such a mixture for the diluted toxin and demonstrated that it induced immunity safely in both animals and man.[44] At the same time it was necessary to know the natural history of diphtheria within the community: How many children of different ages had already acquired immunity, how many were well carriers, and what children were highly susceptible? A simple test for immunity by injecting minute amounts of toxin into the skin was developed by Bela Schick (1877–   ) in 1913.[45] This test made it possible to define more accurately the need for active immunization, as well as the results obtained thereby. Finally, in 1923 G. Ramon showed that toxin treated with formalin (anatoxin) had advantages as an immunizing agent over the earlier toxin-antitoxin mixture.[46] (Anatoxin is now known as toxoid.) Later, alum-precipitated toxoid was found to have still greater antigenic potency.

Knowledge and tools thus became available for a full-scale mass attack on diphtheria. Such an endeavor was first attempted for the protection of children by W. H. Park and Abraham Zingher (1885–1927) in New York City.[47] In 1920 active immunization of school children began, and by 1928 some five hundred thousand had been immunized. Attention was then concentrated on the preschool children, and in 1940 it was estimated that no less than 60 per cent of this group were protected. By this date the disease had been virtually eliminated as a cause of death, with the mortality rate at 1.1 per 100,000. This was in striking contrast to a rate of 785 per 100,000 in 1894. With the adoption of immunization in New York and other large cities such as Toronto, and then progressively in other countries, proof of its efficacy became increasingly evident.[48] During World War II there was a sharp rise in the incidence and severity of diphtheria in Germany as well as in certain countries occupied by the Germans, particularly Norway and the Netherlands. Since 1945, however, diphtheria immunization has been largely accepted in European public health practice, and the incidence of diphtheria has declined sharply.

There has been a steady tendency over the years to immunize at progressively earlier ages. It is now an established fact that a high percentage of susceptible infants responded well to primary immunization against diphtheria when the initial injection is given as early as the second or third month of life.[49] Today, diphtheria toxoid is increasingly being given together with tetanus toxoid and whooping cough vaccine.[50]

That the drop in diphtheria morbidity and mortality is not wholly due to preventive immunization appears to be indicated by the fact that this decline set in actually in the nineteenth century before diphtheria antitoxin began to be used generally, and continued progressively even before preventive immunization became widespread. The death rate among children up to ten years of age in New York City was 785 per 100,000 in 1894, declining to less than 300 in 1900; and in 1920, when active immunization of school children began, it fell below 100. This decline is related to the fact that certain communicable diseases, among them diphtheria, occur in waves with intervening periods during which the disease is either absent or at least significantly rarer. Consequently, it is more difficult to evaluate the effec-

24

tiveness of therapeutic or preventive measures if they are instituted during the waning of an epidemic wave. The German physician Otto-mar Rosenbach recognized this at the end of the nineteenth century and used it as an argument against claims made for the value of diphtheria antitoxin.[51] Nevertheless, whatever the relative weight of the factors that have brought about an almost complete disappearance of diphtheria, it is certain that from a statistical point of view the experience of diphtheria in large communities like New York or Toronto has been significantly better in the postimmunization period than might have been expected from the trend of either morbidity or mortality in the preimmunization period. Certainly, the downward course of diphtheria morbidity and mortality has at least been accelerated by preventive immunization.[52]

One other recent development in the knowledge of diphtheria must be noted because of the possible light it throws on the earlier history, especially epidemics, of diphtheria. An unusual and highly fatal outbreak of diphtheria appeared in 1927 in Germany. This was followed around 1929 and 1930 by the occurrence of unusually severe diphtheria in the north of England. Upon investigation it was found that the diphtheria bacillus is not a single species of microorganism, but consists of three distinct types.[53] A correlation appeared to exist between the types of organism found and the severity of the case, so that they were called *gravis, intermedius,* and *mitis.* Present evidence indicates that severe epidemics with high mortality are due to *gravis* and *intermedius,* while *mitis* is generally responsible for endemic diphtheria. Fatalities with the *mitis* strain are nearly always due to obstruction of the larynx or the trachea. Burnet has suggested that this knowledge might be used to explain epidemiological events prior to the eighteen eighties. Thus, if only *mitis* strains were present in the community, most children would become immune as a result of light infections, and there would be a number of cases of croup, that is, laryngeal diphtheria. With the introduction of virulent *gravis* or *intermedius* strains, there would be an epidemic flare-up, and on the whole the younger children who had not acquired an immunity would be chiefly affected. This does seem to explain the pandemic of 1858 and the ensuing years.[54]

Diphtheria is a disease about which we have a great deal of knowledge. Its cause, mode of transmission, the means by which the disease is caused, therapy, and prevention have all been thoroughly elucidated. Nevertheless, some problems still remain. For example, it is still not possible to outline a definite program for the protection of adult populations. Reactions to diphtheria toxoid in adults are sufficiently severe to interfere seriously with any plan for mass immunization. Fortunately, however, our present modes of prevention and control appear adequate and effective under current conditions.

§ SCARLET FEVER

The story of scarlet fever is more complicated than that of diphtheria; yet the two diseases resemble one another in several ways. Both are caused not by a single organism, but rather by a group of closely related bacteria, each group having in common the capacity to produce a single toxin. In both diseases the poison circulates in the body, attacking various organs. Throughout their history, scarlet fever and diphtheria have been diseases of infancy and childhood—the period during which immunity to the toxin is developed. And, finally, both start with an inflammation of the throat. In fact, scarlet fever may be considered as a sore throat with a diffuse, bright red skin rash in a person infected with streptococci that produce a toxin to which the patient has no effective immunity and which consequently evokes the rash.

On the other hand, there are distinct differences. The various types of diphtheria bacilli have more in common than the streptococci responsible for scarlet fever. Furthermore, in diphtheria the toxin alone accounts for practically all the damage inflicted by the bacillus, while the streptococcus can attack the body not only through the toxin, but also by direct invasion. In addition, no one has yet identified the precise factor which enables some streptococci and not others to produce scarlet fever.

The history of scarlet fever is what might be expected, given these characteristics. Because of the different types of streptococci, the disease has varied greatly in virulence and incidence from time to time. Before the sixteenth century there is no description of a disease which can be recognized with any probability as scarlet fever. Physicians of earlier periods very likely confused scarlet fever with various exanthematic diseases such as measles and German measles on the one hand,

and on the other with acute inflammatory conditions of the throat as indicated in the history of diphtheria.[55] According to Lancellotti, in the spring of 1527 children at Modena were attacked by a disease which he termed *male di scarlatina*. Whether this was scarlet fever is an open question. According to Hirsch, an account of an epidemic of 1543 in Sicily is probably the earliest notice of an outbreak of scarlet fever.[56] In 1553, however, Giovanni Filippo Ingrassia (*ca.* 1510–80), who was concerned with problems of public health and legal medicine, described a disease of children which he differentiated from measles.[57] He stated that it was commonly known as *rossania* or *rossalia,* and described the rash as covering the entire body and consisting of many large and small spots of a fiery red color so that the body appears to be aflame. Although Ingrassia did not mention that the patients suffered from a sore throat, this was evidently scarlet fever. Hecker suggested that this was probably the same disease as the *malum rosatum* of Gentile da Foligno (d. 1348);[58] so that the malady was very likely already present in the fourteenth century.

Generally, however, scarlet fever was still confused with various exanthematic diseases. This is evident from a passage in the *Epidemiorum et ephemeridum libri duo* of Guillaume de Baillou. Among the diseases which occurred in the winter of 1574, he described *Rubiolae* as a condition quite distinct from measles.[59] Nevertheless, one can hardly say what disease in our present terminology was intended. Among the symptoms are fever, hoarseness, sore throat, difficulty in swallowing, and swellings of the glands about the ears. "*Rubiolae,*" wrote Baillou, "comes near to erysipelas in its nature, measles and variola to a papular eruption." Certainly, this is not German measles; it appears to correspond more closely to scarlet fever.

The establishment of scarlet fever as a distinct clinical entity was first accomplished in the seventeenth century. In the earlier part of this period attention seems to have been concentrated on the disease in Germany owing to epidemic outbreaks. There are occasional references to a "red sickness" (*Rotsucht*) in popular writings; and in 1624 Greg. Horst published a book in which he dealt with the red sickness as distinct from smallpox, measles, and *röteln* (possibly rubella). Accounts of epidemics at Wittenberg and Breslau in 1627 by Daniel Sennert (1572–1637) and his brother-in-law Michael Döring (d. 1644) contain the first clear description of scarlet fever with all its distinctive features.[60] In the spring of 1625 Döring had already observed three cases and seems to have called Sennert's attention to the disease. Sennert noted the sequence in which the rash appears and declines— first, the discrete punctate spots, which then merge into a general redness so that the entire body appears as if on fire. The redness in turn fades away, "and wide red spots again appear as in the beginning, which however disappear the seventh or ninth day with the skin falling off like scales." Not only was Sennert the first to note the scaling (desquamation) following the rash, but he was also the first to report serious complications of scarlet fever, particularly the dropsy resulting from inflammation of the kidney and the involvements of the joints (polyarthritis).

For many years thereafter the disease does not appear to have occurred in epidemic form. Not until 1642 is there a report of another outbreak, this time in Brieg, where it returned between 1655 and 1658, the second time in a much more malignant form. Daniel Winkler (d. 1658), a local physician, described the disease as "fiery measles" (*Morbilli ignei*). In 1652 scarlet fever was epidemic for the first time in Schweinfurt, where there were many fatalities among children. The rash appeared on the third or fourth day of the illness, and its disappearance was followed by desquamation. Fehr, the physician who reported the outbreak, designated it as *Rosalia*. An exceedingly malignant epidemic occurred in Thorn in 1664. Many children died on the second day of the illness, some even on the first day; and physicians were unable to decide whether the severe inflammation of the throat or the dropsy was the greater danger.[61]

During the later seventeenth century scarlet fever seems to have been prevalent in various parts of Europe and in the British Isles. Indeed, it was in England that the disease finally received the name by which it has been known to the present. In 1676 Thomas Sydenham (1624–89) introduced into the third edition of his *Observationum medicarum* a short chapter entitled *Febris scarlatina*.[62] This chapter, which is little more than a note, has been much overpraised. Sydenham described it as a very mild disease, which as he put it was hardly more than a name, even though there were occasional fatalities. The disease occurred chiefly in late summer, affecting children more than adults. Sometimes entire families were attacked. It began with a fever, then the skin became covered with small red spots that became broad-

28

er and eventually confluent. The eruption persisted for two or three days and vanished. As the skin returned to its normal condition, it shed fine branny scales. In view of the mildness of the disease, Sydenham advised a conservative regimen of treatment. The patient should be kept indoors, not necessarily in bed, and on a light diet. Bloodletting and heart remedies were unnecessary. Sydenham also differentiated scarlet fever from measles.

Apparently his use of the designation, *Febris scarlatina,* was simply a translation into Latin of a term in common use at the time. This is evident from the notation of Samuel Pepys in his diary on November 10, 1664: "My little girle Susan is fallen sick of the meazles, we fear, or, at least, of a scarlett fevour."[63] Seemingly, the lay public also regarded scarlet fever as a milder disease than measles and in some degree differentiated the two conditions. Interestingly enough, Sydenham, like Sennert before him, does not mention the sore throat of scarlet fever, but unlike his predecessor he does not refer to any complications such as dropsy. It is likely that Sydenham never saw severe scarlet fever. This seems also to have been the experience of Sir Robert Sibbald (1643–1712), professor of medicine at Edinburgh and first president of its College of Physicians. Sibbald described scarlet fever in 1684 as a new disease in Scotland, commenting on its mild character.[64]

This was not the experience of other physicians, however. Richard Morton (1637–98), a contemporary and rival of Sydenham, who practiced in London from about 1667 almost to the end of the century, referred to scarlet fever in the second volume of his *Pyretologia,* published in 1694.[65] In it there are two chapters, one entitled *De morbillis et febre scarlatina,* the other *De febre scarlatina.* Morton believed that measles and scarlet fever were the same disease, the latter being simply a confluent measles. He retained the name "scarlatina," as he put it, out of deference to the common practice of physicians. While most of the cases described by Morton are measles, several cases including that of his own daughter Marcia, aged seven, are clearly cases of scarlet fever. Furthermore, these cases all ran a stormy course and exhibited various complications (adenitis, otitis, throat abscess).

Haeser suggested a social explanation of these discrepant reports. In his opinion, Sydenham's view of scarlet fever as a mild disease probably derived from the circumstance that he practiced almost exclusively in the upper circles of society, while Morton and other physicians who practiced among the poorer classes had an opportunity to become acquainted with the full gravity of the disease.[66] Whether or not this explanation actually throws light on the differing views of Sydenham and Morton, there is no doubt that social conditions and factors have influenced the character of scarlet fever. Observers at various periods have agreed that the children of the lower social classes have been more endangered by scarlet fever and that the complications of the disease have exhibited a more malignant character than in upper-class children.[67] Furthermore, it seems plausible to suggest that the increase in the severity of scarlet fever that set in about the middle of the nineteenth century was related to the social environment and prevailing social attitudes of the period.

Nevertheless, it is clear that this is not the entire story. As a cause of mortality, scarlet fever has varied greatly over relatively short periods of time. Accounts of marked variations in the severity of the disease appear in writings of the past that are almost contemporary. For example, there is small doubt that in England scarlet fever was much more deadly during the later eighteenth century than it had been during the earlier part of the century or during the first decades of the nineteenth century. From the beginning of 1796 to the end of 1800 Robert Willan kept accounts of the cases treated at Carey Street Dispensary in London. Among these scarlet fever was hardly ever missing, and often it was the principal epidemic. In November, 1798, Willan wrote: "The fatal cases of scarlatina were in the month of November, when the disease was more extended, and more virulent than any period within my recollection since the years 1786, 1787."[68] Contrast this with the tone of Thomas Bateman's comment on scarlet fever in the fall of 1814:

The measles and scarlet fever have been very prevalent; and the former, in a few cases, were attended with considerable affections of the chest. The scarlatina has been, in all cases, accompanied by sore throat; in the adults, indeed, in two or three families, the throat, as is usual, was the only seat of the disease, as the rash did not appear on the skin. Under cool treatment, which, however, is often very imperfectly accomplished in the close and crowded apartments of the poor, these cases have uniformly done well.[69]

This passage is noteworthy, not only because of Bateman's obser-

30

vation that scarlet fever patients among the poor did well, indicating that adverse social conditions were compensated by the mild character of the disease. It is equally noteworthy because of his acute clinical observation that when scarlet fever was prevalent, some individuals, particularly adults, had a sore throat without the rash. Bateman intimates that these conditions are really the same disease, and this is now known to be the case. Individuals who are immune to the rash-producing (erythrogenic)toxin of the streptococcus suffer only from a severe sore throat (streptococcal sore throat).

The observations recorded by Willan and Bateman for London are paralleled by those of Robert Graves (1796–1853) for Ireland. Commenting in 1834 on the preceding thirty years, he said:

In the year 1801, in the months of September, October, November, and December, scarlet fever committed great ravages in Dublin and continued its destructive progress during the spring of 1802. It ceased in summer, but returned at intervals during the years 1803–4, when the disease changed its character; and although scarlatina epidemics recurred very frequently during the next twenty-seven years, yet it was always in the simple or mild form, so that I have known an instance where not a single death occurred among eighty boys attacked in a public institution. The epidemic of 1801–2–3–4, on the contrary, was extremely fatal, sometimes terminating in death, as appears by the notes of Dr. Percival, kindly communicated to me so early as the second day. It thinned many families in the middle and upper classes of society, and even left not a few parents childless. Its character seems to have answered to the definition of the *scarlatina maligna* of authors.[70]

An interpretation of these fluctuations in the character of scarlet fever is now possible in terms of our knowledge of bacterial virulence.[71] The virulence of an infective microorganism is not a specific, simple attribute, but rather a complex quality comprising a number of different components such as communicability, resistance to the defense mechanisms of the host, invasiveness or the power to multiply and spread in the host, and the capacity to produce poisonous substances. Such qualities may be found in various combinations in streptococci, so that the results that follow infection may be correspondingly varied. Furthermore, an infection is a relationship of conflict between a given host and a parasitic microorganism in which

31

the outcome is determined not only by the attributes of the invader, but also by the response of the host to invasion. Consequently, any variation in the human host may further affect the character of the disease. A realization of the possibilities inherent in this variability enables us to understand better the wide differences in severity exhibited by scarlet fever at different periods, as well as the confusions and obscurities in the history of scarlet fever epidemics and outbreaks of severe throat infections, particularly before the middle of the nineteenth century.

Epidemics of scarlet fever were described throughout Europe and in the American colonies during the eighteenth century.[72] There were reports from many cities and regions, among them Augsburg (1696, 1705), Breslau (1700), Paris (1702–12), Berlin (1716, 1717), Thuringia and Florence (1717), Scotland (1732–33), Vienna (1740–62), France (1746–51), Sweden (1741, 1763–64), Lausanne (1761), Halle and Würzburg (1763–66), Philadelphia (1764, 1769, 1774), London (1777–78), Göttingen (1780), and Chesham (1788, 1793–94). On the continent of Europe outbreaks of scarlet fever were reported from 1784 on, chiefly in Hungary, northern Germany, along the Rhine, and in Regensburg. These were generally of a mild character. After 1795, however, the disease became more severe in Germany. Between 1795 and 1805 forty thousand children were reported to have succumbed to the disease in Saxony alone.

Many physicians still confused scarlet fever with measles on the one hand and diphtheria on the other. Characteristic in this respect are the accounts of John Fothergill (1748) and John Huxham (1757), previously mentioned. More important in leading to a more precise picture of the disease was the contribution of Nils Rosén von Rosenstein (1706–73). His book on the diseases of children published in 1764 contains a description of scarlet fever based on observations made in 1741 during an epidemic at Uppsala.[73] Rosén gives a detailed, accurate clinical account and mentions the occurrence of dropsy with bloody urine as a consequence of scarlet fever. He also expressed the opinion that the disease was contagious.

Similar clinical observations were made in London 1777–78 by G. Levison, physician to a London charity called the General Medical Asylum, and in 1778 by William Withering (1741–99) of Birmingham, who introduced digitalis into medical practice.[74] Levison described cases which began with shivering and nausea, followed by fever and a crimson red rash over the chest, the extremities, and often the whole body. These patients had a sore throat. The rash scaled off on the sixth or seventh day. He noted that the sore throat and the rash were often encountered separately—the same observation reported by Bateman in 1814. The disease ended suddenly around the eighth or ninth day. In several cases there was suppuration of the glands of the neck. Dropsy was frequent after the acute disease subsided, and some patients died a month later. Withering's account differs little from that of Levison. He noted that in severe cases the rash appeared on the first or second day and that the patient might die as early as the second day. If these patients survived, discharge appeared in great quantities after several days from the nostrils, or the ears, or both. Withering noted that abscesses on both sides of the neck under the ears generally healed in a few days without much trouble. The submaxillary glands were often enlarged. He confirmed Levison's observation on the occurrence of dropsy and reported that in severe cases the patients recovered very slowly. Often they lingered for a month or six weeks from the outbreak of the disease and died eventually of debility.

By the end of the eighteenth century a clinical concept of scarlet fever had been rather generally recognized by physicians. Clinicians were clear about *Scarlatina simplex,* that is, mild scarlet fever without complications. True, there was still some confusion with diphtheria, but then shortly after the turn of the century scarlet fever declined in virulence, and for about the first quarter of the nineteenth century there was small interest in a more precise understanding of scarlatina. In the thirties, however, there was a change for the worse. Scarlet fever began to increase in virulence, culminating in a period of some forty years (1840–80), during which there were frequent and severe epidemics in Europe and America.

In 1831 an outbreak of a very malignant type occurred in Dublin, and in 1834 Ireland was ravaged by the disease which caused as many deaths as cholera had in 1832.[75] The first great epidemic covering all of England occurred in 1840, a second came in 1844, and a third in 1848. The worst epidemics in England occurred during the period 1850–90. In England and Wales the annual average death rates per million population were as follows during this period:[76]

33

Years	Death Rates
1851–60	832
1861–70	972
1871–80	716
1881–90	338

The United States experienced similar outbreaks. In New York City, for example, scarlet fever was very rarely encountered between 1805 and 1822. During these eighteen years there were only 43 reported deaths from scarlet fever. After 1822 this disease gradually assumed an epidemic character, and by the end of 1847 there were 4,874 deaths. During this period the largest number of deaths (579) was recorded in 1837; thereafter there was a progressive decline to 63 in 1845. At this time a second wave began to build up which reached its culmination in 1857 with 1,325 deaths.[77] In 1865, when the Council of Hygiene and Public Health of the Citizens' Association reported on the sanitary condition of New York, scarlet fever was noted as a prevalent and often fatal disease.[78] Chicago in 1844 had 306 deaths due to scarlet fever, and the disease continued to prevail for the next few years.[79] It was again reported in 1856 and was extremely prevalent in 1860 and 1862 in a severe form. Thereafter it disappeared for a time, but in 1868 the Chicago Board of Health reported that scarlet fever was very prevalent, although there were not as many deaths as in other cities. Characteristic is the wide variation in annual death rates. For instance, during the decade 1850–59, scarlet fever showed a maximum mortality rate of 272 per 100,000 and a minimum of 6.[80] Scarlet fever was present in Oregon in 1843. The first definite reference to an epidemic of the disease occurs in a report on epidemic diseases in Portland, in which Dr. W. B. Cardwell states that an outbreak occurred in 1864 and that it was of malignant character. Subsequently it prevailed sporadically, occasionally rising in an epidemic wave.[81] In 1868 scarlet fever was also reported as prevalent among children in Minnesota. Periodic epidemics also occurred in lumber camps of the state. By 1877 the Minnesota State Board of Health was receiving with some degree of regularity reports of scarlet fever cases from local boards. The disease was considered one of the important causes of death among children.[82]

Acute Communicable Diseases

There is no question that a change occurred after 1830, and the disease became, as Charles Creighton noted, "the leading cause of death among the infectious diseases of childhood." It remained so in Europe, in Great Britain, and in the United States until the last decades of the nineteenth century. After 1880 the severity of scarlet fever diminished, and at present it is probably milder than at any period in its history. A review of the experience of Providence, Rhode Island, with regard to scarlet fever from 1865 to 1924 shows that the death rate of children aged two to four decreased during this period from 691 to 28.3 per 100,000 [83] Since the attack rate does not present a corresponding decrease, the decline in the number of deaths cannot be attributed to a lower prevalence or to changes in the population, but must have been due to a diminution in the severity of the disease. From 1886 to 1888 one in every five cases died, while from 1923 to 1924 only one in every 114 cases ended fatally. A similar trend has been demonstrated for England and Wales. [84] The late thirties witnessed an accelerated decline in the case fatality rate. To some extent this probably reflected an improvement in medical care, since it coincided with the introduction of the sulphonamides for the treatment of scarlet fever and its complications.

These trends may be interpreted in terms of our understanding of bacterial virulence, as well as of economic and social developments since the middle of the eighteenth century. Characteristic of the past two hundred years have been the growth of cities and concomitantly a movement of population, either from rural to urban areas or from one country to another. Crowded into the filthy, insanitary environment of the early modern city, these people were inevitably exposed to infections to which they had no immunity. Where this process was not too violent, a temporary equilibrium was established from time to time. It is known, however, that immunity, if not reinforced, tends to disappear after a variable period. This would seem to explain what happened during the first quarter of the nineteenth century. One and possibly two generations of city dwellers had acquired immunity to relatively avirulent streptococci. Such immunity as had been developed to more virulent types during the later eighteenth century disappeared. As the population grew through internal increase as well as recruitment from rural areas, the number of people susceptible to virulent organisms increased. A. G. McKendrick has shown that when the proportion of susceptibles in a population approaches a "threshold density," the situation becomes favorable for an accelerated incidence of cases, that is, an epidemic outbreak.[85] It was probably at some such point around 1830 that a more virulent type of streptococcus was introduced.

The transmissible nature of scarlet fever was in large measure accepted during the nineteenth century.[86] With the development of bacteriology it was at first expected that scarlet fever would be found due to a specific microorganism like diphtheria, typhoid fever, and other communicable diseases. Some fifty years of research, however, were required before the true nature of the mechanism by which the disease is produced became apparent. Streptococci were implicated in the causation of scarlet fever at an early date, but it was not until some twenty-five years ago that the biological activity which enables these organisms to cause disease began to be understood.

Christian Albert Theodor Billroth in 1874 had described streptococci in wound infections and erysipelas, but denied their causative role in these conditions. In 1883 Friedrich Fehleisen grew streptococci in pure culture and produced erysipelas experimentally in human beings. In 1903 H. Schottmüller differentiated streptococci according to their action on red blood cells in vitro. He described three strains—hemolytic, green, and indifferent—and recognized that the hemolytic strains were potentially more virulent than the other varieties.[87] It became evident that the hemolytic streptococci were causally related to scarlet fever. As a result of the researches of Schultz and Charlton, Dochez, and the Dicks, it was recognized that the hemolytic streptococci that caused scarlet fever are distinguished by the ability to produce a specific, rash-producing toxin. In 1918 Werner Schultz and Willy Charlton showed that during the first few days of scarlet fever antitoxic sera have the ability to blanch a scarlatinal rash. This phenomenon is due to neutralization of the toxin in the skin.[88] A streptococcus was isolated as the causal organism of scarlet fever by George and Gladys Dick in 1923. They also demonstrated the existence of the toxin and developed the skin test for immunity, which bears their name.[89] At first an effort was made to use the ability to produce erythrogenic toxin as a means of identifying the scarlet fever organism. It became evident, however, that the capacity to produce the toxin is not peculiar to strains of hemolytic streptococci from scarlet fever alone, but is present also in nonscarlatinal strains. Furthermore, in 1926 Stevens and Alphonse Raymond Dochez definitely established that scarlet fever streptococci could cause throat infections without a rash. Finally, researches on the serologic identification of hemolytic streptococci made possible the determination of the principal pathogenic strains and their subdivision into types. This system was introduced by Rebecca C. Lancefield in 1928 and developed further in 1933.[90] All the strains of hemolytic streptococci that are important as human pathogens fall into one group, Lancefield's Group A. In 1934 F. Griffith independently established twenty-seven or more types of streptococci.[91] All but two or three of these have been found to belong in Lancefield's Group A. Some of these types have been found fairly often in scarlet fever, and together with other types also in such nonscarlatinal conditions as septic sore throat, otitis, tonsillitis, erysipelas, and puerperal sepsis. In short, scarlet fever can no longer be regarded as a specific disease entity, but rather as a clinical manifestation of infection with one of the types of Group A hemolytic streptococci.

This concept of scarlet fever has altered our ideas in several directions. Following the discovery of the erythrogenic toxin, efforts were made to confer artificial immunity, both active and passive. Antitoxic horse serum was produced and used in treatment, as well as to confer temporary passive protection against scarlet fever.[92] A method of active immunization was also developed. This method does provide protection against the clinical condition that we call scarlet fever, but there is no convincing evidence that it protects against infections with Group A hemolytic streptococci that do not produce a rash. As a result, in practice, active immunization is today limited almost entirely to physicians, nurses, and others who may be exposed to infection in institutions. Similarly, the administrative control of scarlet fever has undergone a radical change in American cities during the past twenty years. Up to a decade or two ago most public health authorities in urban areas required that cases of scarlet fever be isolated for twenty-eight to thirty days. Since then it has slowly been realized that this procedure was futile, and more reasonable measures have been adopted. With increased understanding of hemolytic streptococcal infections came a recognition that a considerable proportion of cases were missed or not reported, simply because the patients had no rash.

As a result, the position developed that it was unreasonable to isolate a patient with a rash when an equally infectious patient was not isolated. Current practice emphasizes the need for identifying all infections with Group A hemolytic streptococci by clinical observation and bacteriological culture. Persons suspected of such infection are isolated, and the period of isolation is determined on the basis of clinical recovery. Restrictions on familial and other contacts of a case are made at the discretion of the attending physician and the local health authorities.

Following the discovery in the thirties that sulfonamides were effective in treating streptococcal infections, the idea developed that these drugs could be used prophylactically. During World War II the United States Navy undertook on an extensive scale to check and reduce the spread of hemolytic streptococci throughout various commands by administering sulfonamide drugs to the troops.[93] While this prophylactic experiment was effective in temporarily suppressing the carrier state, certain objectionable consequences appeared. Most significant was the fact that drug resistant strains of hemolytic streptococci developed, and these strains could no longer be controlled by the drugs either for preventive or therapeutic purposes. Mass chemoprophylaxis is, therefore, not to be applied indiscriminately. Under proper supervision it has limited value.

§ MEASLES

Measles is the most widely distributed and the most commonly recognized of all the acute exanthematic diseases to which man is subject. The morbidity is very high in young children, and most people have had the disease by the time they are adults. It seems unlikely that measles was not present in the ancient world; yet it cannot be recognized in any writings before the account of Rhazes (850–923), early in the tenth century.[94] In all probability the disease has been widespread over Europe and Asia since the Middle Ages or earlier. Rhazes distinguished between measles and smallpox, even though he believed that the two conditions were part of one morbid process. This doctrine was followed by physicians of the Middle Ages and persisted well into the eighteenth century. In 1748, for instance, Richard Mead (1673-1754) expressed the opinion that "The measles have a great affinity with the small pox."[95] Nevertheless, beginning in the sixteenth century physicians began to differentiate measles from other acute eruptive fevers. By the early part of the seventeenth century in London the measles had been sufficiently differentiated from smallpox so that the two diseases were reported separately in the bills of mortality after 1629.[96]

The name "measles" is itself apparently a product of semantic and nosographic confusion. During the medieval period, smallpox and measles were coupled together as *variolae* and *morbilli,* the latter term —the diminutive of *morbus*—indicating the status of measles as the little disease in contrast with smallpox. According to Charles Creighton, the English name "measles" was introduced by John of Gaddesden (1280–1361) as the equivalent of the Latin term *morbilli.*[97] The English word was itself derived from the Latin *miselli* and *misellae*— a diminutive of *miser,* and originally referred to the leprous. By some stretch of the imagination, Gaddesden coupled the sores of the legs of "the poor and the wasting," which were called *mesles,* with the *morbilli* of medical authors. Eventually the term "measles" lost its connection with leprosy and became associated with the disease now known by that name.

While measles was distinguished quite clearly and fairly early from smallpox, it continued until the end of the eighteenth century to be confused with scarlet fever. This problem has already been mentioned and will not be discussed here. However, the basis for a clear differentiation of measles from scarlet fever and other diseases was given by Thomas Sydenham in his account of the measles epidemic at London in 1670.[98] More comprehensive than his description of scarlet fever, it covers all the essential clinical features of measles. Sydenham pointed out that young children chiefly are affected, noting that the onset of the disease is marked by fever, malaise, and various catarrhal symptoms such as cough, sneezing, watering of the eyes, and sensitivity to light. He described the eruption as appearing on the fourth or fifth day, first on the forehead and the rest of the face, then rapidly extending over the entire body. Around the sixth day the rash begins to roughen and to scale, and within a day or two, the fever having ceased, the rash disappears, leaving a fine branny desquamation.

Sydenham reported that the measles per se is not fatal, the greatest danger arising rather from other diseases, especially lung conditions, to which the patient may succumb. He did note, however, that adults were much more severely affected by measles and that the prognosis was extremely grave if the disease was of a hemorrhagic character ("the measles are first livid, afterwards black"). Sydenham also described the much severer measles epidemic of 1674, in which there were more deaths. These occurred especially among infants due to lung complications. The importance of measles as an indirect cause of death in childhood had also been recognized by John Graunt.[99] In 1662 he listed measles among the chief causes of death among children under six.

Outbreaks of measles have occurred in all inhabited parts of the world, varying in severity from time to time both in the same and in different places. It is generally endemic in large centers of population and tends to recur at rather regular intervals. In fact, its periodicity is a striking feature of the history of measles. Among populations from which it has been absent for many years, or into which it is introduced for the first time, measles tends to be more severe, especially if such groups live under unhygienic conditions or have no access to proper medical care. All these facets are present in the history of measles from the eighteenth century to the present.

Although there were epidemics of high mortality during the eighteenth century, the disease was generally regarded as moderate in character. William Heberden's remark in 1785 characterizes British opinion. "The measles," he said, "being usually attended with very little danger, it is not often that a physician is employed in this distemper."[100] Medical opinion in Continental Europe appears to have been similar. Tissot in 1762 commented that in France people rarely died of the measles, and when the outcome was fatal it was due to complications.[101] The point of view in Prussia was similar. Commenting on a measles epidemic in 1751, in which almost six hundred children perished, Süssmilch wrote that it was very rare for the disease to be so severe.[102] Toward the end of the century, however, the disease seems to have become a more important cause of mortality. Outbreaks were reported from Erfurt (1778–89), Denmark (1781), Erlangen (1783), around Leipzig (1785), northern Italy (1786), the Hague (1789), Göttingen (1790), Jena (1795), and Erfurt again (1796). For the next few years, until 1801, measles was widely prevalent in Germany, France, and Britain.[103]

Measles reached the New World soon after the arrival of the first European settlers. Outbreaks probably occurred early in the sixteenth century, although it is difficult to identify accurately the eruptive diseases described by the chroniclers of the period. According to Aristides A. Moll, there were probably epidemics of measles as early as 1519 in Santo Domingo, 1523 in Guatemala, and 1531 in Mexico.[104] During the sixteenth and seventeenth centuries there were outbreaks at various times in all the Spanish colonies. Hipólito Unanue (1755–1833), a pioneer of medicine in Latin America, stated that measles was the disease that appeared most often in Lima and from 1628 to 1795 caused serious epidemics all the way from Buenos Aires to Ecuador. In 1785 there was an extremely severe outbreak in Ecuador, with more than twenty-four hundred deaths at Quito.

The disease was also present in the French and English colonies, and while the evidence is limited it is clear that there were a number of epidemics. As early as 1635 a mild epidemic was reported among the French and Indians, and in 1687 a more serious outbreak occurred at Quebec.[105] In New England, measles seems to have appeared soon after the first settlements were founded, and on two occasions reached epidemic proportions.[106] Boston and the surrounding communities were attacked in 1657, and again in the winter of 1687–88, the disease possibly having spread south from Canada, where it prevailed in 1687. This period also saw the publication of the earliest medical document to be printed in America north of Mexico with a specific reference to measles. This was Thomas Thacher's broadside, *A brief rule to guide the common-people of New-England how to order themselves and theirs in the small-pocks or measles,* first printed in Boston in 1677–78, and reprinted in 1702 and 1721–22.[107] Thacher was chiefly concerned with smallpox, and his work will be considered below in relation to the history of that disease. Nevertheless, it is of interest here because Thacher, following the doctrine originated by Rhazes, believed the two diseases to be related: "The Small Pox (whose nature and cure the Measles follows)."

During the eighteenth century there were a number of serious epidemics of measles.[108] From 1713 to 1715 severe attacks affected a number of the colonies, but prevailed chiefly in New England. In Boston there were at least 150 deaths. Measles was again widespread in 1729, although in a milder form. Scattered outbreaks occurred in

New England, New York, and New Jersey from 1739 to 1741, while Connecticut was swept by a severe epidemic in 1740–41. South Carolina, Pennsylvania, New York, Massachusetts, and Connecticut were again visited by the disease in 1747–48, its severity varying widely in different localities. A decade elapsed before the next epidemic visitation of measles. In 1758–59 the disease was epidemic throughout the colonies, with serious fatalities reported from South Carolina. According to Noah Webster, the next widespread outbreak appeared in 1772. At this time there "prevailed in America epidemic catarrh, which was attended or followed by measles in all parts of the country, and of unusual malignancy. In Charlestown, South Carolina, died 8 or 900 children." A malignant outbreak of measles appeared in New York in November, 1788, and soon thereafter spread to Philadelphia.

Apparently measles did not become endemic in America until well into the colonial period. This is indicated by the fact that numerous adults were attacked during the various outbreaks. The intervals between epidemics likewise point in the same direction. The epidemiological history of measles in the English colonies is what might be expected in a thinly populated area, where the population was being replenished and augmented by new births and by immigration. Since measles confers lifelong immunity, once the people in a larger or smaller area had been thoroughly immunized in an epidemic some time had to elapse before a large enough group of susceptibles was again available. It would seem that by the end of the colonial period the population had been quite thoroughly seeded with measles. Later, as the American people began to open the West, the same general pattern tended to repeat itself. Measles followed the westward movement; it appeared first in the Mississippi Valley, spreading quickly through Kentucky and Ohio.[109]

The behavior of measles in colonial America is similar in many respects to the experiences of isolated island communities. Epidemiological happenings tend to be more clean-cut and dramatic in such communities. Much that we know about the epidemiology of measles derives from the classic study made by Peter Ludwig Panum (1820–85) during an epidemic on the Faroe Islands in 1846.[110] After an epidemic prevalence in 1781, measles disappeared completely from the islands for sixty-five years. Reintroduced in 1846, the disease soon became epidemic, attacking a majority of the population. The extent

42

of the epidemic may be judged by the fact that of the 7,864 inhabitants, about 6,100 were ill with measles, and 102 people died of the disease or its complications. Panum, then twenty-six and just out of medical school, was sent to the islands by the Danish government as a member of a medical commission to provide necessary aid to the inhabitants and to make a careful study of the epidemic. His report, published in 1847, established the fundamental epidemiological features of measles, as Sydenham's description had its clinical characteristics. Panum showed that the incubation period of measles was generally thirteen to fourteen days, the rash appearing at that time after previous exposure. He found that all ages were susceptible to the disease and that one attack conferred immunity. Furthermore, Panum showed that the disease is most communicable during the eruption and flourishing of the rash and that it may also be transmitted during the prodromal period, but he found no evidence of transmission in the desquamation state. Finally, he concluded that measles is a purely contagious disease, and therefore that isolation is the surest means of arresting its progress. Many other interesting topics are considered by Panum in his report. In the light of current concern with the question whether simpler societies have less mental illness than highly complex ones, it is interesting to read Panum's discussion of this problem more than a century ago and his conclusion that "there is hardly any country, hardly, indeed, any metropolis, in which mental diseases are so frequent in proportion to the number of people as on the Faroes." One further fact in connection with the Faroe Islands is noteworthy. Another epidemic appeared in 1875, and on this occasion it was shown that only persons under thirty, and who therefore had not been affected by the previous epidemic, were susceptible.

By the latter part of the nineteenth century it was generally accepted that measles was caused by some microscopic *materies morbi,* "that this poison reproduces itself within the diseased organism, and that the spread of the disease from person to person and from place to place takes place solely by the conveyance of the poison."[111] Nevertheless, unequivocal success in experimental demonstration of this doctrine was not achieved until the early twentieth century. The first attempt at transmission of measles had been made in the middle of the eighteenth century. In 1759 Francis Home, whose unfortunate use of the croup concept added to the confusion around diphtheria, reported his experiments with measles.[112] Hoping to emulate the success of variolation as a prophylactic measure against smallpox, he endeavored by so-called *morbillisation* to produce a mild form of the disease that would confer permanent immunity. While dealing with measles at Edinburgh in 1758, Home induced the parents of several children, in return for payment, to allow their children to be inoculated with the disease. He inoculated twelve children, varying in age from seven months to thirteen years, by placing cotton soaked with fresh blood from patients, in the acute stage of the disease, in incisions in the skin. In three trials he placed the blood-soaked cotton in the nose for an hour. Within a week seven children came down with measles. These experiments aroused great interest and hope among Home's contemporaries.[113] On October 27, 1758, Robert Whytt (1714–66), who a decade later published the first clinical description of tuberculous meningitis, wrote to Cadwallader Colden in New York, reported the experiments, and advised the latter to read Home's book, *Medical facts and experiments,* for a fuller account. William Buchan (1729–1805) wrote in 1761 that "no greater boon has ever been discovered for the health of infants than small-pox inoculation; and it is greatly to be hoped that measles, a disease akin to it, may be treated the same way." Tissot referred to the inoculation of measles in 1762, and in 1793 Charles Buxton in a medical dissertation mentioned the practice as a "most powerful means of alleviating the common sequences of measles."

During the nineteenth century a number of other attempts were made to inoculate human subjects with blood and other materials from measles patients. It was not until 1905, however, that the first unequivocally successful transmission of measles was achieved by Ludvig Hektoen (1863–1951).[114] Two persons were injected subcutaneously with blood taken from patients twenty-four and thirty hours after the eruption of the rash; measles appeared eleven to thirteen days later. Transmission of measles to an animal, the monkey, was first indicated in 1898 by Albert Henry Louis Josias, and definitely established in 1911 by John F. Anderson and Joseph Goldberger.[115] Several species of the genus *Macaca* have been shown to be susceptible, but there is no evidence that measles is produced in any mammal other than monkeys. Anderson and Goldberger in 1911 showed that measles is caused by a filterable virus. Since then the

44

virus has been successfully cultivated in tissue culture by Harry Plotz (1938), and in chick embryos by Geoffrey Rake and Morris F. Shaffer (1939, 1940).[116] Based upon these researches, other workers have endeavored to develop a prophylactic vaccine. Up to the present, however, there has not been developed any successful vaccine for active immunization against measles.[117]

The diagnostic importance of the characteristic spots in the mouth was pointed out in 1896 by Henry Koplik (1858–1927), a New York physician.[118] These lesions had been observed by other physicians, among them Nils Fiodorovich Filatov (1847–1902) and Eduard Henoch (1820–1910), but it was Koplik who emphasized the significance of this phenomenon.

The use of serum antibodies for specific prophylaxis and therapy has been developed during the past forty years. In 1918 Charles Nicolle and Ernest Conseil showed that the serum of a child convalescing from an attack of measles protected another child exposed to the disease.[119] Since then other antibody preparations such as adult serum or placental extract have been used.[120] During World War II the availability of large quantities of human plasma as a result of the blood procurement program led to the development of immune serum globulin (gamma globulin) by Edwin J. Cohn and his associates. Gamma globulin is now well established as an effective agent for passive immunization against measles. There is also some evidence that in large doses gamma globulin may modify the severity of the disease when administered early before any rash has appeared.[121]

§ GERMAN MEASLES (*Rubella*)

Rubella is a mild eruptive disease of childhood and has undoubtedly attacked children for many centuries. Nevertheless, because of confusion with other febrile eruptive diseases its true identity was established only comparatively recently. The disease appears to have been described first by Daniel Sennert, who also gave an account of scarlet fever.[122] In 1619 he stated that *röteln* probably belonged to the group of *morbilli,* but that while it began with fever, coughing and other symptoms of measles, the condition was less dangerous. Sennert attributed the name, which appears to have been a popular term, to the red color of the slightly elevated papular eruption. He also differentiated this disease from *rossania,* scarlet fever. The term *"röteln"* was likewise used by Horst in 1624.

Physicians of the seventeenth and eighteenth centuries very probably observed cases of rubella, but it was not until the early nineteenth century that it was separated from measles and scarlet fever as a distinct entity. David Hosack (1769–1835) observed an epidemic of the disease in New York in 1813, designating it as *rubeola sine catarrho* (measles without catarrh).[123] Maton, an English physician, in 1814 described a number of cases that occurred in a London family. In 1829 Wagner, a German physician, gave an account of rubella as a distinct disease entity, retaining the popular designation *"röteln."*[124] For want of another term, the German word was employed also in the English literature until 1866 when Veale proposed the name "rubella," which since then has been generally adopted. The disease was also called German measles because it had been first described by German writers.

Rubella has been found prevalent all over the world and occurs periodically in epidemics. Because of its mild character it did not arouse much clinical interest until recently, and throughout the nineteenth century was undoubtedly confused in many instances with measles. From the point of view of differential diagnosis, Koplik's observation and description in measles of the spots in the mouth that bear his name was clearly an important contribution.

The cause of rubella is a filterable virus. In 1938 Y. Hiro and S. Tasaka reported successful transmission of the disease to children by the inoculation of filtered nasal washings.[125] Habel in 1942 reported successful transmission of rubella to rhesus monkeys. Little is known, however, about the causative agent.

Until 1940 rubella was generally considered a mild, unimportant disease of childhood. Complications were unknown, so that prophylaxis and treatment were not considered necessary. Then in 1941 N. McAlister Gregg, an Australian ophthalmologist, showed that children whose mothers had had rubella during pregnancy, especially during the early months, were likely to be born with congenital damage of some sort.[126] Subsequent studies in Australia, the United States, and England have confirmed this conclusion. Among the more frequent defects are deaf-mutism, cataracts, heart malformations, and microcephaly. Recently Lancaster in a retrospective study showed

46

that deafness had appeared in epidemic form in the past in Australia, particularly among children born in 1899, 1916, 1924, 1925, and during the period 1938–41, and that except for that of 1916 all these epidemics appeared to have been caused by antecedent outbreaks of rubella.[127] In short, congenital damage by rubella in pregnancy had been occurring for at least forty years before Gregg made his brilliant observations.

Unfortunately, there is as yet no established prophylactic procedure. No vaccine for active immunization is presently available. Immune serum globulin as a passive immunizing agent has given contradictory results so far; nevertheless, the use of this substance has been recommended for women exposed to rubella in the first three months of pregnancy. Recently successful results have been reported following the use of the gamma globulin fraction of convalescent German measles serum.[128] It is presently regarded as desirable that every girl should have rubella before reaching the childbearing period.

§ SMALLPOX

Smallpox is an acute eruptive disease which begins suddenly with fever, headache, backache, pains in the limbs, and vomiting. On the second to fifth day the characteristic eruption appears, gradually spreading over the body. The first unambiguous description of smallpox occurs in the well known treatise of Rhazes mentioned above.[129] He referred to the disease as widespread throughout the East, and the same opinion is expressed by Avicenna and other Moslem writers of the tenth and eleventh centuries. It is evident from these accounts that smallpox was a disease well known and established in the Near East before the seventh century. The occurrence of smallpox during earlier periods seems probable, but the evidence is only suggestive. There is, for example, the eruption on the mummy of the Twentieth Dynasty examined by Ruffer and others (mentioned above), but there is no clear-cut proof that the disease was smallpox. Furthermore, there is no account in the Greek and Roman writers before the Christian era of any disease which can be recognized as smallpox. The epidemic described by Eusebius of Caesarea (*ca.* A.D. 260–340) in his *Ecclesiastical history* as having broken out in Syria in A.D. 302 may have been

47

smallpox. According to his account ulcers covered the entire body, even the eyes, so that many became blind, and many of those attacked succumbed to the disease. Other suggestive accounts have also been found in Chinese and Indian medical works dating from the period between the third and the sixth centuries. There seems to be rather general agreement among students of the history of smallpox that the disease became epidemic in Arabia toward the end of the sixth century, and then spread through the Mediterranean area into Europe. Epidemics reported for Italy and France in A.D. 570 by Marius, Bishop of Avenches, and by Gregory of Tours (in A.D. 581) for that city after A.D. 573 were probably outbreaks of smallpox. The term "variola," which now designates smallpox, occurs for the first time in the report of Marius, where it simply means "spotted."

Of the existence of smallpox in the Middle Ages there is no doubt. Almost all the medical writers of the period refer to the disease, and for the most part the Western authors base their accounts on the writings of Rhazes, Avicenna, and other Moslem physicians. Smallpox was known in England during the Middle Ages, but from the few existing references it is impossible to infer anything concerning the prevalence of the disease. With the end of the medieval period smallpox seems to have become more widely prevalent in Europe as well as in Asia, Africa, and the Americas, where it was introduced by European explorers and settlers.

From the fifteenth century onward, as treatises on the diseases of children became more numerous, most of them included a discussion of smallpox and measles. On the whole, the disease seems to have been mild and infrequently fatal. In his treatise on contagion published in 1546, Girolamo Fracastoro (1483–1553) treats smallpox rather lightly as a disease to which almost everyone was subject.[130] There are, however, several reports of epidemics in Italy in the sixteenth century, as for instance at Mantua in 1567, and at Brescia in 1570, 1577, and 1588.[131] Ambroise Paré refers to smallpox in France, describing cases he had seen in 1586 as well as at other times.

The term "smallpox" appeared in England early in the sixteenth century as the counterpart of the French term *la petite vérole*. The latter was employed in contradistinction to *la grosse vérole,* which was used to designate syphilis. The terms indicate an implied recognition of some superficial similarity between the two conditions. The common element is, of course, the eruption which occurs in both diseases. It is interesting to note a somewhat similar terminological development in German. During the fifteenth, sixteenth, and seventeenth centuries the word *Blattern* was used to designate syphilis, but by the eighteenth century it had become applied to smallpox. These terminological shifts naturally tend to obscure still further the vague picture of smallpox during this period.

Smallpox was noted in England during the earlier sixteenth century, but it was only toward the end of the Elizabethan period that it began to receive recognition as a common disease. In 1629 the first printed bills of mortality for London listed smallpox as a separate disease, and it remained a regular entry from year to year. A few years before his death in 1631, John Donne, poet and dean of St. Paul's, referred to smallpox in London.[132] Throughout the Stuart period there are frequent references to smallpox in England, particularly in London, and the increasing severity of the disease is reflected in the rising figures of the bills of mortality. By the end of the seventeenth century, smallpox had come to be regarded almost as an inevitable part of childhood. Infants and young children were reported as having the disease in a milder form, while it was more often fatal in older children and adults. By the beginning of the eighteenth century, smallpox was endemic in the cities and towns of Great Britain, and a leading cause of death. Queen Mary died in 1694 during a smallpox epidemic, and Thomas Babington Macaulay in discussing this event gives a vividly colored picture of the impact of the disease:

> That disease over which science has since achieved a succession of glorious and beneficient victories, was then the most terrible of all the ministers of death. The havoc of the plague had been far more rapid; but the plague had visited our shores only once or twice within living memory; and the smallpox was always present, filling the churchyards with corpses, tormenting with constant fears all whom it had not yet stricken, leaving on those whose lives it spared the hideous traces of its power, turning the babe into a changeling at which the mother shuddered, and making the eyes and cheeks of the betrothed maiden objects of horror to the lover.[133]

While Charles Creighton showed convincingly that the actual incidence of facial disfigurement was greatly exaggerated, there is no

doubt that Macaulay does picture accurately the psychological reaction to the disease.

The clinical appearance of the disease was carefully studied by a
number of English physicians during the later seventeenth century,
among them Thomas Sydenham, Richard Morton, Thomas Willis
(1621–75), and Walter Harris (1647–1732). In his *Observationes
medicae circa morborum acutorum historium et curationem,* Sydenham dealt with the epidemics of smallpox during the years 1667–72.
He distinguished between discrete and confluent forms of the disease,
advising a conservative and expectant regimen of treatment in the
former, but active interference in the latter. His active treatment consisted in administering a vomit and a purge to the patient and then
having him bled. Thereafter the patient was put on a cooling regimen.
Sydenham's practice is described by Thomas Dover (1660–1742),
buccaneer and physician, who studied with him:

> Whilst I lived with Dr. Sydenham, I had myself the smallpox, and fell
> ill on the twelfth day. In the beginning I lost twenty ounces of blood. He
> gave me a vomit, but I find by experience purging much better. I went
> abroad, by his direction, till I was blind, and then took to my bed. I had
> no fire allowed in my room, my windows were constantly open, my bed-
> clothes were ordered to be laid no higher than my waist. He made me take
> twelve bottles of small beer, acidulated with spirit of vitriol, every twenty-
> four hours. I had of this anomalous kind to a very great degree, yet never
> lost my senses one moment.[134]

This treatment found opposition among Sydenham's contemporaries. His rival Richard Morton preferred a heating regimen, and
other physicians objected to bloodletting and purging in smallpox.
These controversies continued throughout the eighteenth century,
leading in one instance to a duel between Richard Mead and John
Woodward in 1719.

On the Continent, as in Great Britain, smallpox was a continuing
threat to public health throughout the eighteenth century. It smol-
dered endemically in city and town, flaring up recurrently into epidemic outbreaks. The impact of the disease is reflected in various statements and estimates dealing with smallpox mortality and its effects
on the population. In 1723 James Jurin (1684–1750), first physician
to Guy's Hospital and secretary of the Royal Society, published in the

Philosophical Transactions "A comparison between the mortality of the natural small pox and that given by inoculation."[135] From a study of the London bills of mortality he showed that one-fourteenth of the population in and near London had died of smallpox during the preceding forty-two years. According to William Douglass, writing in 1760, smallpox was a chief cause of the high infant mortality in Europe. What this meant may be seen from Rosén von Rosenstein's statement in 1765 that "the smallpox carries off yearly the tenth part of Swedish children."[136] In Berlin from 1758 to 1774 there were 6,705 deaths from smallpox. Of these 5,876 were in the first five years of life.[137] The London bills of mortality show that 50 per cent of all deaths occurred among children under the age of five.

In the light of this situation it was no accident that when a practical possibility of preventing smallpox was suggested it was tried. London suffered severe epidemics in 1710, 1714, and 1720; and public opinion was strongly sensitive to the need for some new method of dealing with smallpox. This possibility was first suggested in England in 1714. It had been known for centuries that an attack of smallpox almost always conferred immunity to subsequent infections. Based on this principle an effective prophylactic procedure against smallpox had been developed and had long been used in various parts of the world, especially in the East. In this method smallpox matter from a mild case was inoculated into a healthy individual so that a mild attack would occur; this would then provide protection against any severe attack in the future. The practice was first brought to the attention of English physicians by Emanuel Timoni (d. 1718), a Greek of Constantinople.[138] In 1713 he sent a letter containing an extensive description of inoculation to Dr. John Woodward, Gresham professor of physic, who had it printed in the *Philosophical Transactions* of the Royal Society for 1714. A year later, in 1715, Peter Kennedy, a Scottish practitioner, who had spent some time in Constantinople and then became an ophthalmic surgeon in London, published *An essay on external remedies* in which a chapter is devoted to "the variolae or small pox, the manner of ingrafting or giving them, and of their cure." While Kennedy's account aroused no great interest, Timoni's letter had repercussions both in England and New England. With the impact on New England we shall deal below. In England, Sir Hans Sloane (1660–1753) was stimulated to make further inquiries into the matter, and he obtained information on the practice of inoculation from Giacomo Pylarini (1659–1718), a Venetian physician who had formerly practiced at Constantinople. This account was published at Venice in 1715, and reprinted in the *Philosophical Transactions* for 1716, arousing further interest among physicians and scientists. Medical men recognized the importance of these accounts, but to the public at large they were "virtuoso amusements."

There the matter stood until 1721 when the operation was popularized by Lady Mary Wortley Montagu (1689–1762). While living in Constantinople, where her husband was the British ambassador, she had had her small son inoculated in March, 1718. In the spring of 1721, three years after her return from the Levant, a severe smallpox epidemic broke out in England. Lady Mary decided to have her five-year-old daughter inoculated, and had the operation performed in the presence of several physicians, who were tremendously impressed by the result.[139] Popular interest was not slow in following and was further heightened when the royal family became actively interested. Before having the children of Caroline, Princess of Wales, inoculated, George I arranged to have the method tried first on six volunteers from among the prisoners at Newgate condemned to death, and then on eleven charity children of varying ages. The results were successful, and in April, 1722, the royal children were inoculated.

With royalty setting the fashion, further impetus was given to the practice of inoculation. Despite such influential endorsement, however, the subject was soon embroiled in violent controversy. Two opposing factions developed, sermons were preached for and against the new procedure, and a bitter pamphlet war ensued. While most of the opposition was essentially irrational, the claim that inoculation could spread the smallpox was correct. In addition to the danger of spread, there was also the disquieting fact that some inoculated individuals came down with severe attacks, some of them fatal. Thus, after some initial successes, the method fell into disrepute from about 1728 to 1743. In that year (1743) a physician named James Kilpatrick arrived in London from Charleston, South Carolina, and published an account of the severe smallpox epidemic which ravaged that city in 1738. According to Kilpatrick, this murderous outbreak seemed to have been stopped by the use of inoculation. In addition, he described some improvements in the method used, for example, the arm-to-arm method, as well as shallow scarifications. Partly through Kilpatrick's influence, and also because of the increased prevalence and severity of smallpox during the latter part of the century, inoculation became a well-established practice. Other modifications were introduced by Robert Sutton, who began his work in 1755 and became one of the best-known inoculators of the period. It was his second son, Daniel Sutton (1735–1819), who made the Suttonian system a household word throughout the world. His most famous competitor was Thomas Dimsdale (1712–1800), who in 1768 inoculated Catherine II of Russia as well as numerous members of the Imperial Court. Dimsdale was paid £10,000—one of the largest fees on record—and in addition £2,000 for his expenses as well as an annuity of £500 for life. Furthermore, Catherine made him a Baron of the Russian Empire.

Voltaire was the most ardent exponent of inoculation in France, and it was he who first aroused the interest of Catherine the Great. Despite his agitation, however, inoculation did not become a general practice in France until after 1750. The spread of inoculation to other parts of Europe followed a similar chronological pattern. Inoculation was introduced in Sweden and Denmark around 1754–56, in the former country by the king. Because of its close relations to England the method was introduced early into Hanover, where the first inoculation was carried out in 1722. However, it was not introduced into the other German states until later in the century. Frederick II of Prussia arranged in 1775 for William Baylies to teach the practice of inoculation to fourteen provincial physicians. Inoculation was not unopposed, however. In 1797, for example, the philosopher Immanuel Kant expressed the opinion that anyone who permitted himself to be inoculated against smallpox endangered his life.[140]

While the practice of inoculation was being developed, the first efforts were made to determine by statistical means its value as a prophylactic measure. Johann Peter Süssmilch (1707–67) discussed the burning problem of inoculation in his work, *Die göttliche Ordnung* (1765), and endeavored to demonstrate the value of the method by calculating that an inoculated individual is twenty-five times less likely to die of smallpox than one who has not submitted to variolation.[141] A more significant contribution to this aspect of the inoculation problem was made in 1760 by the mathematician Daniel Bernoulli (1700–82). In an essay communicated to the Royal Academy of Science in Paris he undertook to analyze the mortality caused by smallpox and to show the advantages of inoculation as a preventive measure.[142] Bernoulli endeavored to do this by applying the calculus of probability. It is interesting to note that this paper was criticized by D'Alembert, who argued that for an individual the risk of dying as a result of inoculation may seem greater.[143]

As the practice of inoculation gradually came into favor in England and then spread over Continental Europe, a parallel drama was being enacted independently in the American colonies. Smallpox was introduced into the New World soon after its discovery. Thereafter it appeared in waves from time to time in one or more localities, but its prevalence was never comparable to that in Britain or Europe. Nevertheless, the terror evoked by the disease was equally vivid. It was the need for informing the public regarding the nature of the disease and the means for dealing with it that led to the publication in 1677–78 of Thomas Thacher's *Brief rule* .... As in England, the need for an effective preventive was recognized, so that when the reports of Timoni and Pylarini appeared the seed fell on a receptive soil in America. Two men, the Reverend Cotton Mather (1662–1728) and the physician Zabdiel Boylston (1680–1766), both of Boston, introduced the practice. Mather had learned about inoculation not only from the communications in the *Philosophical Transactions,* but also from slaves brought from Africa. In April, 1721, ships from the West Indies brought smallpox to Boston. Mather proposed to the physicians of Boston that they undertake inoculation. Only Boylston responded by inoculating his son Thomas, aged six, and two Negro slaves, a man and a boy. The result of the trial was successful, and Boylston proceeded to inoculate others. By September he had inoculated thirty-five persons with no deaths. These events touched off a bitter controversy in Boston. Nevertheless, despite prolonged opposition the practice was gradually accepted, and when Boylston died in 1766 he had seen inoculation come into general use, not only in Boston, but elsewhere in the colonies. As early at 1722 the selectmen of Boston had insisted that Boylston should not inoculate without licence and the consent of the authorities. By 1760 legal safeguards regulating the conditions under which inoculation could be performed had been set up. During the Revolution inoculation was practiced widely, and General George Washington ordered the entire American army to be inoculated. In this he was no doubt influenced by John Morgan, physician-in-chief of the American armies, who in 1776 wrote a *Recommendation of inoculation according to Baron Dimsdale's method*. Inoculation hospitals were established at various points for this purpose.

There is no question that inoculation had been shown to be of value in preventing smallpox. It was relatively effective in the American colonies where the population was less dense and proper precautions against spread could be taken. This was not the case in Great Britain. Except for the rich who could go to special isolation hospitals, it was agreed that the method could not easily be applied on a mass basis. To be sure, physicians such as John Coakley Lettsom (1744–1815) and John Haygarth (1774–1827) proposed means for making inoculation available to poor people. In 1798, however, Edward Jenner (1749–1823) published his revolutionary discovery of vaccination, and the need to solve these problems disappeared.

Edward Jenner was a country practitioner who had studied under John Hunter, the celebrated surgeon, and had then returned to his native Berkeley. According to his own statement Jenner had long been interested in the relation between cowpox vaccinia and smallpox. As a country doctor he also practiced inoculation. In the course of his work he found patients in whom inoculation would not take since they had already had the cowpox. Taking this as a point of departure, Jenner had the idea that it might be possible to inoculate an individual with cowpox matter from another person who had contracted the disease naturally; and then that matter from this individual might be used to inoculate other individuals, and so on. In 1796 an opportunity to try out this idea presented itself. Jenner inoculated a boy, James Phipps, with cowpox matter taken from the hand of a milkmaid, Sarah Nelmes, who had acquired the infection naturally. Then after several weeks he inoculated the boy with smallpox, but it failed to take—James Phipps was immune to smallpox. Jenner first offered his observations to the Royal Society, but the paper was refused. He then published his work in 1798 under the modest title, *An inquiry into the causes and effects of the variolae vaccinae, a disease discovered in some of the western counties of England, particularly Gloucestershire, and known by the name of the Cow pox.*

While the initial reception accorded to the *Inquiry* was not promising, it was not neglected for long. Confirmation soon came from Henry Cline, a London surgeon who was a friend of Jenner. Further confirmation came from George Pearson (1751–1828), a physician to St. Thomas's Hospital, who later opened the first dispensary for public vaccination. The new practice was rapidly adopted, and by 1801 at least one hundred thousand persons had been vaccinated in England alone. The spread of vaccination all over the world was astonishingly rapid, and within a few years Jenner's *Inquiry* had been translated into the principal European languages. C. F. Stromeyer and G. F. Ballhorn in 1799 began to vaccinate in Hanover and by 1801 had performed two thousand operations. In 1799, Benjamin Waterhouse (1754–1846), first professor of the theory and practice of physic at the Harvard Medical School, received a copy of Jenner's *Inquiry*. Impressed with the new method of vaccination, he secured some matter from England and vaccinated his children as well as several domestics, seven persons in all. They were then inoculated with smallpox, but all proved resistant. Waterhouse then extended the practice to others and in 1800 published an account of his work under the title *A prospect of exterminating the small-pox*. Thomas Jefferson was an active supporter of Waterhouse and contributed considerably in establishing vaccination as a public health procedure. In New York, Valentine Seaman was the first advocate of the new practice and in 1802 organized an "Institute for the Inoculation of the Kine Pox." Its purpose was to provide free vaccination for the poor.

Although vaccination was generally accepted, acceptance did not occur without opposition.[144] Some opposition was due to vested interests such as the established inoculators. Other opponents had valid scientific objections. Some claimed that vaccination transmitted other diseases. Still others objected on religious grounds. Finally, when an attempt was made in England to render vaccination compulsory, the argument was raised that this would be an infringement upon individual liberty by the state. In the face of all this, however, vaccination fought its way to general acceptance.

One of the most serious objections to vaccination, the danger of transmitting other diseases such as syphilis, has long been eliminated. In 1845 Negri of Naples began to propagate virus in cows, thus eliminating the dangers inherent in the use of humanized virus. The practice spread from Italy to France in 1866, and then to Germany and other parts of Europe. Virus obtained from France was introduced into a herd of cows near Boston in 1870, and this was the beginning of the use of calf lymph in the United States. The use of sterilized glycerine for the preservation of lymph was first recommended by Robert Koch.

Today three major types of the variola-vaccinia virus group are recognized: *variola major,* smallpox; *variola minor,* alastrim; and *vaccinia,* cowpox. These three diseases are closely related and have basically the same physical characteristics, yet they produce distinctive reactions in human beings and experimental animals. Until the end of the nineteenth century, virulent smallpox was the prevalent disease in most countries of the world. Gradually, however, the milder alastrim (*variola minor*) has become more and more widely disseminated.[145] Virulent smallpox is today restricted to limited geographic areas such as India, China, and Mexico. From time to time, however, cases of this type are imported elsewhere and lead to sharp outbreaks characterized by a high fatality rate. In 1947 a traveler coming from Mexico introduced a virulent strain into New York City and produced an outbreak. It was quickly brought under control, however, by rapid action on the part of the municipal health authorities. In the course of this campaign a large part of the population of New York was vaccinated. Public health authorities must still be alert to smallpox and the possibility of its spread.

The cause of variola is still not definitely known. However, fluid from variola lesions contains numerous elementary bodies, which are small and spherical, with a diameter of 200 m μ. These were first described in 1887 by John Buist of Edinburgh, who believed that they represented the contagium of smallpox and cowpox. In 1906 they were described by Enrique Paschen, after whom they are now named.[146] Neither report was widely accepted at the time of its appearance. Information has now accumulated, however, which indicates the soundness of the original hypothesis of these early workers.

§ CHICKEN POX (*Varicella*)

Chicken pox is a mild communicable disease caused by a virus. It is characterized by a febrile onset, followed after twenty-four hours by an itching vesicular eruption of the skin, and spreading in some cases to the mouth and the pharynx. While chicken pox was not definitely separated as a distinct disease entity until the later eighteenth century, hints of its existence are to be found in earlier clinical descriptions, particularly those of smallpox. Rhazes refers to a weak smallpox, which may have been varicella, and for centuries it was considered merely a variety of smallpox.

The first indication that chicken pox is a separate disease seems to have come from Ingrassias,[147] who in 1553 described a condition which he called *crystalli,* evidently translating a popular name into Latin. According to Ingrassias, the common people believed it to be of the same nature as smallpox and measles, but he did not share this opinion, distinguishing *crystalli* and *variolae.* From this account he seems to be describing chicken pox. Guido Guidi (1500–69), a contemporary of Ingrassias, also referred to *crystalli,* but he was uncertain as to their specific nature. He did say, however, that the condition was commonly called *ravaglione,* which is suggestive as it is the present Italian term for chicken pox.

Throughout the sixteenth and seventeenth centuries and a good part of the eighteenth, varicella continued to masquerade as a variety of smallpox. Richard Morton in 1694 spoke of "chicken pocks" as if it was simply a form of smallpox. In 1760 an anonymous work appeared at Amsterdam under the title *Tractatus duo pathologici.*[148] The author was François Boissier de Sauvages (1706–67), physician and botanist. The volume contained two treatises—one on diseases of children, the other on skin diseases. In the last chapter of the work on children's diseases De Sauvages describes a variety of smallpox which he called lymphatic variola or, in French, *la vérole volante* (fleeting variola). He even noted that true variola might occur while the patient was recovering from the milder disease. From his description it is clear that De Sauvages observed varicella, but he did not take the decisive step in differentiating it from smallpox.

This step was taken in 1767 by William Heberden the Elder (1710–1801). On August 11 he read a paper "On the chicken pox" before the College of Physicians in London,[149] in which he definitely stated that chicken pox is a different disease from smallpox.

The principal marks by which the chicken pox may be distinguished from the smallpox are (1) the appearance on the second or third day from the eruption of that vesicle full of serum upon the top of the pocks; (2) the crust which covers the pocks on the fifth day, at which time those of the smallpox are not at the height of their suppuration.

Nevertheless, this view was not immediately adopted. Rosén von Rosenstein in 1765 described a "water smallpox" which he recognized as something quite distinct from true smallpox, and that the one disease did not protect against the other. Yet he still used the same name for both. R. A. Vogel in 1772 dealt with chicken pox and smallpox together under the heading *Febris variolosa.*[150] He called it *variolae spuriae* or *varicella,* a term which he was the first to employ. This term was soon adopted, as is indicated by the circumstance that it is used by Thomas Bateman in his reports on the diseases of London from 1804 to 1816. The relationship between varicella and smallpox continued to be argued throughout most of the nineteenth century. As late as 1866 the famous dermatologist Ferdinand von Hebra (1816–80) maintained the unitary view of the two diseases. Perhaps the last important exponent of this theory was Max Kassowitz (1843–1913), who in 1873 published a paper in which he maintained that varicella and variola are manifestations of the same disease.[151]

Some physicians did not regard chicken pox as infectious and considered it instead as a skin disease. However, in 1875 Johann Steiner (1832–76), through deliberate inoculation with varicella virus, demonstrated that the disease is infectious.[152] In 1909 János von Bókay (1858–1937) suggested that varicella and *herpes zoster* (shingles) were etiologically related.[153] Elementary bodies like the Paschen bodies in smallpox were described as occurring in varicella in 1911 by Aragao and by Enrique Paschen in 1917.[154] Since von Bókay's original observations, evidence has accumulated that the virus which causes chicken pox is closely related to that which produces *herpes zoster,* but there is still no conclusive evidence that they are identical. There is no method of prevention. Vaccination with chicken pox virus has been proposed, but has not been practical.

§ MUMPS

As already indicated, mumps had been recognized as a discrete clinical entity in the Hippocratic work *Epidemics I*. It was described as a mild epidemic ailment characterized by large, diffuse, nonsuppurative swellings near the ears that subsided gradually. Young men particularly were attacked, and sometimes the disease was complicated by painful swelling of the testes (orchitis). Cases were recorded by medical writers at various times, but little attention was given to the study of the disease. Guillaume de Baillou recorded outbreaks of mumps in sixteenth-century Paris. The disease was described in 1755 by Richard Russell, who expressed the opinion that it was communicable. In 1790 attention was drawn to mumps by a very full description presented by Robert Hamilton (1721–93) to the Royal Society of Edinburgh.[155] According to Michael Underwood, evidence of encephalitis as a complication of mumps appears to have been noted by American physicians.[156] Mumps nephritis was reported in 1884 by E. O. Croner (1838–1905).[157]

While most authors in the nineteenth century recognized that mumps was contagious, this was not conclusively demonstrated until some two decades ago. In 1913 Nicolle and Conseil punctured human parotid glands and injected the fluid thus obtained into the parotids of bonnet monkeys. By this method a suggestive reaction was produced. Then in 1921 Martha Wollstein demonstrated that in mumps the salivary fluid contains a virus which, when injected into cats, produced inflammation of the parotids, the testes, and the membranes of the brain. It was not until 1934, however, that C. D. Johnson and E. W. Goodpasture conclusively proved the causative agent of mumps to be a filterable virus.[158] More recently reagents have been prepared that elicit a skin reaction in persons who have had mumps. It is thus possible to distinguish those individuals who are immune from those who are susceptible. Attempts have been made to develop a vaccine for active immunization, and a vaccine is now available which will produce a temporary immunity against the disease in most cases. Gamma globulin from mumps convalescent serum has been found to be highly effective in reducing the incidence of complications, particularly orchitis.

Usually outbreaks of mumps are small and localized. However, the disease has often appeared in larger epidemics in armies in time of war. During World War I, among 4,000,000 men in the United States Army there were 230,356 cases of mumps, as compared with 96,817 cases of measles. The noneffective rate for mumps was the third highest for all diseases. Mumps was considerably less important among American troops during World War II.[159] Epidemics occurred principally among soldiers from rural areas.

§ WHOOPING COUGH

The history of whooping cough begins in the sixteenth century. It is more than probable, however, that the disease had been recognized much earlier by the common people, if not by the medical profession. The existence of colloquial names when the condition first began to be described is presumptive evidence of popular recognition. In England the name "chin cough" was employed, while the equivalent Scottish term was "kink." These terms occur early in the sixteenth century, for example, in 1519 in Horman's *Vulgaria* and in Moulton's *This is the myrror or glass of helth.*

The first detailed description, however, is contained in an account by Baillou of an epidemic which occurred in 1578 in Paris:

> Fevers attacked children of four months, ten months, and a little older, and carried off an enormous number. Especially that common cough which is popularly called Quinta or Quintana, of which mention has been made before. The symptoms of this are severe. The lung is so irritated that in its struggle to drive out by utmost effort the cause of irritation, it can neither inspire, nor with any ease expire. The patient seems to swell up, and as if on the verge of suffocation with his breathing obstructed in midthroat.

Baillou goes on to explain the possible origins of the term *quinta* and points out that some attribute it to the fact the cough "repeats at certain hours; and experience shows this is true, for they are free from this distress of coughing sometimes for an interval of four or five hours, then the paroxysm of coughing repeats, sometimes so distressing that blood is driven out by its violence, through nose and mouth. Very frequently the stomach empties its contents."[160]

Baillou states that he had "never yet read any author who gives any account of this cough," but it is clear that the disease was well known to the lay public. This is borne out by the statement of Thomas Willis almost a hundred years later that "whooping cough is left to the management of old women and empirics." Lack of medical interest in whooping cough during this period is probably due to this situation. Johann Schenck von Grafenberg (1530–98) refers in passing to the epidemic described by Baillou. Otherwise the medical writers of the sixteenth century are silent on the subject.

However, there are several accounts of whooping cough in the seventeenth century, and it received the attention of many eighteenth-century writers. In 1600 Herome Reusner, a German physician about whom little is known, published a book on scurvy, which also contains information on many other subjects. Speaking of whooping cough, he indicated that the disease was known as *coqueluche* in France. (It may be noted in passing that the term *coqueluche* was first applied to influenza and then transferred to whooping cough. In England, Thomas Willis discussed the disease in 1675 and pointed out the age and seasonal incidence. "This disease," he stated, "attacks chiefly children and infants, and at particular seasons, to wit, especially in spring and autumn."[161]

Sydenham mentioned the disease in passing in his *Observationes medicae,* but the reference is noteworthy because it contains the first appearance in English of the names "pertussis" and "whooping cough." In Germany, Michael Etmüller (1644–83) gave a clear account of whooping cough.

Numerous physicians dealt with the disease in the eighteenth century. Two early monographs on the subject were published by Michael Alberti in 1728 and by Friedrich Hoffmann (1660–1742) in 1732.[162] A number of whooping cough epidemics were reported during this period. Theodor Zuinger (1658– 1724), professor of medicine at Basel, described an epidemic that occurred in 1712. John Huxham (1692–1768) described an outbreak in England in 1724. According to Rosén von Rosenstein, an epidemic swept Sweden and the neighboring countries from 1745 to 1748. He expressed the opinion that the disease is communicable. Other epidemics were described in Switzerland in 1755 and in Brunswick in 1770. Whooping cough also occurred in epidemic form in the American colonies, particularly in South Carolina, where it was widespread and virulent. It is small wonder that Lionel Chalmers in 1776 referred to it as "that dangerous and obstinate complaint." One of the early American descriptions after Chalmers was that of Benjamin Waterhouse entitled *An essay concerning tussis convulsiva, or whooping cough,* which appeared in Boston in 1822.

62

By the end of the eighteenth century, whooping cough had become a well-recognized clinical entity. In the nineteenth century attention was turned to the discovery of its cause. It was not until the beginning of the twentieth century, however, that the causative organism *Hemophilus pertussis* was first observed and cultivated. This was accomplished by Jules Bordet (1870–1939) and Octave Gengou and reported in 1906.[163] In 1916 Ingeborg Chievitz and Adolph H. Meyer introduced the cough-plate method for bacteriologic diagnosis of whooping cough.[164]

Active immunization for the prevention of whooping cough was undertaken soon after Bordet and Gengou described *H. pertussis*. Von Bókay (1914) used a vaccine obtained from the cough plates of patients. In 1931 P. H. Leslie and A. D. Gardner classified *H. pertussis* cultures into four types. Types III and IV were found to be ineffective for vaccines. This established an experimental basis for the development of an effective vaccine.[165]

In 1938 Harrison introduced alum-precipitated pertussis vaccine. This led to the general use of pertussis vaccine mixed with diphtheria toxoid. L. W. Sauer has been the leading exponent in the United States of active immunization. Passive immunization is possible through the use of pertussis human immune serum or of the gamma globulin fraction of this serum. Pertussis mortality on the decline in the United States for many years, has been decreasing more rapidly in recent years, owing perhaps to immunization and specific therapy for complications.

§ REFERENCES

[1] Ruffer, Sir M. A. (1921): *Studies in the palaeopathology of Egypt*. Chicago, University of Chicago Press. P. 32.
[2] Thucydides (1910): *History of the Peloponnesian War*. (Everyman's Library.) London and Toronto, J. M. Dent; New York, E. P. Dutton. Pp. 128–35.
[3] Hippocrates (1923): With an English translation by W. H. S. Jones. (Loeb Classical Library.) Cambridge, Mass., Harvard University Press; London, William Heinemann, Ltd. Vol. I, pp. 147–49.
[4] *Ibid.*, pp. lv–lxi.
[5] See, for example, Celsus (1935): *De medicina*. (Loeb Classical Library.) Cambridge, Mass., Harvard University Press; London, William Heine-

mann, Ltd. Vol. I, pp. 381–82; Caelius Aurelianus (1950): *On acute and on chronic diseases*. Chicago, University of Chicago Press. Pp. 299–305.

[6] Hippocrates, *op. cit.*, Vol. II, pp. 327–29.

[7] Aretaeus, the Cappadocian (1856): *The extant works of*. London, Sydenham Society. Pp. 253–55.

[8] Medical Research Council (1923): *Diphtheria: its bacteriology, pathology and immunology*. London, His Majesty's Stationery Office. P. 15.

[9] Newsholme, A. (1898): *Epidemic diphtheria*. London, Swan Sonnenschein & Co. P. 110.

[10] Haeser, H. (1865): *Geschichte der Epidemischen Krankheiten*. Jena, Friedrich Mauke. P. 387.

[11] Goodall, E. W. (1934): *A short history of the epidemic infectious diseases*. London, John Bale, Sons and Danielsson.

[12] Newsholme, *op. cit.*, p. 111.

[13] Webster, N. (1800): *A brief history of epidemic and pestilential diseases*. London, G. G. and J. Robinson. Vol. I, p. 226.

[14] Hecker, J. F. C. (1834): *Der Englische Schweiss*. Berlin, T. C. F. Enslin. Pp. 64–68.

[15] Newsholme, *op. cit.*, p. 111.

[16] Haeser, *op. cit.*, p. 392; Mansa, F. V. (1873): *Bidrag til falkesygdommenes og sundhedpleiens historie i Danmark*. Copenhagen. Pp. 192–97.

[17] Medical Research Council (1923): *Diphtheria*, p. 16.

[18] Major, R. H. (1945): *Classical descriptions of disease*. 3rd ed. Springfield, Illinois, Charles C. Thomas. P. 139.

[19] Haeser, *op. cit.*, pp. 392–94; Hecker, J. F. C. (1839): *Geschichte der neueren Heilkunde*. Berlin, T. C. F. Enslin. Pp. 239–47; Morejon, A. H. (1843–46): *Historia bibliográfica de la medicina española*. Madrid. Vol. II, p. 124; Vol. IV, pp. 62, 107–64, 304–5; Medical Research Council (1923): *Diphtheria*, pp. 16–20.

[20] Medical Research Council (1923): *Diphtheria*, pp. 19–20.

[21] Still, G. F. (1931): *The history of paediatrics*. London, Humphrey Milford; Oxford University Press. Pp. 229–34.

[22] Hecker, *op. cit.*, p. 247; Hirsch, A. (1886): *Handbook of geographical and historical pathology*. London, New Sydenham Society. Vol. III, p. 78.

[23] Hirsch, *op. cit.*, p. 80; Creighton, C. (1894): A history of epidemics in *Britain*. Cambridge, Cambridge University Press. Vol. II, pp. 685–91; Webster, *op. cit.*, Vol. I. pp. 378–84; Caulfield, E. (1939): *A true history of the terrible epidemic vulgarly called the throat distemper which occurred in His Majesty's New England colonies between the years 1735 and 1740*. New Haven, Connecticut; Duffy, J. (1953): *Epidemics in Colonial America*. Baton Rouge, Louisiana State University Press. Pp. 115–29.

[24] Webster, *op. cit.*, p. 310.

[25] Major, *op. cit.*, pp. 155–57.

[26] Chalmers, L. (1776): *An account of the weather and diseases of South Carolina.* London, Edward and Charles Dilly. Vol. II, pp. 91, 93, 207.

[27] Hirsch, *op. cit.,* pp. 78–81; Süssmilch, J. P. (1765): *Die Göttliche Ordnung* .... Berlin. Vol. I, pp. 525–29.

[28] Duffy, *op. cit.,* pp. 132–33.

[29] Still, *op. cit.,* p. 429.

[30] Bateman, T. (1819): *Reports on the diseases of London and the state of the weather from 1804 to 1816.* ... London, Longman, Hurst, Rees, Orme, and Brown. P. 191.

[31] Semple, H. R. (1859): *Memoirs on diphtheria. From the writings of Bretonneau, Guersant, Trousseau* .... London, New Sydenham Society; Major, *op. cit.,* pp. 157–61.

[32] Haeser, *op. cit.,* pp. 660–64; Hirsch, *op. cit.,* pp. 81–100; Creighton, *op. cit.,* pp. 734–44; Newsholme, *op. cit.,* pp. 117–20, 121–22.

[33] Oertel, M. (1871): *Dtsch. Arch. klin. Med., 8,* 242–354; Trendelenburg (1869): *Arch. klin. Chir., 10,* 720–42.

[34] Klebs (1883): *Verhandl. Congr. inn. Med.,* pp. 139–54.

[35] Loeffler, F. (1884): *Mitth. kaiserl. Gesundheitsamte, 2,* 421–99.

[36] Roux, E., and A. Yersin (1888): *Ann. Inst. Pasteur, 2,* 629–61; (1889): *Ibid., 3,* 273–88; and (1890): *Ibid., 4,* 385–426.

[37] Fraenkel, C. (1890): *Berl. klin. Wschr., 27,* 1133–35.

[38] Behring, E., and S. Kitasato (1890): *Dtsch. med. Wschr., 16,* 113–14; Behring (1890): *Ibid.,* 1145–48.

[39] Wright, J. (1914): *A history of laryngology and rhinology.* 2nd ed. Philadelphia, Lea and Febiger. P. 228.

[40] Winslow, C. E. A. (1929): *The life of Hermann M. Biggs.* Philadelphia, Lea and Febiger. Pp. 91–100.

[41] Biggs, H. M., W. H. Park, and A. L. Beebe, (1895): *Report on bacteriological investigations and diagnosis of diphtheria, from May 4, 1893 to May 4, 1894.* (Scientific Bulletin No. 1, Health Department, City of New York.) New York.
This report was reproduced in facsimile by the New York City Health Department on the occasion of the eighty-first annual meeting of the American Public Health Association in New York City in November, 1953.

[42] Goodall, *op. cit.,* p. 75.

[43] Smith, T. (1909): *J. exp. Med., 11,* 241–56.

[44] Behring, E. von (1913): *Dtsch. med. Wschr., 39,* 873–76.

[45] Schick, B. (1913): *Münch. med. Wschr., 60,* 2608–10.

[46] Ramon, G. (1923): *C. R. Acad. Sci., 177,* 1338–40.

[47] Park, W. H. (1922): *J. Amer. med. Ass., 79,* 1584–91; Zingher, A. (1921): *Arch. Pediat., 38,* 336–39; Zingher, A. (1923): *J. Amer. med Ass., 80,* 456–60.

[48] Russell, W. T. (1943): *Spec. Rep. Ser. Med. Res. Coun., Lond.,* No. 247; O'Hara, D. (1943): *Air-borne infection. Some observations on its decline.*

New York, Commonwealth Fund. Pp. 23–24; Burnet, M. (1953): *Natural history of infectious disease.* Cambridge, Cambridge University Press. Pp. 269–70.

(49) Bradford, W. L., E. Day, and F. Martin, (1949): *Pediatrics, 4,* 711–18.

(50) McGuinness, A. C. (1952): *J. Amer. med. Ass., 148,* 261–65.

(51) Rosenbach, O. (1904): *Physician versus Bacteriologist.* New York and London, Funk and Wagnalls. Pp. 413–48.

(52) Burnet, *op. cit.,* pp. 269–71.

(53) Anderson, J. S., *et al.* (1931): *J. Path. Bact., 34,* 667–81; McLeod, J. W. (1943): *Bact. Rev., 7,* 1–41.

(54) Burnet, *op. cit.,* p. 274.

(55) Haeser, *op. cit.,* pp. 63 ff.; Hirsch, *op. cit.,* Vol. I, p. 171.

(56) Hirsch, *op. cit.,* Vol. I, pp. 172–73.

(57) Haeser, *op. cit.,* pp. 380–81.

(58) Hecker, *op. cit.,* p. 219.

(59) Still, *op. cit.,* pp. 197–98.

(60) Haeser, *op. cit.,* pp. 380–81; Major, *op. cit.,* pp. 193–94.

(61) Hecker, *op. cit.,* pp. 225–26.

(62) Sydenham, T. (1844): *Opera omnia.* London, *Impensis Societatis Sydenhamianae.* Pp. 243–44.

(63) Pepys, S. (1927): *Diary of.* (Everyman's Library) London and Toronto, J. M. Dent; New York, E. P. Dutton. Vol. I, p. 532.

(64) Creighton, *op. cit.,* p. 681.

(65) *Ibid.,* pp. 682–83.

(66) Haeser, *op. cit.,* p. 380.

(67) Kaiser (1885): *Eulenbergs Vierteljahresschrift, 42,* 353; Neefe, M. (1897): *Z. Hyg., 24,* 247–88; Grotjahn, A. (1915): *Soziale Pathologie.* 2nd ed. Berlin, August Hirschwald. Pp. 270–1; Sydenstricker, E. (1933): *Health and environment.* New York, McGraw-Hill. Pp. 177–85; Rudder, B. de (1934): *Die akuten Zivilisationsseuchen.* Leipzig, Georg Thieme Verlag. Pp. 188–94.

(68) Creighton, *op. cit.,* pp. 719–20; Greenwood, M. (1935): *Epidemics and crowd diseases.* London, Williams and Norgate, Ltd. P. 212.

(69) Greenwood, *op. cit.,* p. 212.

(70) Graves, R. J. (1843): *A system of clinical medicine.* Dublin, Fannin and Co. P. 493. Cited by Creighton, *op. cit.,* Vol. I, p. 722.

(71) Dubos, R. J. (1945): *The bacterial cell.* Cambridge, Massachusetts, Harvard University Press. Pp. 188–228.

(72) Hecker, *op. cit.,* pp. 228–34; Haeser, *op. cit.,* pp. 488–89; Duffy, *op. cit.,* pp. 133–37.

(73) Still, *op. cit.,* p. 437.

(74) Creighton, *op. cit.,* pp. 708–11.

(75) Scott, H. H. (1934): *Some notable epidemics.* London, Edward Arnold and Co. P. 166.

(76) Creighton, *op. cit.,* pp. 726–27.

(77) *Annual report of the deaths and interments in the city and county of New York, for the year 1848.* Document No. 43, Board of Aldermen, March 5, 1849. Pp. 886–90; Smith, J. M. (1860): *Report on the medical topography and epidemics of the state of New York.* Philadelphia, Collins. P. 103.

(78) *Report of the Council of Hygiene and Public Health of the Citizens Association of New York upon the sanitary condition of the city.* New York, D. Appleton and Company. 1865. Pp. 29, 72, 113, 139, 179, 183, 237, 248, 319.

(79) Webb, C. B. (1940): *A history of contagious disease care in Chicago before the Great Fire.* Chicago, University of Chicago Press. Pp. 37–8, 59, 82, 99, 106, 119, 133.

(80) Sydenstricker, *op. cit.,* p. 181.

(81) Larsell, O. (1947): *The doctor in Oregon.* Portland, Oregon, Binfords and Mort. Pp. 24, 120, 266, 426, 428, 609.

(82) Jordan, P. D. (1953): *The people's health. A history of public health in Minnesota to 1948.* Saint Paul, Minnesota Historical Society. Pp. 6, 7, 15, 46, 109.

(83) Pope, A. S. (1926): *Amer. J. Hyg., 6,* 389–430.

(84) Woods, H. M. (1933): *Spec. Rep. Ser. Med. Res. Coun., Lond.,* No. 180.

(85) McKendrick, A. G. (1940): *Edinb. med. J., N. S. 47,* 117–36.

(86) Hirsch (1883): *op. cit.,* Vol. I, pp. 194–96; Scott, *op. cit.,* pp. 165–93; Henle, J. (1910): *Von den Miasmen und Kontagien.* Leipzig, Johann Ambrosius Barth.

(87) Schottmüller, H. (1903): *Münch. med. Wschr., 50,* 849–53, 909–12.

(88) Schultz, W., and W. Charlton (1918): *Z. Kinderheilk., 17,* 328–33.

(89) Dick, G. F., and G. H. (1924): *J. Amer. med. Ass., 82,* 265–66.

(90) Lancefield, R. C. (1928): *J. exp. Med., 47,* 91–103, 481–91; (1933) *Ibid., 57,* 571–95.

(91) Griffith, F. (1934): *J. Hyg., 34,* 542–84.

(92) Dochez, A. R., and L. Sherman (1924): *J. Amer. med. Ass., 82,* 542–44.

(93) Coburn, A. F., and D. C. Young (1949): *The epidemiology of hemolytic streptococcus.* Baltimore, Williams and Wilkins.

(94) Major, *op. cit.,* pp. 196–98.

(95) Mead, R. (1748): *A discourse on the small pox and measles, to which is annexed, A treatise on the same diseases by the celebrated Arabian physician Abu-Beker Rhazes.* London, John Brindley. P. 99.

(96) Graunt, J. (1899): *Natural and political observations upon the Bills of Mortality, in the economic writings of Sir William Petty.* Edited by C. H. Hull. Cambridge, Cambridge University Press. Vol. II, pp. 342–43, 406.

(97) Creighton, *op. cit.,* pp. 632–3.

(98) Sydenham, *op. cit.,* pp. 183–8.

(99) Graunt, *op. cit.,* p. 349.

(100) Cited by Creighton, *op. cit.,* p. 647.

(101) Tissot (1762): *Avis au peuple sur sa santé, ou traité des maladies les plus fréquentes.* Paris. P. 195.

[102] Süssmilch, *op. cit.*, pp. 523–25.

[103] Haeser, *op. cit.*, p. 488.

[104] Moll, A. A. (1944): *Aesculapius in Latin America.* Philadelphia, W. B. Saunders. P. 507.

[105] Duffy, *op. cit.*, p. 166.

[106] Caulfield, E. (1943): *Yale J. Biol. Med., 15,* 531–56.

[107] Thacher, T. (1937): *A brief rule to guide the common-people of New-England how to order themselves and theirs in the small-pocks or measles.* Facsimile reproductions of the three known editions with an introductory note by Henry R. Viets. Baltimore, Johns Hopkins Press.

[108] Webster, *op. cit.*, pp. 362, 374, 384, 467; Duffy, *op. cit.*, pp. 166–77; Packard, F. R. (1931): *History of medicine in the United States.* 2nd ed. New York, Paul B. Hoeber. Vol. I, pp. 94–5.

[109] Drake, D. (1850–55): *A systematic treatise, historical, etiological, and practical, on the principal diseases of the interior valley of North America.* Vol. II, p. 586.

[110] Panum, P. L. (1847): *Bibliot. Laeg.,* 3R., *1,* 270–344. English translation by A. S. Hatcher (1939): *Med. Class., 3,* 829–86.

[111] Hirsch, *op. cit.*, Vol. I, p. 169.

[112] Home, F. (1759): *Medical facts and experiments.* London, A. Millar. P. 266.

[113] Duffy, *op. cit.*, p. 178, n. 29; Still, *op. cit.*, p. 412; Tissot, *op. cit.*, p. 202.

[114] Hektoen, L. (1905): *J. infect. Dis., 2,* 238–55.

[115] Josias, A. H. L. (1898): *Méd. moderne, 9,* 153–54; Anderson, J. F., and J. Goldberger (1911): *Publ. Hlth Rep., Wash., 25,* 847–48.

[116] Anderson, J. F., and J. Goldberger (1911): *J. Amer. med. Ass., 57,* 113–14; Plotz, H. (1938): *Bull. Acad. Méd. Paris, 119,* 598–601; Rake, G., and M. F. Shaffer (1939): *Nature, Lond., 144,* 672–73; (1940): *J. Immunol., 38,* 177–200.

[117] Maris, E. P., et al. (1943): *J. Pediat., 22,* 17–29; (1949): *Pediatrics, 4,* 1–8.

[118] Koplik, H. (1896): *Arch. Pediat., 13,* 918–22.

[119] Nicolle, C., and E. Conseil (1918): *Bull. Soc. méd. Hôp. Paris, 3,* sér., t. *42,* 336–38.

[120] Rietschel (1921): *Z. Kinderheilk., 29,* 127–32; McKhann, C. F., and F. T. Chu (1933): *Amer. J. Dis. Child., 45,* 475–79.

[121] Cohn, E. J., et al. (1944): *J. clin. Invest., 23,* 417–32; Enders, J. F. (1944): *Ibid., 23,* 510–30; Stokes, Jr., J.; E. P. Maris and S. S. Gellis (1944): *Ibid., 23,* 531–40.

[122] Goodall, *op. cit.*, p. 63.

[123] Hosack, D. (1824): *Essays on various subjects of medical science.* New York, J. Seymour. Vol. II, pp. 334–463.

[124] Wagner (1829): *Litt. Ann. ges. Heilk., 13,* 420–28.

[125] Hiro, Y., and S. Tasaka (1938): *Mschr. Kinderheilk., 76,* 328–32.

[126] Gregg, N. M. (1941): *Trans. ophthal. Soc. Aust., 3,* 35–46.

[127] Lancaster, H. O. (1951): *Brit. med J., ii,* 1429–32.

[128] Aycock, W. L., and T. H. Ingalls (1946): *Amer. J. med. Sci., 212,* 366–79; McLorinan, H. (1950): *Med. J. Aust., ii,* 390–92.

[129] For the early and largely conjectural history of smallpox, see Creighton, *op. cit.,* Vol. I, pp. 439–45; Goodall, *op. cit.,* pp. 51–4. Hirsch, *op. cit.,* Vol. I, pp. 123–27.

[130] Fracastoro, G. (1930): *De contagione et contagiosis morbis et eorum curatione, libri III.* Translation and notes by Wilmer Cave Wright. New York, G. P. Putnam's Sons. Pp. 72–5.

[131] Haeser, *op. cit.,* p. 347.

[132] Creighton, *op. cit.,* Vol. I, p. 463.

[133] Macaulay, T.B. (1906): *The history of England from the accession of James II.* (Everyman's Library.) London, J. M. Dent; New York, E. P. Dutton, Vol. III, 320.

[134] Dover, T. (1732): *The ancient physician's legacy to his country.* London. P. 114. Cited by Creighton, *op. cit.,* Vol. II, p. 446, n. 1.

[135] Wilkes, S., and G. T. Bettany (1892): *A biographical history of Guy's Hospital.* London, Ward, Lock, Bowden and Co. Pp. 99–104; Duffy, *op. cit.,* p. 20.

[136] Still, *op. cit.,* p. 324.

[137] Fischer, A. (1933): *Geschichte des deutschen Gesundheitswesens.* Berlin, F. A. Herbig. Vol. II, p. 266.

[138] For the history of smallpox inoculation see Creighton, *op. cit.,* Vol. II, pp. 463–516; Leikind, M. C. (1942): *Ciba Symposia, 3,* 1090–101, 1124; Stearns, R. P., and G. Pasti, Jr. (1950): *Bull. Hist. Med., 24,* 103–22; Kittredge, G. L. (1921): *Introduction to Increase Mather: Several reasons proving that inoculating or transplanting the small pox is a lawful practice.* Cleveland. Pp. 1–67. Blake, J. B. (1952): *New Engl. Quart., 25,* 489–506; Blake, J. B. (1953): *J. Hist. Med., 8,* 284–300.

[139] Halsband, R. (1953): *J. Hist. Med., 8,* 390–405.

[140] Fischer, *op. cit.,* p. 267.

[141] Süssmilch, *op. cit.,* Vol. II, p. 440.

[142] Bernoulli, D. (1766): *"Essai d'une nouvelle analyse de la mortalité causée par la petite vérole et les avantages de l'inoculation pour la prevenir." Histoire de l'Académie royale des sciences, année 1760, avec les mémoires de mathématique et de physique pour la même année.* Paris.

[143] D'Alembert (1761): *"Sur l'application du calcul des probabilités à l'inoculation de la petite vérole." Opuscules Mathématiques,* II. Cited by Harald Westergaard (1932): *Contributions to the history of statistics.* London, P. S. King and Son. P. 93.

[144] For an analysis of the opposition to vaccination, see Stern, B. J. (1927): *Should we be vaccinated? A survey of the controversy in its historical and scientific aspects.* New York and London, Harper and Brothers.

[145] Hedrich, A. W. (1936): *Publ. Hlth Rep., Wash., 51,* 363–92.

[146] Gordon, M. (1937): *Edinb. med. J., N. S. 44,* 65–71; Paschen, E. (1906). *Münch. med. Wschr., 53,* 2391–93.

[147] Goodall, *op. cit.,* pp. 56–7.

[148] Still, *op. cit.,* p. 403.

[149] Heberden, W. (1767): *Med. Trans. Coll. Phys.* 3rd ed., *1,* 427–36; Still, *op. cit.,* pp. 439–42.

[150] Goodall, *op. cit.,* pp. 57–8.

[151] Kassowitz (1873): *Jb. Kinderheilk., 6,* 160–75.

[152] Steiner (1875): *Wien. med. Wschr., 25,* 305–8.

[153] Bókay, J. von (1909): *Wien. klin. Wschr., 22,* 1323–26.

[154] Goodall, *op. cit.,* p. 58; Paschen, E. (1917): *Dtsch. med. Wschr., 43,* 746–47.

[155] Hamilton, R. (1790): *Trans. roy. soc. Edinb., 2,* 59–72.

[156] Mettler, C. C. (1947): *History of medicine.* Philadelphia, Blakiston Company. P. 744.

[157] Croner (1884): *Dtsch. med. Wschr., 10,* 138.

[158] Johnson, C. D., and E. W. Goodpasture (1934): *J. exp. Med., 59,* 1–19.

[159] McGuinness, A. C., and E. A. Gall (1944): *War Medicine, 5,* 95–104.

[160] Still, *op. cit.,* p. 197.

[161] *Ibid.,* p. 284.

[162] Hirsch, *op. cit.,* Vol. III, p. 29.

[163] Bordet, J., and O. Gengou (1906): *Ann. Inst. Pasteur, 20,* 731–41.

[164] Chievitz, I., and A. H. Meyer: *Ibid., 30,* 503–24.

[165] Leslie, P. H., and A. D. Gardner (1931): *J. Hyg., Camb., 31,* 423–34.

BY C. H. STUART-HARRIS
M. D., F. R. C. P.*

chapter 2 / influenza

> "Many important events were attributed to the
> influence of the stars: storms, earthquakes, famines
> and epidemics. If Florence was in the grip of an
> epidemic of colds, coughs and fevers, astrologers were
> consulted, and they declared that it was caused by the
> influence of an unusual conjunction of planets. This
> sickness, which kept recurring from time to time in hard
> winters, came gradually to be known as 'influenza.'"
> Ginevra Niccolini di Camugliano: *The chronicles
> of a Florentine family, 1200–1470.*

MANY HAVE SOUGHT by a description of the epidemiological behavior
of influenza to answer the riddle of its causation. The recorded history
of epidemics is thus strewn with hypothesis and fancy. But the discovery of the causative viruses of influenza in the recent past has
warned against too speculative an approach to the many problems
associated with this disease. Who, for instance, can argue concerning
the reason for the periodical recurrences of influenza without knowledge concerning the different viruses and the mechanism of resistance
to their attack? It is a special characteristic of this group of viruses to
produce only temporary immunity, in contrast to many other viruses
such as those of measles, smallpox, or yellow fever, whose attack leads
to a permanent change in the attitude of the host. For the historian
the discovery of the causative viruses marks a new approach to the
epidemiology of the disease. Yet there are still uncharted diseases of
the respiratory tract that resemble influenza clinically, and the problem stated so succinctly by Otto Leichtenstern (1896) is still apparent:

* Professor of medicine, University of Sheffield, England, he is author of *Influenza
and other virus infections of the respiratory tract* (1953).

71

If we carefully analyze the influenza epochs compiled by historians, and especially the description by A. Hirsch, comprising the years from 1173 to 1875, we shall see that in the last century, which was characterized by increasing facilities for the distribution of news, scarcely a year passed in which the epidemic prevalence of influenza in some part of the world is not recorded. Many of these local and limited epidemics were nothing more than late sequels of the great pandemics, often separated by long intervals, the germs of the disease planted by these epidemics having remained alive for years. We must speak of influenza-epochs and not of influenza-years. Many of the other epidemics described as influenza have very probably nothing in common with "influenza vera." They are epidemics of local "catarrhal fever."

The identification of the influenza virus A occurred in 1933; influenza virus B was first recovered in 1940; and the newest influenza virus of all, that of virus C, was found only six years ago. The first serious laboratory attempt to study epidemics on a global scale was made in 1949, and the chain of reference laboratories organized by the World Health Organization is still far from complete in all corners of the globe. But the information at present available clearly indicates the major importance of influenza virus A in the pandemic experience of influenza, with a lesser role of influenza virus B in more localized outbreaks. The significance of influenza virus C cannot be appreciated as yet, but it is quite certain that localized outbreaks of respiratory disease resembling influenza clinically, but occurring independently of country-wide epidemicity, are not related to any known virus of the influenza group. Under these circumstances one may question the validity of many of the historical records of influenza in terms of relationship to the modern disease. Providing, however, that influenza is identified not solely by clinical evidence, but by reason of its explosive outburst and almost simultaneous occurrence in widely separated geographical areas, then the older historical records are descriptive of something familiar in the eighteenth century and afterwards, and for which the term "influenza" is certainly justified.

§ HISTORY OF INFLUENZA EPIDEMICS

(a) *Before the nineteenth century*. No one can with certainty discern the earliest recorded epidemics of influenza. August Hirsch (1883) considered the first outbreak which could reasonably be regarded as influenza occurred in 1173, when a "certain evil and unheard-of cough" affected Italy, Germany, and England. There were, however, earlier epidemics in which a cough was a principal symptom, epidemics that could have been the same disease, but information is too scanty for judgment to be passed. Outbreaks in the fourteenth and fifteenth centuries due to influenza are mentioned by Hirsch, but many give the epidemic of 1510 first place, while that of 1580 is sometimes termed the first pandemic. It seems certain that the word "influenza" was first used in Italy, either because of the supposed influence of the stars or because of the classical term for catarrh—*influxio,* whose Italian form was *influsso.* The term did not, however, reach England until 1743, and a host of phrases such as "the new burning ague," "the new acquaintance," "the gentle correction," "the strange fever," and the "jolly rant" accompany descriptions of outbreaks in the sixteenth and seventeenth centuries. It is likely that influenza was often forgotten in the intervals between its periodic recurrences, and each renewal of the disease was thought to be a new phenomenon until resemblance to former experience became apparent.

The "malignant epidemic catarrh" of 1580 occurred in a century when plagues, agues, and the sweating sicknesses all vied with respiratory disease. Yet this epidemic was widespread in Europe and Africa, and clinical accounts are very similar to those by Thomas Willis and Thomas Sydenham of the later outbreaks in the seventeenth century. Other epidemics mentioned in letters are often quoted because of their reference to the illness of notable persons, such as the Edinburgh outbreak of the "newe acquayntance" of 1562 in the Court of Mary Queen of Scots, mentioned in Thomas Randolph's letter to William Cecil, Lord Burghley (Creighton, 1894). But Willis' account of "catarrhal fever," though of a more strictly medical character, is befogged by reference to the state of the air and effervescence of the blood in spring. Sydenham's account of the epidemic cough of 1675 and afterwards is also involved with the doctrine of epidemic constitution and replacement of one constitution by another with change of seasons. Most early authors were also more concerned with portraying the fearful ravages of disease than with facts, and one turns with relief to the straightforward description by John Huxham (Thompson, 1852) of the epidemic of 1743 as he saw it in Plymouth:

73

Towards the end of April, a kind of fever, in general slight, but sometimes not a little fatal to old men and children who had weak lungs, raged
throughout all this country. At once, and at the same time, innumerable
persons were seized with a wandering kind of shiver and heaviness in the
head; presently also came on a pain therein, and also in the joints and back;
several, however, were troubled with a universal lassitude. Immediately a
very great and acrid defluxion from the eyes, nostrils and fauces, and very
often falling upon the lungs, which occasion almost perpetual sneezings,
and commonly a violent cough.

The epidemic of 1743 was widespread in Europe and particularly
in Italy, where there were approximately eighty thousand affected
persons in Rome alone, and five hundred deaths in one day. Germany
and England were affected some weeks later, and the London weekly
mortality rate was trebled in one week. It is clear, however, from this
and earlier outbreaks that influenza was, and is, a disease of variable
mortality, and one cannot but sympathize with the confusion of the
chronicler whose superstitions or beliefs were given full rein in at-
tempting to explain the vagaries of this disease.

There were many recorded epidemics in the eighteenth century,
and the one in 1782 which affected the world from China to Europe
and America created an abundant literature. The report of the Royal
College of Physicians mentions an observation, since noted repeatedly,
which was particularly puzzling. On the one hand, it was observed
many times that influenza broke out in certain localities shortly after
the arrival of persons coming from places previously attacked by the
disease. But the crew of the East Indiaman *Atlas,* sailing in 1780 from
Malacca to Canton, suffered an outbreak when they were in the China
Seas, though there had been no cases in the former port. When the
ship arrived at Canton, the sailors were astonished to learn that an
outbreak had occurred there at almost the same time as the epidemic
aboard ship. Edward Gray's account (Thompson, 1852) of the 1782
epidemic, which was very detailed, mentions similar experiences of
influenza on board ships many miles at sea, but unfortunately he
concludes his account with reference to the annual epidemic at St.
Kilda following the arrival of the steward and his party. These epidemics are clearly outbreaks of common colds, though influenza in
island communities has often been observed elsewhere to follow the

74

calling of ships and the disembarkation of apparently healthy individuals. (Isaacs *et al.*, 1950.)

(b) *The nineteenth century and afterwards.* The first half of the nineteenth century experienced the same pattern of epidemics as the eighteenth century, and there were pandemics in 1830, 1837, and 1847. The last caused a particularly sharp outbreak in London in December; a new system of registration had been introduced, and an excess of five thousand deaths in the six weeks of the epidemic was recorded. A minor epidemic occurred in England in 1855, and then came a lull for forty years during which no epidemics were prevalent in Western Europe and which preceded the violent disturbances of 1889 to 1893. The 1890 pandemic, as it is sometimes called, actually began with a mild outbreak in 1889, and this was followed by two further epidemics in 1891 and 1892, which were successively more violent and productive of increasing mortality. The fourth epidemic in 1893 was again milder, but from this time to the present day the periodic recurrences of influenza have been apparently more severe than in the pre-1890 period, and the intervening troughs of mortality have also been altered. The available records of mortality in the nineteenth century for England and Wales show clearly the almost complete absence of influenza from 1860 until the sudden outburst in 1890. The base line of annual mortality subsequent to this year is then elevated to a point much higher than that previously reached, and one has to follow the records as far as 1948 to find any figure comparable with the pre-1890 epoch. Much the same experience is recorded in Australia, as pointed out by F. M. Burnet and E. Clark (1942), although the pre-1890 period was not so deceptively peaceful as in England. These authors suggest that a "virus reservoir" in the Siberian and northern Asiatic areas was established after the Russian epidemics of 1886 and 1887 and that the 1889–93 pandemic originated from this source. There is in fact no solid evidence for the view that an influenza virus reservoir in a fixed location is ever established, and one must not forget that the first invasion of Western Europe after the period of quiescence was in 1889–90 and that this was not the most lethal outbreak of the pandemic. The more fatal epidemics of 1891 and 1892 showed, moreover, what is sometimes termed the "normal" age distribution of mortality. Influenza, both before 1890 as in Huxham's

75

time and in recent years, has usually caused deaths primarily in the older age groups, and this was certainly the case in the later waves of the 1889–93 pandemic. In only the initial epidemic was an appreciable share of the mortality (25 per cent) borne by those aged twenty to forty, and as no figures are available for the incidence of the disease, the true mortality rate is unknown.

Following this pandemic, the base line between epidemics and the height of the recurrent epidemics were increased—compared with the period before 1890. Then in 1916 and 1917 influenza epidemics with an unusual number of pneumonic complications were experienced both in Europe and America. From out of this threatening sky there came the first deceptively mild wave of the greatest pandemic in recorded history. This summer wave, as it is sometimes called, apparently began in various army camps in the United States of America in March and April and then appeared in Europe at the ports of disembarkation of American troops in France. Though mild almost everywhere, the morbidity was often high, and by June, 1918, the experience in England indicated an unusual tendency to pneumonia with 38.9 per cent of all the deaths in those aged twenty to forty. The second and third waves of this colossal epidemic, which were experienced in November, 1918, and March, 1919, were worldwide and highly lethal; it has been estimated that fifteen million people died. The young adults between twenty and forty contributed about 50 per cent of the total deaths, though the actual incidence of the disease was greatest between the ages of five and fifteen and least in those aged fifty-five and over. The mortality rate in those attacked rose steadily with increasing age, and the fearful slaughter of young adults was due to the exceptionally high attack rate and remarkable tendency to pneumonic involvement. The heliotrope cyanosis seen in those smitten with pneumonia has become a classical description of fulminating influenzal pneumonia, and though occasional cases of this type have been seen both before and since 1918, nothing comparable with the numbers of those affected has ever been observed. The havoc of this pandemic was so fearful that for years afterwards the name influenza carried an implied threat both to lay and medical people. As Major Greenwood (1935) says, one has to turn back to the pestilence of 1348–49 for any parallel experience in history.

The accounts of the 1918 pandemic which have appeared in the form of several monographs must be read by those interested in detail, for it is impossible in this chapter to give more than a token description. The main features in addition to the mortality were first, the widespread geographical dispersion and synchronous development of epidemics in places separated by thousands of miles, second, the relatively slow spread from one town to another near by, and third, the apparent protection of some groups affected severely in one wave from the effects of a later wave and apparent absence of protection in other groups. In fact, the 1918 pandemic exhibited so many paradoxes that the epidemiologist has found it a most suitable subject for speculation and development of theories concerning the causation of influenza. Moreover, the fact that its etiology remained at the time unsolved has furnished a constant stimulus to laboratory workers on influenza ever since.

For a few years after the pandemic, exceptionally large epidemics of influenza continued to be experienced, particularly in 1922, 1927, and 1929. Since 1929, both in Europe and America, the peaks of the major epidemics have fallen, and the troughs of intervening mortality have been at a steadily lower level. In 1948 a nadir was reached in England and Wales, which was actually comparable with the level of deaths from influenza in the pre-1890 epoch, but moderate epidemics have since been experienced in 1949, 1951, and 1953. It is difficult to assess the significance of the fall in mortality in the past twenty years. An acceleration of this fall set in after 1937, which may have been due to chemotherapy of the pneumonic complications, but periodic rises and falls in influenza mortality have occurred before, and the present phase may be due to a combination of circumstances favoring the host. The most important feature of this post-1918 period is the fact that in successive epidemics the percentage of the mortality in those over fifty-five has steadily risen from the 1918 figure of 25 per cent to 88 per cent in 1951. Even in the sharp Liverpool outbreak of the latter year, when more deaths occurred in the city than in 1918, almost all the mortality was borne by the older age groups. A greater share of the excess mortality from influenza during recent outbreaks has also been borne by chronic conditions other than respiratory ones, of which heart disease was the largest contributor.

§ ETIOLOGY AND INTERPRETATION OF
THE EPIDEMIOLOGY OF INFLUENZA

Studies on the etiological agent concerned in influenza may be said to have begun with the 1890 pandemic, when R. F. J. Pfeiffer (1892) described the bacillus now known as *Hemophilus influenzae* (Pfeiffer's bacillus). Failure to recover this organism from certain outbreaks and particularly during the summer wave in 1918 cast doubt upon its importance, but the virus theory, though unproven, began to be widely held. In 1933, Wilson Smith, C. H. Andrewes, and Sir Patrick P. Laidlaw recovered the virus now known as influenza virus A from throat washings of patients during the epidemic of 1932–33. There is no longer any possible doubt that this virus alone, and without any bacterial accompaniment, is the causative agent of the majority of country-wide epidemics of influenza and of most pandemics since 1933. It is an occasional cause of localized outbreaks, and sporadic cases of infection have also been identified. In general, however, influenza virus A does not behave as an identifiable cause of endemic respiratory disease, and the reason for its sudden appearance in epidemic form has thus far defied all attempts at revelation. Observations of epidemics in England, the United States, and Australia have now shown that influenza A recurs in epidemic form, though in variable intensity, every two years and rarely annually. Major outbreaks in any one country are usually at least four years and occasionally as long as seven years apart. Entirely independently of influenza A, the infection caused by the influenza virus B, which was simultaneously recovered in New York by T. Francis, Jr., and T. P. Magill in 1940, recurs in the population at two, four, or more years' intervals in the form of local outbreaks or less often of moderate country-wide epidemics. Pandemic experience of influenza B is a long drawn-out affair with successive foci of infection lighting up and burning out in different areas. Influenza B appears also as a cause of sporadic infection in the population between epidemics to a greater extent than influenza A.

Experimental work on these two viruses has confirmed the temporary character of the immunity which they engender and which is probably due to the surface character of the infection and lack of systemic invasion. Added to this, however, significant antigenic differences have been found between the viruses recovered from different epidemics, and this modification is also a possible weapon which enables the virus to break through the barrier of partial immunity created by its previous epidemic attack upon the human population. The entire lack of cross-immunity between the viruses of the influenza A and B groups is a further reason for epidemic recurrences of influenza in the population at annual or irregular intervals. Subclinical infection is another striking characteristic of infection by either viruses experimentally and in man, and the discovery that at least double the number of individuals in a group show serological changes as develop clinical attacks during an epidemic is an important factor in herd immunity. Meanwhile, the role of bacteria of the nasopharyngeal tract such as pneumococci, hemolytic streptococci, and staphylococci, has been shown to be concerned with the development of pneumonic complications, while *hemophilus influenzae* may be similarly concerned with the bronchitic complications of the disease. The mortality experienced in an epidemic cannot, however, be simply a matter of the number of pneumonic complications as shown by T. Anderson and the co-authors' account of recent epidemics in Glasgow (1953). The virulence of the influenza virus, which affects its ability to attack the lower respiratory tract, to create conditions favoring secondary bacterial infection, and also to weaken the circulatory system, is probably of a variable character. So far, however, the virulence of different influenza virus strains has not proved susceptible to experimental study in the laboratory.

Finally, experimental observations upon swine influenza by R. E. Shope (1944) have shown that in this species an influenza virus serologically related to influenza virus A co-operates with an organism of the *hemophilus* group—*Hemophilus influenzae suis*—in the production of an explosively epidemic disease with high incidence of pneumonia. The virus survives from one epidemic to the next by a complicated cycle of events involving a common lung parasite of pigs—swine lungworm. An entire herd of pigs may thus be seeded with virus in a masked form, and after a provocative stimulus either of a meteorological or shock-like character, the virus is enabled to emerge in its normal infective form and to produce clinical phenomena. Such a complex life cycle is highly unlikely in the case of human influenza virus. No evidence of virus surviving between epidemics in a latent phase has yet been uncovered, though many consider this to be a likely event. The alternative reservoir is that of a continual chain of infection in one or other area of the globe, which is difficult to reconcile with the almost simultaneous involvement in an epidemic of widely separated areas.

All these important laboratory studies can now be applied to the interpretation of the epidemiological character of human influenza. Probably the most important characteristic of the influenza virus A, which is significant in relation to the extraordinary variability of behavior of the human disease, is its biological plasticity. As it is possible to modify the virus in the alternate directions of enhanced virulence or attenuation for an experimental host, it cannot be doubted that similar variations can occur under the conditions of natural passage from man to man. In addition to variations in virulence, this virus can modify its antigenicity, which is the chief factor against which antibody protection is attempted by the infected host, and this may well account for the apparent success of the parasite in its recurrent attacks upon man.

Apart from the characteristic of periodic recurrence of influenza, there are certain major puzzles which have been mentioned in the description of historical outbreaks. The first of these is the property of explosiveness or rapid building up of large numbers of cases of influenza in a previously healthy group. So far there is no completely satisfactory explanation of this from the virus standpoint, for populations have usually been studied after the epidemic has occurred and not before the event. Either the pre-epidemic phase is one of intensive spread of the virus in such a form that it is present in the majority of individuals in a latent phase (on the analogy of swine influenza), or else it spreads by causing largely subclinical infections to a selected few individuals from which the whole group can be rapidly involved. One must not forget that an incubation period as short as forty-eight hours could enable rapid spread throughout a group of individuals in close contact, and explosive influenza outbreaks are usually found in a school, a regiment, or other group in close residential contact. Meanwhile, it is important to stress that, although direct spread of virus from one individual to another cannot be doubted, the transmission of the disease from town to town or country to country is not much faster in these days of rapid transport than in the days before the automobile and the airplane. The full story of how influenza virus spreads is still unknown; we must have a fuller knowledge of its natural history.

Then there is the problem of the apparent escape of a community from infection during one epidemic and yet the fact that the next wave may cause no more severe an outbreak than in an originally more involved neighboring group. The fact that subclinical infection is a major phenomenon may possibly explain this form of herd immunity, for the visible cases of influenza are exceeded in number by those invisibly infected.

The sudden changes in behavior of influenza, and particularly its absence during the forty years before 1890 and its changed behavior since that date, furnish the virus worker with a major challenge. All that can be said at present is that until the viruses have been studied for a longer period of time, there is no real explanation but only conjecture. Some feel that the pre-1890 epoch was associated with widespread infection of an exceptionally benign type of virus and that the change from this to a more virulent organism introduced that form of virus known now as influenza virus A. C. H. Andrewes (1942) argued that the high interepidemic level of mortality attributed to influenza which has been seen ever since 1890 until recently is due to infection with a basic form of virus devoid of its characteristic antigenic and pathogenic properties and from which the recognizable A and B viruses periodically regenerate. Others believe the background of respiratory infection to be a composite of various virus infections totally unrelated to the influenza viruses. This brings in the fact that knowledge of the various virus infections of the respiratory tract, of the common cold, and of febrile catarrh is still rudimentary. Few will doubt the bearing of this knowledge ultimately upon the influenza problem, if only because the influenza epidemic is just as often superimposed upon a background of epidemicity of colds and catarrhs as it is depicted as descending from a cloudless sky. One may perhaps be forgiven for referring to the possible changes in virulence or antigenicity of viruses by the mechanism of hybridization of two strains with different properties shown to be possible in the laboratory (Burnet and Lind, 1951) and, therefore, probable in nature. The question as to whether or not pandemic influenza of the 1918 type is due to the sudden origin of a novel type of virus of high virulence or of unique antigenicity by mutation or by genetic recombination will not be solved by armchair speculation or laboratory experiment alone, and it may be that a future historian will report the solution of the problem as the result of study of a further human devastation. Meanwhile, evidence exists for believing that the virus responsible for the 1918 pandemic may have passed into an animal host and that it survives to this day as the swine influenza virus already mentioned.

Finally, the laboratory has so far given a negative answer to those who have believed in the variable clinical characters of influenza. Gastro-intestinal outbreaks occurring alongside outbreaks of influenza were often attributed to this disease, but the laboratory has shown no such relationship. Past epidemiologists also referred to nervous forms of influenza as typified by cases of encephalitis or even to the mysterious epidemic of *encephalitis lethargica* that appeared in the years following the 1918 pandemic and which has since disappeared. No positive link between influenza virus and human encephalitis has been discovered, though laboratory strains of influenza virus with neurotropic properties for mice have been artificially developed. It seems in general unlikely that influenza viruses of the types known so far are related to the infection of the human nervous system, but no one can utterly discount the possibility.

§ REFERENCES

Anderson, T., N. R. Grist, J. B. Landsman, S. I. A. Laidlaw, and I. B. L. Weir (1953): "An epidemic of influenza due to virus B." *Brit. med. J., i,* 7–11.

Andrewes, C. H. (1942): "Thoughts on the origin of influenza epidemics." *Proc. R. Soc. Med., Sect. Pathol., 36,* 1–10.

Burnet, F. M., and E. Clark (1942): *Influenza.* Walter & Eliza Hall Institute of Research, Melbourne. Monograph 4. Melbourne, Macmillan & Co., Ltd.

Burnet, F. M., and P. E. Lind (1951): "A genetic approach to variation in influenza viruses." *J. gen. Microbiol., 5,* 59–66, 67–82.

Creighton, C. (1891–94): *A history of epidemics in Britain.* 2 vols. Cambridge, Cambridge University Press.

Deutschman, Z. (1953): "Trend of influenza mortality during the period 1920–51." *Bull. World Hlth Org., 8,* 633–45.

Francis, Jr., T. (1940): "A new type of virus from epidemic influenza." *Science, 92,* 405–8.

Greenwood, M. (1935): *Epidemics and crowd diseases.* London, Williams & Norgate, Ltd.

Influenza

Hirsch, A. (1883): *Handbook of geographical and historical pathology.* Translated and edited by Charles Creighton. London, New Sydenham Society. Vol. I.

Isaacs, A., M. Edney, M. Donnelley, and M. W. Ingram (1950): "Influenza in an isolated community: an epidemic on Ocean Island." *Lancet, i,* 64–6.

Leichtenstern, O. (1896): *"Influenza und Dengue."* In *Nothnagel's Spezielle Pathologie und Therapie.* Vienna, A. Hölder. Authorized translation from the German, under the editorial supervision of Alfred Stengel (1905): Philadelphia & London, W. B. Saunders & Company.

Magill, T. P. (1940): "A virus from cases of influenza-like upper-respiratory infection." *Proc. Soc. exp. Biol., N. Y., 45,* 162–64.

Pfeiffer, R. (1892): *"Vorläufige Mittheilungen über die Erreger der Influenza."* *Dtsch. med. Wschr., 18,* 28.

Shope, R. E. (1944): "Old, intermediate, and contemporary contributions to our knowledge of pandemic influenza." *Medicine, Baltimore, 23,* 415–55.

Smith, W., C. H. Andrewes, and P. P. Laidlaw (1933): "A virus obtained from influenza patients." *Lancet, ii,* 66–8.

Thompson, T. (1852): *Annals of influenza or epidemic catarrhal fever in Great Britain.* London, Sydenham Society.

Reports concerning the 1918 pandemic:

Frost, W. H. (1941): *Papers of: a contribution to epidemiological method.* Edited by K. F. Maxcy. New York, Commonwealth Fund; London, Oxford University Press. Pp. 321, 340.

Jordan, E. O. (1927): "The influenza epidemic of 1918." *J. Amer. med. Ass., 89,* 1603–6, 1689–93, 1779–83.

Rep. publ. Hlth med. Subj., Lond. (1920): *Report on the pandemic of Influenza, 1918–1919.* No. 4. London, H. M. Stationery Office.

Thomson, D., and R. Thomson (1933): "Influenza." *Ann. Pickett-Thompson Res. Lab., 9,* 1–640.

Vaughan, W. T. (1921): "Influenza: an epidemiological study." *Amer. J. Hyg.,* Monograph *1.*

BY E. M. BROCKBANK

M. B. E., M. D., F. R. C. P.*

and WILLIAM BROCKBANK

M. A., M. D., F. R. C. P.†

chapter 3 / pneumonia

IT IS DIFFICULT to collect information about pneumonia, as we understand it now, from the works of the early physicians. The methods of
diagnosis were very primitive and unsatisfactory until the end of
the eighteenth century. All inflammatory conditions of the respiratory
organs, including the pleura, were looked upon as of the same nature
and origin, and were called "peripneumonia." Many physicians wrote
on the subject, but we can only refer to a few of the chief stages in the
substitution of scientific methods for empiricism in the investigation,
diagnosis, and treatment of the disease.

In the history of any disorder it is of interest to read the first definite reference to it in medical literature. As regards pneumonia, this
occurs in the writings of Hippocrates, the "Father of Medicine," who
lived between 460 and 370 B.C. Like other early writers, he included
all acute diseases of the chest which were accompanied with pain in
the side under the term "peripneumonia"—a term which persisted
for over two thousand years.

If the fever be acute, and if there be pains on either side, or in both, and
if expiration be attended with pain, if cough be present, and the sputa
expectorated be of a blond or livid colour, or likewise thin and frothy, and
florid, or having any other character different from the common, in such a
case the physician should proceed thus: if the pain pass upward to the

---

* Hon. Consulting Physician, Manchester Royal Infirmary, England, he has written numerous books and papers on medicine and medical history.

† Son of E. M. Brockbank, he is Hon. Physician to the Manchester Royal Infirmary,
the history of which he wrote in 1952.

clavicle ... the inner vein in the arm should be opened on the side affected, and the blood abstracted according to the habit, age, and color of the patient, and the season of the year, and that largely and boldly if the pain be acute.

The pain could also be eased by means of hot water in a bottle or bladder, or with a sponge squeezed out of hot water and covered up to keep in the heat, or by a cataplasm of linseed applied to the hypochondrium as far up as the breasts. The bowels were to be kept open by clysters or by a purge when the fever was at its height. A linctus was prescribed containing galbanum and pine fruit in Attic honey; or southernwood in oxymel. It was also a good thing to give as a drink opoponax (bitter resin with a garlic taste) in oxymel. Ptisan, made of husked barley, sometimes with oxymel, was ordered as a drink.

Aretaeus, in the second century, gave an even clearer account of peripneumonia and referred to the cause of the pain:

This is what we call peripneumonia, being an inflammation of the lungs, with acute fever, when they are attended with heaviness of the chest, freedom from pain, provided the lungs alone are inflamed; for they are naturally insensible, being of loose texture, like wool. . . . But if any of the membranes, by which the lung is connected with the chest, be inflamed, pain also is present; respiration bad, and hot; [the patients] wish to get up into an erect posture, as being the easiest of all postures for the respiration . . . ; there is thirst, dryness of the tongue, desire of cold air, aberration of mind; cough mostly dry, but if anything be brought up it is a frothy phlegm, or slightly tinged with bile, or with a very florid tinge of blood. The blood-stained is, of all others, the worst.

Aretaeus gave excellent directions for the application of his remedies which were much the same as those in use at the beginning of the present century, namely copious bleeding from both arms simultaneously (but so as to avoid unconsciousness), purging, attenuant and diluent drinks, rubefacients containing mustard applied to the chest, alkaline substances such as soda given in the decoction of hyssop, and, when the fever had subsided, wine devoid of astringency.

There was no evidence in any of the early writings of the physical examination of the sick. The methods of diagnosis were the inspection

85

of the patient and his excreta, of the blood withdrawn by venesection, and estimation of the temperature by touch. The pulse was felt, and conclusions were drawn from its characters before Harvey discovered its physiological significance.

No progress was made in medieval times. Thomas Sydenham (1624–89) gave the first good account in English of the disease, but thought that the true peripneumonia was of the same nature as a pleurisy, except that it affected the lungs more universally. His description of a pleurisy is more like that of pneumonia. He refers to a "bastard peripneumony," which affected the stout and fat beyond adult life, and those who had been overaddicted to spirituous liquors, more especially to brandy. Fever was absent. Hermann Boerhaave's pupil John Huxham (1692–1768), who practiced in Totnes and Plymouth, combined first-rate ability as an original observer and practitioner with the posings of the quacks of his time. He invented the formula of the compound tincture of cinchona, known as Huxham's tincture, as a tonic for treatment of the disease.

In *Essays on fevers* (1755), Huxham described pleurisies, peripneumonias, and pleuroperipneumonia. He was a great advocate of bleeding, as might be expected from his methods of attracting patients, and he valued the evidence obtainable from the appearance of the blood drawn at different stages of these diseases. He recognized the *Peripneumonia Notha* of Sydenham by its sluggish course and slight degree of fever. Pleuroperipneumonia was characterized by a severe pain in the breast, acute fever, heaviness at the breast, cough, difficulty of breathing, and spitting of blood. He referred to the dangers of peripneumonia which followed catarrhal fevers and quoted Hippocrates to the same effect, with a warning against venesection as a part of its treatment. His account is very like the type of pneumonia met with in an influenza epidemic. He considered that wet cupping over the shoulders could be done with safety and gave good relief. He found setons and issues very serviceable.

Most of the writers until this time followed Hippocrates closely. Paracelsus in 1527 actually burnt Galen's works publicly because he differed from the Father of Medicine. Consequently, little progress was made in unraveling the problem of pneumonia until anatomy was studied more carefully on the continent, and the changes met with in dissections began to be noted by the more observant. Thus we find Hermann Boerhaave in 1709 describing in his *Aphorisms* two kinds of peripneumonia:

The Seat of the one is in the Extremities of the *Arteria Pulmonalis,* and of t'other in the Productions of the Windpipe call'd *Bronchia* ... A Pleurisy is said to be present when the Patient is afflicted with an acute continual Fever with a hard Pulse, an acute inflammatory Pain and Stitch much increased upon breathing in the Air.

This was possibly a recognition of lobar and of lobular pneumonia: " ... hence the lungs grow weighty, unable to unfold themselves and livid. ... *It terminates into Health.* ... By causing the Patient as soon as possible *to spit* freely, abundantly yellowish with a little mixture of blood." Boerhaave placed the seat of pain in the pleura.

Giovanni Battista Morgagni (1682–1771) went farther and described the post-mortem appearance of the lung as a consolidation, the texture being like that of solid flesh. He noticed also the adhesion of the surfaces of the two pleurae.

Even the great William Cullen (1712–90), founder of the Glasgow Medical School, who was the first to give clinical lectures in Great Britain, thought that inflammation of the thorax constituted but one genus and placed it under the name of pneumonia: "Though sometimes distinct, yet, in general, no accurate limits could be placed between pleuritis and pneumonia, and to distinguish between them was a refinement of little or no use in the practice of medicine."

§ TREATMENT BY BLEEDING

Cullen believed that the most important method of treatment was bleeding, and he set about the job with an energy and enthusiasm that is frightening to the twentieth-century mind:

The remedy chiefly to be depended upon, is that of bleeding at the arm, which will be performed with most advantage in the arm of the side affected, but may be done in either arm, as may be most convenient for the patient or the surgeon. The quantity drawn must be suited to the violence of the disease, and to the vigour of the patient, and generally ought to be as large as this last circumstance will allow. The remission of pain, and the relief of respiration, during the flowing of the blood, may limit the quantity to be then drawn; but if these symptoms of relief do not appear, the bleeding should be continued till the symptoms of a beginning syncope come on. It is seldom that one bleeding, however large, will prove a cure of this disease; and although the pain and difficulty of breathing may be much relieved by the first bleeding, these symptoms commonly, and after no long interval, recur, often with as much violence as before. In the event of such recurrence, the bleeding is to be repeated, even in the course of the same day, and perhaps to the same quantity as before.

Sometimes the second bleeding may be larger than the first. There are persons who, by their constitution, are ready to faint even upon a small bleeding; and, in such persons, this may prevent the drawing so much blood at first as a pneumonic inflammation might require; but, as the same persons are sometimes found to bear after-bleedings better than the first, this allows the second and subsequent bleeding to be larger, and to such a quantity as the symptoms of the disease may seem to demand.

It is according to the state of the symptoms that bleedings are to be repeated, and they will be more effectual when practised in the course of the first three days, than afterwards; but they are not to be omitted, although four days of the disease may have already elapsed. If the physician shall not have been called in sooner, or if the bleedings practised during the first days shall not have been large enough, or even although these bleedings shall have procured some remission; yet, upon the recurrence of the urgent symptoms the bleeding should be repeated at any period of the disease, especially within the first fortnight; and even afterwards, if a tendency to suppuration be not evident, or if, after a seeming solution, the disease shall have again returned.

§ HEPATIZATION OF LUNGS

The darkness began to be less dense with the first accurate description of hepatization of the lungs in pneumonia, which was given by John Hunter's nephew, Matthew Baillie (1761–1823). He was the first British physician to treat pathology as a subject in itself and to connect the case history with the post-mortem findings:

Inflammation of the substance of the lungs, I believe, seldom takes place without some similar affection of the pleura; at least in the instances which I have seen, this has been most frequently the case. When a portion of the lungs is inflamed, its spongy structure appears much redder than usual, the colour being chiefly florid, but partly of a darker hue. This arises

88

from a great number of the small vessels distributed upon the cells of the lungs, being so enlarged as to admit the red globules of the blood. There is also an extravasation of the coagulable lymph into the substance of the lungs, and sometimes of blood. The extravasated blood has been said upon some occasions to be in very large quantity; but this has never fallen under my own observation. That portion of the lungs which is inflamed becomes considerably heavier than in the natural state, from the accumulation of blood in its vessels, and the extravasation of the coagulable lymph; it therefore commonly sinks in water. . . .

The pleura covering the inflamed portion of the lungs is also commonly affected with inflammation; it is crowded with fine red vessels, and has generally lying upon it a layer of coagulable lymph.

§ AUENBRUGGER AND LAËNNEC

The first step towards improving methods of clinical observation was taken by Leopold Auenbrugger in 1761 when he advanced the means of diagnosis of consolidation of the lungs by his discovery of the different notes obtained by percussion over air-containing and airless lung or fluid. Romance, or truth, says that he got the idea when a boy by tapping on the wine barrels of his father, who was an innkeeper, to see how much liquid they contained. At any rate he mentioned the note obtained in this way in his work on percussion, but this discovery was not noticed or accepted as of any value for fifty years, when Jean-Nicolas Corvisart, physician to Napoleon I, drew attention to its importance and Laënnec used it in support of his own observations with the stethoscope.

It was left to the genius of the short-lived René Théophile Hyacinthe Laënnec (1781–1826) to place our modern conception of pneumonia, pleurisy, pulmonary tuberculosis, and other lung affections on a sound basis and to describe how to diagnose pneumonia in the early stage and to differentiate it from pleuritic affections. In this he was greatly assisted by his epoch-making discovery of the value of auscultation in the diagnosis of affections of the chest and his invention of the stethoscope. In 1819 he published his classical work under the title *De l'auscultation médiate, ou traité du diagnostic des maladies des poumons et du coeur, fondé principalement sur ce nouveau moyen d'exploration.* His new method was auscultation by means of something intervening between the ear and the chest, namely the stetho-

scope. He defined pleurisy as being inflammation of the pleurae themselves and not, as was thought, an affection of the pulmonary tissue.
He was particularly definite about pleurisy occurring with pneumonia, which he called pleuropneumonia.

Acute pneumonia, he said, "presents three degrees, or stages . . .
*engorgement or inflammatory congestion—hepatization—and puru-
lent infiltration.*" Other writers had noticed these changes of the lungs
in peripneumonia, but Laënnec was probably the first to fix their true
characters as different stages in the disease. He also described how
some portions of the lungs were hepatized, while those immediately
surrounding them were perfectly sound. This variety, he said, had
been called lobular and had arisen in several different points at the
same time.

He knew and recognized the importance of Auenbrugger's work,
though others did not, but his own chief contribution to the diagnosis
of diseases of the lungs was the information gained by the use of the
stethoscope. He looked upon the fine crepitous *râles* as the definite
sign of the earliest stage of pneumonia and also of the resolving stages.
He described puerile breathing, moist *râles,* pectoriloquy (meaning
the voice sound), and aegophony, and showed their value in the diagnosis of pulmonary disease. Some of Laënnec's paragraphs are well
worth reading:

Peripneumony is one of the longest-known diseases: its diagnostic symptoms are not, however, on this account, unequivocal. Impeded respiration,
deep pain in the side affected, incapacity of lying on the opposite one, fever,
cough, viscid sputa, sometimes mixed with blood, the urine of a deep red
are the principal symptoms assigned to this disease by authors. There is,
however, not one of these but may be absent in the most violent cases, while,
on the other hand, they are almost all common to many other diseases. . . .
The percussion of the chest, according to the method of Auenbrugger, is a
much surer means of ascertaining this disease, in all its stages, than the
examination of the external symptoms only. The little time and trouble
required by it, and the certainty of its results, would exclude the necessity
of any other mode of exploration, if it were applicable in all cases; but . . .
this is not the case. The exploration by the cylinder has not this disadvan-
tage: it indicates the pulmonary inflammation in every possible case, and
points out, moreover, the degree of it, with much greater precision than
percussion. In the first degree of peripneumony, the respiratory murmur

is still heard in the part affected, whether percussion affords any sensible alteration of sound or not; and it is, further, accompanied by that species of *rattle* of which I give the name of *crepitous rattle,* and which is the pathognomonic sign of this first degree of Peripneumony. This species of rattle resembles the crepitation of solid salts in a heated vessel, or it may be said to be very analogous to the noise emitted by the healthy lungs when compressed in the hand—only stronger. The only other diseases in which this species of rattle is found, are edema of the lungs and haemoptysis. The second and third varieties of peripneumony are distinguished by the total absence of the respiratory murmur. On the patient making a deep inspiration we see and feel the motion of the thoracic parietes, but we hear no sound whatever. Sometimes, however, in place of the natural sound of respiration we hear the *mucous rattle.* This is particularly the case when a pulmonary catarrh is conjoined with the peripneumony, or when the viscid mucous sputa of the early stage are changed, towards its latter stage, into a thicker and more opaque expectoration. We commonly observe, also, in all varieties of the disease, but especially in the two first, that the respiration acquires the character which we have named *puerile* in the parts of the lung which have remained sound.

It will be noticed that no mention is made of bronchial breathing. The nearest Laënnec advanced to the recognition of this important sign of consolidation is the reference to puerile breathing. His definition of this in an earlier part of the book is not as clear as might be wished.

These extracts have been taken from the translation made by John Forbes, M. D., physician to the Penzance Dispensary. Forbes in his preface to the first edition was guilty of one of the famous false prophecies in medicine. Dealing with the newly invented stethoscope he wrote:

I have no doubt whatever, from my own experience of its value, that it will be acknowledged to be one of the greatest discoveries in medicine by all those who are of a temper, and in circumstances, that will enable them to give it a fair trial. That it will ever come into general use, notwithstanding its value, I am extremely doubtful; because its beneficial application requires much time, and gives a good deal of trouble both to the patient and the practitioner; and because its whole hue and character is foreign, and opposed to all our habits and associations. It must be confessed that there is something even ludicrous in the picture of a grave physician formally listening through a long tube applied to the patient's thorax, as if the disease within were a living being that could communicate its condition to the sense without. Besides, there is in this method a sort of bold claim and pretension to certainty and precision of diagnosis, which cannot, at first sight, but be somewhat startling to a mind deeply versed in the knowledge and uncertainties of our art, and to the calm and cautious habits of philosophising to which the English physician is accustomed. On all these accounts, and others that might be mentioned, I conclude, that the new method will only in a few cases be speedily adopted, and never generally.

This paragraph was omitted from subsequent editions.

Thomas Addison, in his *Observations on pneumonia* (1843), made an important contribution to knowledge. He laid particular stress on his opinion that pneumonia had its origin and essential seat in the air cells of the lungs and that the ordinary pneumonic deposits all poured into these cells. In this way he upset a long cherished notion that pneumonia had its seat in a supposed parenchyma of the lungs and that the products of pneumonic inflammation were poured out into that tissue. He described "lobular pneumonia," which he found to occur in persons of bad cachectic habits of body and especially towards the end of various chronic diseases and after surgical operations.

During the nineteenth century much progress was made in clinical investigation and diagnosis in Continental Europe.

Josef Skoda described a useful diagnostic point in his work on percussion and auscultation published in 1839:

A partial emphysema in the midst of the lung deprived of air (as happens in pneumonia, where, not infrequently the tissue around the hepatized portion and especially at the borders of the lung, is emphysematous) generally produces a tympanitic sound; . . . . The sound is, moreover, in many cases remarkably tympanitic, even when the diminution of the quantity of air in the lung is the effect of an increase in its fluid or solid constituents.

This form resonance is known as "Skodaic resonance" and may be found in cases of lobar pneumonia over an air-containing upper lobe above a large patch of consolidation.

Carl von Rokitansky in 1849 first described the pathological differences between lobar and lobular pneumonia; and the terms "croupous" and "fibrinous" were applied about the same time to lobar pneumonia by Julius Cohnheim, because the exudation of the pleura was like that of membranous croup.

§ BACTERIOLOGY

A very great advance in the comprehension of the nature and cause of pneumonia was made in 1881 when Pasteur isolated the pneumococcus from saliva, but it was not until three years later that Albert Fränkel associated the organism with the disease. Meanwhile, in 1883 Carl Friedländer had noticed that the lungs in certain kinds of pneumonia contained bacilli, but he did not appreciate their exact significance at the time.

Anton Weichselbaum in 1886 investigated various types of pneumonia and isolated organisms which corresponded to those found by the former workers. It became generally recognized that Fränkel's organism, known as the pneumococcus, was by far the commonest cause of lobar pneumonia, that of Friedländer occurring alone in only about 1 per cent of cases and producing a severe form of the disease.

Other organisms were sometimes responsible. Hemolytic streptococci usually caused a bronchopneumonia, but the distribution could be lobar. Streptococcal pneumonia occurred in epidemics of measles or influenza. Staphylococci, *hemophilus influenzae,* and a whole range of viruses could also cause the trouble. Because of this the term "atypical pneumonia" was recently produced to cover all forms of the disease which differed clinically from the classical pneumococcal lobar pneumonia. The term has found more favor in America than in Britain, where the word pneumonia is prefaced by an adjective indicating the cause and the underlying pathology, for example, staphylococcal pneumonia. The rapid success of modern chemotherapy has tended to cut out the differentiation between lobar and bronchopneumonia.

In the last twenty years much work has been done on the different strains of pneumococcus. At first three and a heterogeneous fourth group were recognized, but this number has been increased to more than seventy. Types I, II, and III are responsible between them for half the cases of pneumococcal pneumonia. Types I and II are commonly responsible for the classical lobar pneumonia of young adults.

Type III, a virulent strain, is frequently found in old and debilitated patients. Type XIV is particularly prone to cause pneumonia in infants.

§ TREATMENT OF PNEUMONIA

Treatment changed down the ages as conceptions of the nature of the disease altered, but two methods persisted from ancient days until the last few years—bleeding and wet cupping. James Gregory of Edinburgh is credited with the aphorism that "the danger of a large bleeding is less than the danger of the disease," and Laënnec thought it an excellent saying. This so-called "antiphlogistic" treatment had for its object the reduction of the inflammation in the chest, which was thought to be the cause of the pneumonia.

Cupping has persisted particularly in France. Mr. George Orwell, to his intense disgust, was wet-cupped for pneumonia in a Paris hospital in 1929. It was a favorite treatment for the disease in the French army as recently as 1939.

Of the older methods, leeches were frequently used, and counter-irritation was a great stand-by. Setons, issues, the cautery, and the burning moxa all had staunch supporters among the most distinguished physicians. Not all the case notes carry conviction to the modern mind. For example, one recorded by Marshall Hall of St. Thomas's Hospital in the middle of the nineteenth century in praise of setons:

Two years ago, I was consulted by Mr. P——, a barrister, affected with pneumonia of the middle and upper lobes of the right lung. A seton was inserted and Mr. P—— went to Madeira. On his return, the physical signs and the symptoms of the pneumonia had disappeared.

It is odd to find the emetics, especially tartarated antimony, were freely employed by some physicians in the eighteenth century as being able alone to cure pneumonia.

Alteratives were used to effect the "resolution of any obstruction of an inflammatory nature" by "stimulating the lymphatic system." Calomel and opium in small doses, with plenty of barley water to drink, had their advocates. But tartar emetic was the most widely used drug given in small doses to induce tolerance. Laënnec used it this way

94

and claimed considerable success, without his patients being either "vomited or purged." He met with few who could not bear the treatment.

When antipyrin and other coal-tar antipyretic preparations were put on the market last century they were tried in pneumonia in the hope that by reducing the temperature the course of the illness would be shortened. It was accepted that they, like quinine, did actually reduce the temperature; even if they did so and caused no harm, they did no real good. Some physicians felt that the raised temperature itself was one of Nature's means of combating the disease. Sponging was a much more satisfactory and pleasant method of alleviating the discomforts of fever.

In the nineteen twenties the treatment of pneumonia was quite a formidable business. It began with three grains of calomel to make sure the bowels were well opened. An expectorant mixture containing a number of gastric irritants was prescribed every four hours, even if the sputum was coming up freely. Many physicians used in addition a digitalis preparation to strengthen the heart muscle. The safest was a fresh infusion given every four hours and alternating with the cough mixture. A hypnotic was essential. In the early days of the illness Dover's powder was thought to be particularly effective, but after the third day morphia or any preparation containing it was regarded as dangerous. Chloral and bromides were then used until the barbiturates became fashionable. Antiphlogistine helped to relieve any pleural pain, and brandy and oxygen were useful stand-bys; the latter often bubbled through the former. It was not unusual for a patient to be kept mildly intoxicated until the crisis came. Lastly it was essential that stimulants should be handy, the most effective being strychnine, coramine, and hypodermic injections of ether. The three were sometimes used in rotation at hourly intervals. The careful resident would put all these substances down on the patient's bedticket, and the nursing staff, embued with the knowledge that nursing was the real answer to the problem, would see that the patient drank as much fluid as he wanted and even more, and generally minister to his needs. One of the old school of ward sisters taught her nurses never to pass a patient with pneumonia without giving him a drink. A patient could take as much as fifteen pints of fluid in twenty-four hours. The idea was to flush the toxins out of the system, and certainly a patient with a moist tongue did much better than one with a dry tongue.

The time of crisis was anxiously awaited. Many a patient was helped through the crisis, so it was thought, by frequent injections of some form of stimulant. The least thing would tip a patient over the brink. Some relatives visiting a woman at the height of the crisis laid a bunch of white lilies reverently on her chest. She opened her eyes, looked at the waxy whiteness of the flowers, and said, "Am I as ill as that?" Within a few minutes she was dead, and the lilies were put to their proper purpose.

No disease gave more anxiety—but all that has gone. In the early thirties a new and accurate method of rapid typing of pneumococci coupled with the administration of the appropriate antiserum in the shortest possible time became a highly developed technique. The effectiveness of this treatment varied with the types, type I giving good results and type III poor. It was about to become universally applied when a new drug, prontosil, was brought into use in 1935. It belonged to the sulphonamide group and had magical properties in dealing with the hemolytic streptococcus. It was followed in a year or two by "M and B 693," sulphapyridine, a drug that was particularly effective against the pneumococcus, probably saving Winston Churchill's life at a critical stage of the war. The treatment of pneumococcal pneumonia changed in a flash. The moment the diagnosis was made, the drug was given by mouth, and within twenty-four hours the infection was killed. No longer was there anxiety. The crisis of pneumonia became a legend of the past. There were difficulties with the drug. It was apt to cause nausea. It could cause anuria by blocking the renal tubules with crystals unless the old practice of giving plenty of fluid was continued. It could cause an alarming agranulocytosis. These difficulties, once they were recognized, were easily surmounted, and with the passage of time less toxic and even more effective members of the sulphonamide family were evolved—sulphathiazole, sulpha-diazine, sulphamezathine, and sulphatriad being the most important.

Then came penicillin. In 1944 it was found that doses of ten thousand units injected every three hours for twenty-four hours were sufficient to produce a marked effect on symptoms and on the pyrexia. Various workers began to assess the relative merits of sulphonamides and penicillin. It appeared that the latter was slightly more effective, mainly because there were fewer toxic symptoms and a smaller incidence of empyema. But the patients were burdened with eight injections in twenty-four hours. On the whole the newer sulphonamides won the battle at first, but when larger doses of penicillin given at eight-hour intervals were found to be equally effective the pendulum swung back. Some preferred one, some preferred the other. The faint-hearted used both at the start of the illness. One large group of statistics showed that with penicillin alone the death rate from pneumococcal pneumonia was 6.4 per cent; with penicillin and sulphonamide 7.5 per cent, and with sulphonamide alone 14.3 per cent. Nevertheless, a drug that could be given orally had obvious advantages. In the days before chemotherapy the mortality was in the region of 30 per cent.

Chloromycetin, aureomycin, and terramycin also proved effective forms of treatment, but far more expensive than the sulphonamides. They are used in the main when sulphonamides and penicillin have failed or when the predominant organism in a specimen of sputum is shown to be particularly sensitive to one or other of them.

The effectiveness of modern treatment has led to an anomalous position. Accurate clinical diagnosis, is no longer necessary. The moment there is the slightest suggestion of pneumonia the patient is given a course of chemotherapy. There is no doubt that much respiratory disablement is avoided by this policy, but the underlying disease is masked and an accurate diagnosis is often impossible. Most patients suffering from pneumonia are now treated at home by the general practitioner. Hence, the clinical diagnosis of pneumonia is often no longer bacterial, pathological, or anatomical. It is almost confined to those cases that respond to chemotherapy and those that do not. In the cases of those that fail to respond, the bacteriological diagnosis and sensitivities are of the greatest possible importance.

§ REFERENCES

Baillie, M. (1833): *The morbid anatomy of some of the most important parts of the human body.* 8th ed. London, J. T. Cox and E. Portwine. Pp. 38–9.
Brockbank, W. (1954): *Ancient therapeutic arts.* London, William Heinemann.
Cullen, W. (1816): *First lines of the practice of physic.* London, Longman & Co. Vol. I, pp. 141–42, 151–52.
Florey, M. E. (1952): *The clinical application of antibiotics.* (*Penicillin*). London, Oxford University Press.

Garrison, F. H. (1929): *An introduction to the history of medicine*. 4th ed. Philadelphia, W. B. Saunders.

Hall, M. (1845): *Practical observations and suggestions in medicine*. London, John Churchill. P. 47.

Horder, Lord (1952): *The British encyclopaedia of medical practice*. 2nd ed. London, Butterworth & Co. Vol. X.

Laënnec, R. T. H. (1821): *A treatise on the diseases of the chest in which they are described according to their anatomical characters and their diagnosis established on a new principle by means of acoustic instruments*. London, T. and G. Underwood. Pp. xviii–ix, 311–13.

Major, R. H. (1945): *Classic descriptions of disease*. 3rd ed. Springfield, Charles C. Thomas.

Sturges, O. (1876): *The natural history and relations of pneumonia*. London, Smith, Elder & Co.

BY LEWIS J. MOORMAN
M. D., B. S., F. A. C. P.*

chapteR 4 / TUBERCULOSIS

AT ITS BEST, history is fragmentary. Many important events escape the record. Like the future, much of the past is unknown, though it impinges with significant import upon our very existence. Who would not like to know when the first tubercle bacillus entered the body of the first human host? And what would one not give to know the full weight of its impact upon our civilization? It was Allen Kramer Krause (1881–1941) who said: "Some day a man will write a new kind of history. Its keynote will be the shaping of human destiny by disease. . . ." In part, this brief historical sketch reveals the meaning of this significant assertion.

Confidently, we may say that long before the Sumerians assembled their clans between the Tigris and the Euphrates and left the first recorded history in books of clay, the crafty tubercle bacillus was pursuing its deadly course and leaving its own historic record in the less perishable portions of the human body. Exhumed prehistoric skeletons show the angular spines of hunchbacks literally appearing as intriguing question marks. In time it was learned that they represent victims of tuberculosis with bodies bowed in obeisance to the tubercle bacillus.

These angular spines represent only one of the varied manifestations of this disease which may attack any one of, or all, the organs of the body. This obvious example of the destructive and deforming evidence of the malady is mentioned in order to give the reader a per-

* Emeritus professor of medicine, University of Oklahoma; editor-in-chief, *Journal of the Oklahoma State Medical Association;* and author of *Tuberculosis and genius* (1940) and *Pioneer doctor* (1951). He was president of the National Tuberculosis Association in 1932 and president of the American Trudeau Society in 1940.

spective that reaches beyond the outposts of recorded history and to emphasize the fact that the tubercle bacillus, with a long and success-ful career, is humanity's most experienced adversary. It knows man's habits, his weaknesses, his inherent and acquired defenses, and his fluctuating resistance as influenced by the exigencies of his existence. Throughout the civilized world, this microscopic trouper has success-fully participated in all recorded wars with its major offensive in the wake of death, pyramiding the silent suffering of those left behind. Likewise, it has capitalized the depleting effects of famine and other catastrophic events. It has ravished primitive races wherever strange new people have suddenly appeared in their midst with the tubercle bacillus as one of the occult gifts of civilization.

With such an insidious enemy ever ready to crash the physical defenses of the body, it behooves every human being to be armed with all available knowledge.

§ FIRST RECORDED REFERENCES

Although certain mythological references with vague symptomatic pictures are found in the songs of Orpheus, as far as can be determined the first obvious recorded references to the ravages of tuberculosis appear in the Code of Hammurabi earlier than 2000 B.C.

Homer refers to a "grievous consumption that separates soul and body," and in Deuteronomy (seventh century B.C.) it is said: "The Lord shall smite thee with a consumption, and with a fever, and with an inflammation." Lawrason Brown (1871–1937) believed that the Indo-Aryans (1500 B.C.) were acquainted with the pulmonary type of the disease, phthisis (wasting of the body), and that it was caused by "over fatigue, sorrow, fasting, pregnancy and chest wounds." Treat-ment was administered by the priests who exhorted: "Oh Fever, with thy Brother Consumption, with thy Sister Cough, go to the people below!" In addition, they practiced outdoor living, walking, riding, and life in the mountains or in goat stables. The latter is in keeping with the cow-stable therapy practiced in England at a much later date.

The early Jews seemed to have little knowledge of the disease; yet their relatively high immunity has been attributed to contact through many generations. While it was prevalent in Egypt, little is known regarding the Egyptians' approach to diagnosis and treatment. The

Persians, through the distinguished physicians, Rhazes (A.D. 850–923) and Avicenna (A.D. 980–1037), contributed asses' milk and powdered crab shells (no doubt for calcium). In China phthisis was known as *lao-ting* and affected the lungs, causing cough and physical depletion. A Chinese philosopher said: "The physician can control the disease, but not destiny." In early Greece phthisis was treated in the temples where the patients had the additional advantages of diet, climate, gymnastics, milk, and occasionally, sea voyages.

§ HIPPOCRATES AND GALEN

Of succeeding significance is the remarkable understanding of Hippocrates in the fifth century B.C. His writings showed a surprising knowledge of phthisis. He recognized its symptoms and recommended treatment similar to that employed in modern times. He discussed the association of the angular spine with ulceration of the lung, also glandular affections such as scrofula and struma.

After a long period of silence, Galen (A.D. 130–200), the last of the Greek physicians in Rome, revived the teachings of Hippocrates and added his own voluminous account of "ulcer of the trachea"— known to Hippocrates as phthisis, subsequently called consumption and today, tuberculosis (the later name derived from the word "tubercle," meaning a small nodule or tumor mass).

Galen suspected contagion and warned against the danger of contact. He believed in change of climate and sent his jaded Roman citizens to Stabia, opposite the Isle of Capri, considered the most beautiful beach in the world. Perhaps he should have credit for establishing the first institutional management of tuberculosis. In this delightful setting, his patients rested in the balmy atmosphere of Vesuvius, with warm milk from cows grazing on the salubrious slopes of Milk Mountain, where, according to Galen, the favorable herbiage produced the best therapeutic milk in the world.

Though less well known, Galen's contemporary Aretaeus of Cappadocia, an acute clinical observer, left a classical account of the disease tuberculosis. He was one of the first to recognize the relationship of empyema and phthisis. These two men of Greek lineage, reviving the teachings of Hippocrates, laid the foundation for our modern understanding of tuberculosis. This was fitting since the disease obviously was carried from Greece to Rome and thence throughout the Roman empire and to European countries as a result of Roman conquests.

For at least twelve centuries medical thought moved in narrow channels fixed by the teachings of Galen, but when the awakening of the Renaissance came, it was animated by the sleepless critical Greek spirit. The incentive for scientific investigation and animal experimentation came through the writings of Aristotle, Hippocrates, Galen, and Aretaeus. It was said that "Greece arose from the dead with the New Testament in one hand and Aristotle in the other."

§ THE KING'S EVIL

During this long, scientifically arid period, the tubercle bacillus was not idle. Uncurbed, it wrought its ravages wherever civilized people congregated. Only an occasional dim light came from various parts of the world. In the early part of the sixteenth century the iconoclastic Paracelsus (1493–1541) described "miners' phthisis." Later, Richard Wiseman (1622–76) wrote about tuberculosis of the joints with the accumulation of fluid, and he coined the term *tumor albus* (white swelling). It is interesting to note that in England scrofula (tuberculosis in the glands) was known for centuries as the "King's Evil" and treated by the "royal touch." Dr. Samuel Johnson (1709–84) as a child during the reign of Queen Anne (1665–1714) was one of the last to receive the "touch." Spurning the divine right of kings, this condition thrived in England, and in 1791 the Royal Sea Bathing Infirmary for Scrofula was founded.

Finally, Franciscus Sylvius (1614–72) gathered up some of the loose threads and further clarified the pathology of tuberculosis by establishing a more specific meaning of the term "tubercle" and divining the direct relationship of scrofula and phthisis.

He pointed the way for all great clinical teachers in that he led his "pupils by the hand to medical practice. . . . Together with me they have seen the happy results of treatment when God has granted to our cases a restoration of health; or they have assisted in examining the body when the patient has paid the inevitable tribute to death."

Tuberculosis

At the beginning of the Renaissance the commendable spirit of curiosity took root in England and, in the field of tuberculosis, stimulated by the anatomical studies of Vesalius (1514–64) and the discovery of the circulation of blood by William Harvey (1578–1657), such men as Christopher Bennet (1617–55), Thomas Willis (1621–75), Thomas Sydenham (1624–89), Richard Morton (1637–98), Benjamin Marten (1704–82), William Stark (1740–70), William Withering (1741–99), James Carson (1772–1843), George Boddington (1799–1882), Matthew Baillie (1761–1823), and William Budd (1811–80) worked toward a better understanding of the clinical and pathological aspects of the disease, and Boddington initiated methods approaching modern sanatorium care.

Christopher Bennet, a victim of tuberculosis in the midst of the confusion characterizing available knowledge, presented practical ideas about therapy in his book *The nature and cure of consumption*. Thomas Willis, his contemporary, made meticulous studies of the anatomy and physiology of the lungs and decided that consumption arose "from a Fault of the Lungs." Interestingly he wrote: "For in the Lungs rather than in the Heart or Brain the threads of Life are spun and there they are oftenest broken." Sydenham believed in fresh air and recommended persistent horseback riding as a method of cure. Richard Morton agreed with Sylvius concerning the meaning of tubercle. He commanded much attention and exerted great influence through his voluminous work on consumption entitled *Phthisiologia*. Significantly, he wrote: "I cannot sufficiently admire that any one, at least after he comes to the Flower of his Youth, can dye without a touch of a Consumption." The high incidence and shocking mortality in the midst of universal confusion about the cause and manifestations of the disease were coincident with rapidly increasing facilities for the acquisition of knowledge and may have inspired the dawning urge for more specific investigations.

According to S. Lyle Cummins, Professor Charles Singer in *Janus* (1911) referred to Marten as "a neglected predecessor of Louis Pasteur." In his book, *A new theory of consumptions, more especially of a phthisis or consumption of the lungs,* he expresses the belief that phthisis is very contagious, and his discussions are in line with the

modern germ theory as the cause of many diseases. Cummins is of
the opinion that his conception of infectivity of man, means of transmission, and the importance of contact represents "almost an inspired statement."

William Stark, who apparently developed miliary tuberculosis
from a scratch on his hand at the autopsy table, made valuable contributions to the existing knowledge of tuberculosis before his death at
the age of thirty. His unpublished work shows that he had reached
sound conclusions with reference to the pathology of the disease and
the nature of tubercle.

William Withering, another victim of tuberculosis, manifested a
rare understanding of the disease. He observed and recorded occupational influences in terms which have been confirmed by modern
studies. He believed tuberculosis to be infectious, and while depre-
cating the practice of sending patients to far away climates, he considered the Isle of Wight a favorable resort. He observed classical
symptoms of pulmonary tuberculosis in his pet monkeys, typifying
tuberculosis in man. He followed them to autopsy in order to confirm his observations.

In addition to his monumental work on the foxglove and his
scientific investigations and publications in other fields, it may be
said that Withering anticipated Pasteur when, in connection with
his study of scarlet fever, he suggested the possibility of causative "ani-
malcules capable of generating their kind."

James Carson recommended artificial therapeutic pneumothorax
and directed a surgical incision of the chest wall in a case of advanced
pulmonary tuberculosis to produce collapse of the lungs, thus antici-
pating the work of Carlo Forlanini by seventy years.

George Boddington wrote intelligently about tuberculosis and
practiced institutional management before Hermann Brehmer (1826–
99) achieved credit for the establishment of the first sanatorium a
decade later in Germany.

Matthew Baillie's work in pathology at St. George's Hospital
London, may have been inspired by William Stark. For eighteen
years Baillie studied the pathology of diseases of the chest and added
much valuable data. He likewise received an autopsy wound, supposedly the source of his tuberculous infection, which apparently ran
a chronic course and took his life when he was sixty-two. He pub-

Tuberculosis

lished the first orderly treatise on morbid anatomy based upon clinical and autopsy studies.

William Budd and his contemporary, Jean-Antoine Villemin, simultaneously developed the conviction that tuberculosis is a specific infection; but Budd, bent upon the duties of general practice, was too busy with his patients to vitalize his conviction. Villemin, a professor with opportunity and facilities unknown to Budd, pursued his belief that "the phthisical soldier is to his messmate what the glandered horse is to his yokefellow." He proved that tuberculosis is "transmissible by inoculation from man to the lower animals."

With both patient and disease in mind, physicians made rapid progress. Thus our modern concepts of tuberculosis were taking form. For three centuries in England this interest paralleled the exceptionally high mortality. John Locke (1632–1704) said that in London one death out of every five was due to tuberculosis. The tubercle bacillus had had many centuries of unopposed progress. It was high time for the British physicians to seek all possible knowledge, throw up their defenses, and devise new weapons.

Climaxing this period, Leopold Auenbrugger (1722–1809) made his original investigation and published his monograph on percussion (tapping the surface of the body for information about the underlying structures). Unfortunately, his discovery was not widely accepted and did not come into general use until Jean Nicolas Corvisart (1755–1821) popularized it with a second French translation and the combined force of his approval, his position, and his personality.

Maximilian Stoll (1742–88) at the University of Vienna made valuable contributions to our knowledge before he died a victim of the disease which he sought to conquer. It was through his aphorisms that Corvisart learned of Auenbrugger's work. Benjamin Rush (1745–1813) was the first to give the study of tuberculosis a prominent place in the annals of American medicine.

§ FRENCH PIONEERS

At the turn of the eighteenth century French physicians were keenly aware of tuberculosis, and Paris became the center of bedside and autopsy investigations, which had been so assiduously pursued by Stark and Baillie in England.

105

Marie François Xavier Bichat (1771–1802), dying of tuberculosis at the age of thirty-one, made a great contribution to medical science in that he progressed from Morgagni's organ pathology to tissue pathology within the organ. He applied his inquiring mind to the pathology of tuberculosis and pointed the way for succeeding students of the disease.

Gaspard Laurent Bayle (1774–1816) devoted much of his short but remarkable professional life to the study of tuberculosis. His book on research in pulmonary phthisis presents the results of clinical studies with autopsy reports on nine hundred individuals dying of tuberculosis. Perhaps he knew more about the disease in all its phases than any one who had gone before.

Bayle's illustrious contemporary, René Théophile Hyacinthe Laënnec (1781–1826) was equally avid in his study of this disease, fatal to so many of his own generation. Likewise, he was interested in checking every symptom observed at the bedside with the pathological findings at autopsy. More truly than any one else he assembled in orderly fashion all existing knowledge concerning the various clinical and pathological manifestations of tuberculosis and in rapid succession made phenomenal additions. He was able to show that no matter whether circumscribed in one organ or widely distributed through the body, the various pathological manifestations were due to a single disease. His studies took into account not only the possible wide distribution of the disease, but also the various stages giving rise to lesions very different in appearance, yet to him representing changes due to a common cause. In time he received credit for establishing the unity of tuberculosis and forever bringing to an end the confusing speculations which had troubled students of the disease throughout the ages. There were many doubting Thomases, but with few exceptions Laënnec's conclusions were accepted and ultimately confirmed by the discovery of the tubercle bacillus in 1882.

Of no less significance was his interest in auscultation, his invention of the stethoscope, and his ever-increasing pursuit of physical diagnosis. This implies the use of the five senses in the acquisition of knowledge concerning the condition of the organs of the body and the changes resulting from disease. Through the application of these natural methods of examination, Laënnec's discernment was incredibly keen. In half the time required to teach the average medical student these methods, Laënnec, without chart or compass, conceived, observed, recorded, tabulated, and communicated virtually all that is now known about physical diagnosis as applied to the chest. His remarkable work, *A treatise on the diseases of the chest and on mediate auscultation,* was published in 1819 and translated into English by John Forbes in 1821. Suffering from advanced tuberculosis and dying from exhaustion at forty-five, Laënnec left unlearned the one lesson that might have prolonged his own life. He never knew how to conserve energy and build resistance until it was too late.

Among Laënnec's contemporaries was Pierre Charles Alexander Louis (1787–1872), who deserves special consideration. He supported Laënnec's claims concerning the unity of tuberculosis and devoted much of his long life to the study of its varied manifestations. He believed that tuberculosis of the lungs preceded tuberculosis in other parts of the body. He attempted to introduce mathematical accuracy in medicine through statistical studies. The results of his untiring efforts were published in *Recherches anatomico-pathologiques sur la phthisie* (Paris, 1825) and translated into English by Walter Hayle Walshe and published in London in 1843.

Rudolf Virchow, who established cellular pathology on a secure basis, made valuable contributions toward the study of tuberculosis, but to his dying day he opposed the unitarian theory of phthisis. He agreed with Johann Lukas Schönlein, who coined the word "tuberculosis," in order to differentiate erroneously the nodular tubercles from the cheesy patch and the ulcerated area characterizing what he recognized as phthisis. In 1865 Villemin proved through animal inoculation that tuberculosis is a specific infectious disease. Five years later A. C. Gerlach proved that milk from tuberculous cows conveyed the disease. In 1873 Edwin Klebs proved the existence of bovine tuberculosis by feeding experiments. Later, in the United States, Theobald Smith (1859–1934) through animal experimentation isolated and cultivated bovine tubercle bacilli and differentiated them from the human type.

§ DISCOVERY OF THE TUBERCLE BACILLUS

Through clinical, anatomical, physiological, pathological, and bacteriological studies with the aid of animal experimentation, medicine moved into a new era productive of great advances in our knowledge of tuberculosis. In the midst of confusion and controversy, Robert Koch, whose researches had been stimulated by Pasteur, announced the discovery of the tubercle bacillus as the specific cause of the disease.

This discovery represents one of the most significant events, not only in the history of tuberculosis, but in the history of medicine. To emphasize the importance of this meticulous bit of research, Allen K. Krause said: "Given the same circumstances, the same pioneer quest, the same limited knowledge of possibilities, the same imperfection of initial media, and the view is almost compelling that only the rarest of investigators would have maintained the prolonged and heartbreaking vigil for the earliest showing through the minutest particles that belonged, as yet, only to the shadowy realm of a 'working hypothesis.' "

This remarkable performance and the dramatic presentation of his work at the Berlin Physiological Society shattered the convictions of the great Virchow, leaving the old war horse of pathology speechless. Again quoting Allen K. Krause: "When, full of years and every honor that a man of medicine can accumulate, he passed on to eternal peace, he could not reconcile himself to the idea of the all-embracing and unified cause of that appalling diversity of effect that tuberculosis comprehends."

While five types of tubercle bacilli have been discovered, with rare exceptions only the human and bovine strains cause tuberculosis in man. In those countries where tuberculosis is being eliminated from the dairy herds there is very little bovine tuberculosis. In the United States, aside from educational support, the National Tuberculosis Association left the control of bovine tuberculosis largely in the hands of the dairy and livestock interests. The Bureau of Animal Husbandry initiated the program of eradication of tuberculous cattle in 1917, and the federal government reimbursed the owners of cattle slaughtered because of positive tuberculin reactions. The combination of public opinion, business expediency, and government support has resulted in phenomenal control.

During the past few decades accredited (tuberculosis-free) herds, accredited counties, and finally accredited states have been developed. Compulsory pasteurization of milk has helped reduce the incidence of bovine tuberculosis. Because of this concerted effort, many lives have been saved and many deformities and crippling effects, especially among children, have been prevented. The veterinarians deserve great credit for their untiring effort in this fight against bovine tuberculosis. Since it was Theobald Smith who surprised Robert Koch by making the distinction between the bovine and the human types, it is not strange that the United States lead in the eradication of bovine tuberculosis.

Growing knowledge of the specific cause and the common channels of infection in the human being resulted in a great awakening with the initiation of concerted efforts toward prevention and control. For the first time in the history of the world, it was possible to organize antituberculosis campaigns on a scientific basis with the postulate that the tubercle bacillus is the specific preventable cause.

Gradually the knowledge that tuberculosis is preventable spread throughout all enlightened communities with a crystallization of opinion that methods of control should be instituted with full cooperation of the people. In 1882 Robert Koch, in the last paragraph of his historic treatise on *The etiology of tuberculosis,* made this prophetic statement: "When the conviction that tuberculosis is a specific infectious disease has become firmly established among physicians, the question of an adequate campaign against tuberculosis will certainly come under discussion and it will develop by itself."

Sixteen years (1898) after the cause was discovered, the British National Association for the Prevention of Tuberculosis was founded. Its sound principles were based upon Koch's discovery of the specific cause and a conviction that tuberculosis should be prevented. Thirty-five years later Sir Robert Philip spoke as follows:

The view was voiced at a meeting convened at Marlborough House by King Edward VII—then Prince of Wales—on 20 December, 1898, both by His Royal Highness, who became president of the Association, and by Sir William Broadbent, Bt, who was first chairman of its council. The proposal was supported influentially by laymen and doctors alike.

In 1885 Edward Livingston Trudeau (1848–1915) founded the Adirondack Cottage Sanatorium, which is now the Trudeau Sanatorium. Though Boddington, Brehmer, and Peter Dettweiler (1837–1904) preceded Trudeau in the field of sanatorium management, they had not conceived the idea of prevention based upon a specific cause.

In his improvised backwoods laboratory at Saranac Lake, Trudeau succeeded in culturing the tubercle bacillus and tried to develop immunity "in my animals by dead germs, or preventive inoculations of substances derived from the liquid cultures from which the bacilli had been filtered. I published this work in the *New York Medical Record* as early as November, 1890 . . . ." He was disappointed to find that his experiments did not confer immunity against subsequent inoculations. Nevertheless he anticipated Koch's published methods of making tuberculin by at least one year. In spite of this failure, Trudeau "saw the glorious hope of future relief to humanity from sickness, suffering and death which lay in the study of disease at the bedside, and of infection and germs and sick animals in the laboratory."

In his interesting book, *Tuberculosis in history,* S. Lyle Cummins after discussing Trudeau's remarkable career says that he "left American physicians the secret of how to manage and how to begin to treat the most formidable of all foes to humanity. They have taken his advice and there is no place where the tuberculous are so well 'managed' and treated as in America today."

In 1887 Robert Philip (later Sir Robert) opened the Edinburgh Dispensary for tuberculosis control and initiated his educational program. Under the same stimulus and in the same year, Hermann Biggs (1859–1923) in New York published the first popular educational pamphlet on tuberculosis. In 1892 Lawrence F. Flick organized the Pennsylvania Society for the Prevention of Tuberculosis, engaging the interest and co-operation of the people as well as of the profession. Guided by these principles, the National Association of Tuberculosis was founded in 1904.

§ CHRISTMAS SEAL

From these pioneer ventures all volunteer and government agencies, including a number of international organizations, have sprung with world-wide recognition of the heavy toll in morbidity and mortality, the socioeconomic significance of the disease, and the desirability of universal participation in its control. Soon after the turn of the century Einar Holboell, a postal clerk in Denmark, conceived the idea of the Christmas-stamp sale. In 1907 Miss Emily P. Bissell, hard pressed for funds, instituted the stamp sale in the state of Delaware. Promptly, the American Red Cross, realizing the educational and financial potentialities of Miss Bissell's experiment, developed the Christmas Seal sale, which was transferred to the National Tuberculosis Association in 1919. Since that time the Christmas Seal has touched the pocketbooks of millions, rich and poor, throughout the nation, and today it reaches round the world. In recent years in the United States the annual Christmas Seal sale has amounted to more than twenty million dollars. Never before did a penny's worth go so far and give so much satisfaction. Encircling the globe, the Christmas Seal carries incalculable spiritual, educational, and financial values.

In Great Britain the National Association for the Prevention of Tuberculosis largely parallels the work of the National Tuberculosis Association in the United States, and the progress of the Christmas Seal sale in the two countries is similar.

Tuberculosis associations are working for prevention and control in nearly all civilized countries and the International Union against Tuberculosis, the World Health Organization, the World Medical Association, and other international groups are interested in global control, so important as we look toward the ultimate elimination of this disease from the face of the earth. This is perhaps not too much to expect when the course of the disease for four thousand years is compared with the progress made since the discovery of the tubercle bacillus less than a hundred years ago. For decades the importance of prevention has been driven home by the educational campaigns of various agencies, carefully prepared pamphlets and circulars, magazine and newspaper articles, strip films, lectures, personal instruction in tuberculosis dispensaries, sanatoria and hospitals by physicians, nurses, and trained public health educators.

§ THE PURSUIT OF CURE

Today even gross illiteracy cannot wholly prevent the acquisition of knowledge about the prevention of tuberculosis. Lack of knowledge on the part of any intelligent citizen is a reflection upon the community in which he lives. The truth of this assertion and the obligations resting upon each responsible individual in any enlightened community are emphasized by the recent advances in management and treatment, both medical and surgical. Recent progress in the methods of discovery of the disease, its prevention, and control have been phenomenal. Though many of these developments are too recent to warrant historical appraisal, they have captured public interest which should be encouraged. In spite of the fact that history in the field of medical science should be fifty to one hundred years old before it is recorded, the following advances deserve consideration. Though Koch was disappointed in his efforts to prevent or cure tuberculosis with his tuberculin, in the hands of Clemens von Pirquet and others, it became a most useful diagnostic agent. The tuberculin test is widely employed throughout the world in diagnostic studies and case-finding campaigns.

The development of surgical collapse and surgical section of the lungs has almost revolutionized treatment, thus restoring physical competency in many otherwise hopeless cases, and materially limiting the spread of infection. Progress continues, and while much has been accomplished, the estimate of ultimate results rests upon "the crutch of time."

Shortly before the turn of the last century Wilhelm Konrad Roentgen accidentally discovered the cathode ray, properly called the Roentgen ray. This discovery opened a vast new field in diagnosis, particularly in connection with examination of the lungs. Because of this, we now see as man never saw before. The influence of this discovery in the control of tuberculosis staggers description. It serves as a valuable diagnostic aid, and its importance in mass case-finding campaigns is incalculable. It has definitely contributed to the rapid decline in mortality.

Today B.C.G.,[†] representing an attenuated strain of tubercle bacilli, is being widely employed in many countries as a protection (vaccine) against the development of tuberculosis. In the United States, where control along universally accepted lines has been so successful, it is recommended only in selected groups where exposure is great.

† Bacille Calmette-Guérin, named after Léon Charles Albert Calmette (1863–1933) and Camille Guérin (1872–   ).

§ DISCOVERY OF STREPTOMYCIN

Finally chemotherapy deserves conservative consideration without definite prognostic conclusions. René Jules Dubos, of the Rockefeller Institute for Medical Research, should have credit for preparing a culture medium upon which tubercle bacilli could be grown and thus facilitating the development of the therapeutic use of the antibiotics. The discovery in 1943 of streptomycin by Selman A. Waksman of Rutgers University, New Jersey, and its hopeful employment in the treatment of tuberculosis in the human being with the succeeding concerted efforts in clinical and laboratory research and the sustained acquisition of knowledge concerning the use of the new drugs singly and combined have resulted in unprecedented progress and enthusiasm. By the end of 1952 the literature on streptomycin alone contained six thousand references. Soon after the discovery of streptomycin and its hopeful employment in the treatment of tuberculosis, isonicotinic acid hydrazide (isoniazid) was being employed with great enthusiasm, and its premature announcement caused unwarranted excitement in the wards of tuberculosis hospitals and unfortunate newspaper publicity. The psychological spree has passed, and isoniazid has taken its place in the therapeutic program virtually parallelling streptomycin in usefulness. The true merits of other chemotherapeutic agents now under consideration are still undetermined. At this moment of historic significance, phthisiologists, rich in knowledge, constantly on the verge of discovery, remain speechless, while the world awaits the answer. Millions of dollars are being spent in research. Thousands of scientific investigators follow the devious ways of Koch's enigmatic little bacillus with the hope of finding a truly specific therapeutic agent.

As at the beginning of this sketch, the limitations of history posed puzzling queries; so an uncertain future troubles the reader with another intriguing question: Who would not like to know when the last tubercle bacillus will be eradicated from the last human host?

§ REFERENCES

Brown, Lawrason (1941): *The story of clinical pulmonary tuberculosis.* Baltimore, Williams & Wilkins Co.

Burke, Richard M. (1938): *A historical chronology of tuberculosis.* Springfield, Illinois, and Baltimore, Maryland, Charles C. Thomas.

Cummins, S. Lyle (1949): *Tuberculosis in history from the 17th century to our own times.* London, Baillière, Tindall & Cox.

Dubos, René and Jean (1952): *The white plague, tuberculosis man and society.* Boston, Little, Brown & Co.

Flick, Lawrence F. (1925): Development of our knowledge of tuberculosis. Lancaster, Pennsylvania, Wickersham Printing Company.

Krause, Allen K. (1928): "Tuberculosis and public health." *Amer. Rev. Tuberc., 18,* 271.

Moorman, Lewis J. (1940): *Tuberculosis and genius.* Chicago, University of Chicago Press.

Moorman, Lewis J. (1944): "Our knowledge of tuberculosis: 4,000 years accumulation—40 years application." Presidential Address. *Trans. 40th Annual Meeting, National Tuberculosis Association.* New York, National Tuberculosis Association.

Moorman, Lewis J. (1947): *The American Sanatorium Association—A brief historical sketch. Historical Series No. 3.* New York, National Tuberculosis Association.

Moorman, Lewis J. (1951): *Pioneer doctor.* Norman, University of Oklahoma Press.

Perkins, James E., Floyd M. Feldman, in collaboration with Ruth Carson (1952): *You and tuberculosis.* New York, Alfred A. Knopf.

Solomon, Saul (1952): *Tuberculosis.* New York, Coward-McCann.

BY W. S. C. COPEMAN
O. B. E., M. D., F. R. C. P.*

chapter 5 / Rheumatism

THE TERM "rheumatism" is one of very considerable antiquity, as it goes back to the era of Galen, if not before. It was not used in its modern sense, however, until the seventeenth century. The "rheum" was regarded in those early days as a "peccant humour" which flowed from the brain to all parts of the body, stirring up pain in the soft tissues which it traversed and swelling the joints into which it flowed. This rheumatism (or catarrh) was considered to be a distillate from one of the four humors, which were believed, until as late as the middle of the seventeenth century, to compose the body.

There is little evidence that the ancient physicians separated the conditions of rheumatism and gout, although the fact that Ralph Bocking (Radulphus), confessor to St. Richard of Wyche, Bishop of Chichester, writing in the thirteenth century, discerned a need to coin the word "gout" does suggest that some difference must have been recognized by then. He thought both to be due to the same cause, however, and it was this idea of a fluid dropping into the cavities of certain joints which gave rise to his term "gout," from the French word *goutte,* meaning a drop. Gout and rheumatism were studied and written about by Hippocrates under the generic name of "arthritis" four hundred years before the Christian era, although knowledge concerning their cause was candidly summed up by the physician Aretaeus of Cappadocia in the second century A.D., when he said that none but the gods understood it!

* Physician to the rheumatism department, West London Hospital, and to the Arthur Stanley Institute for Rheumatic Diseases, Middlesex Hospital, London; president of the European League against Rheumatism; chairman of the Empire Rheumatism Council; and author of *Textbook of the rheumatic diseases* (1948).

115

§ GUILLAUME DE BAILLOU AND THOMAS SYDENHAM

The difference between gout and rheumatism was first discerned by a French court physician named Guillaume de Baillou, or Ballonius, in a posthumous work called *Liber de rheumatismo et pleuritide dorsale* (1642). (This book was translated into English by C. C. Barnard [*Brit. J. Rheumat.*, 1940, *ii*, 141–62].) He used the word "rheumatism" for the first time in its modern sense of an acute polyarthritis which is not connected with gout. De Baillou was evidently an outstanding man and has been called "the first epidemiologist of modern times," as it was he who first opposed the medieval scholastic system of "pigeonholing" the phenomena of disease, and drew attention to the evolution and natural history of disease processes. He also was the first to describe whooping cough as a separate disease. His views strongly influenced the great English physician Thomas Sydenham (1624–89), who revived the old Greek ideal of personal medical observation and experience as opposed to the authoritarianism which had lasted for a thousand years and completely barred any progress in medicine. He was essentially a man of action (he fought for Cromwell) and was considered by contemporaries to be rich in the Saxon's special gift of manly independence and saving common sense. He was called, in admiration, the "English Hippocrates." Following the lead of Baillou he wrote a brilliant account of acute rheumatism (1683) and contrasted it with gout. It would be difficult to improve upon his description of the onset of this disease even today:

This disease may come on at any time. It is commonest, however, during the autumn, chiefly attacking the young and vigorous. . . . The sad list of symptoms begins with chills and shivers; these are followed immediately by heat, disquietude, thirst, and the other concomitants of fever. One or two days after this (sometimes sooner) the patient is attacked by severe pains in the joints, sometimes in one and sometimes in another, sometimes in his wrist, sometimes in his shoulder, sometimes in the knee—this last joint oftenest. This pain changes its place from time to time, takes the joints in turns, and affects the one that it attacks last with redness and swelling. . . .

This disease, when separate from the fever, is often called *arthritis* (*gout*). Nevertheless, it differs essentially from that disease, as every one knows who knows the two diseases well.

Sydenham's treatise on gout, of which he himself was a victim, is generally thought to be his masterwork and is also much quoted still in books on this subject. He also sensed that there were other forms of rheumatism, and he coined the term "scorbutical rheumatism" in an attempt to separate those cases which he believed to be due to neither gout nor rheumatic fever. The disease groups which he was probably trying to cover under this designation were rheumatoid arthritis and osteoarthritis. In 1686 he also carefully described that curious variant of acute rheumatism known previously as St. Vitus's dance and subsequently as Sydenham's chorea, which he differentiated from hysteria.

The next chapter in the story of rheumatism was opened by the great Dutch physician Hermann Boerhaave, who was addicted to aphorisms, of which he published several volumes. In one of these aphorisms he points out that not only are the joints affected by acute rheumatism, but also "invading sometimes the Brain, Lungs and Bowels," while his pupil Baron Antonius Störck of Vienna not only described such involvement of the internal organs clinically, but confirmed its existence by post-mortem examinations. It was left to the English physician David Pitcairn, however, to point out the most important visceral manifestation of rheumatism, namely that heart disease could be caused by this affliction. This fact was briefly noted in the second edition of the book on *Morbid anatomy* published by John Hunter's nephew, Matthew Baillie, in 1793, while on July 29 of the next year the minutes of the "Fleece Medical Society" in Gloucestershire recorded that "Mr. Jenner favoured the Society with Remarks on a Disease of the Heart following Acute Rheumatism, illustrated by Dissections." (*Brit. med. J.*, 1816, *i*, 1297.)

In 1812 William Charles Wells, an American high Tory, who emigrated to England for political reasons and later became physician to St. Thomas's Hospital, published a paper in which he confirmed Pitcairn's observation "that persons subject to rheumatism were attacked more frequently than others, with symptoms of an organic disease of the heart ... he [Pitcairn] concluded, that these two diseases depend upon a common cause, and in such instances, therefore, called the latter disease rheumatism of the heart." He also described the occurrence and nature of rheumatic nodules for the first time, although the importance of these as a sign of activity in this disease was not generally appreciated until this was pointed out many years later by Sir Thomas Barlow (1882).

§ MALADIE DE BOUILLAUD

Seventeen years after the invention of the stethoscope by the brilliant young French physician Laënnec, Jean Baptiste Bouillaud, who was on the staff of the Children's Hospital in Paris, stressed this association on clinical grounds and showed the frequent occurrence of lesions of the endocardium as well as those of the pericardium, which had previously been described. In 1836 he enunciated his long famous "law of coincidence" in which he stated that "In the majority of cases of diffuse articular rheumatism with fever there exists in a variable degree a rheumatism of the sero-fibrinous tissue of the heart. The coincidence is the rule and non-coincidence the exception." (*Proc. R. Soc. Med., Sect. Hist. Med.,* 1931, 24, 1257.) Rheumatic fever associated with heart disease is called *maladie de Bouillaud* in France to this day. Sir Thomas Watson (1843) stated, however, that "One law respecting the connexion between the cardiac and the arthritic symptoms may be stated with confidence, namely, that the *younger* the patient is who suffers acute rheumatism (and I have seen it so early as the third or fourth year) the more likely will he be to have rheumatic carditis. The chance of the combination appears to diminish, after puberty, as life advances."

It was as the result of the observations of men such as these that the way was prepared for the work of those great English clinicians who staffed the Hospital for Sick Children in Great Ormond Street, London, at the end of the last century—W. B. Cheadle, Thomas Barlow, David B. Lees, A. E. Garrod, Frederic Still, F. J. Poynton, and C. F. Coombs—who all studied, and added their respective contributions to, this subject. They showed that the lesions of rheumatism involve every layer of the heart, that rheumatic carditis should be considered as the most serious of all diseases of childhood and adolescence, that the hemolytic streptococcus was almost certainly involved in its causation, and that prolonged rest was the essential and most effective element in the prevention and treatment of rheumatic heart disease. In 1904 Ludwig Aschoff, professor of pathology at Marburg in Germany, demonstrated the special kind of microscopic inflammatory nodule characteristic of the cardiac rheumatic process that still bears his name, and which Alvin Frederick Coburn (1931) and others have shown to represent a late reaction to hemorrhage and necrosis in the early stages of the disease.

§ THE VIRTUES OF COLCHICUM

The only advance which was made during this period in the story of gout was the rediscovery by Antonius Störck of the virtue of colchicum, the corm of the autumn crocus, in its treatment. This remedy had been known to the Greeks, but since it had always been included as a minor item in a prescription containing many other ingredients, and since it was known to be a violent purgative, it had been eliminated as a constituent of this traditional prescription during the Middle Ages. This remedy still remained the most effective in our possession until a few years ago, when it became possible to synthesize the active principle, colchicine, which is now used in preference.

§ FIRST DESCRIPTION OF RHEUMATOID ARTHRITIS

Soon after the inauguration of the First French Republic a young medical man named Augustin Jacob Landré-Beauvais published a thesis for his doctorate at the University of Paris entitled *Doit-on admettre une nouvelle espèce de goutte sous la denomination de goutte asthénique primitive?* in which he describes sufficiently accurately, for the first time under that name, the condition which is now known as rheumatoid arthritis; about the same time (1805) John Haygarth, a distinguished Bath physician, also wrote of his conviction "that there is one painful and troublesome disease of the joints of a peculiar nature, and clearly distinguishable from all others by symptoms manifestly different from the gout, and from both acute and chronic rheumatism." In 1859 Alfred Baring Garrod, who was at that time physician to the West London Hospital, proposed the name "rheumatoid arthritis" to replace the many "aliases," in addition to those already mentioned, under which this disease had hitherto been spoken of; these included rheumatic gout, chronic rheumatic arthritis, *"rhumatisme nouveaux,"* and many others. His reasons for proposing this name, by which the disease has been known ever since, are of

119

interest and may be quoted. After stating that the term "rheumatic gout" and the other synonyms bore no relation to the etiological facts as he knew them, he said: "Although unwilling to add to the number of names, I cannot help expressing a desire that one might be found for this disease. . . . Perhaps *Rheumatoid Arthritis* would answer the object, by which term I should wish to imply an inflammatory affection of the joints not unlike rheumatism . . . but differing materially from it." In 1896 G. A. Bannatyne, another physician who lived and practiced in Bath, published a small book on the pathological changes found in this disease, and in the fourth edition (1906) he finally differentiated it from osteoarthritis.

Although Sydenham had pointed out that painful joints might be one of the sequelae of dysentery, the French physician C. Bouchard seems to have been one of the first to suggest that rheumatoid arthritis might be a result of infection elsewhere in the body when in 1891 he pointed out that polyarthritis might follow a number of common infections, including scarlet fever. This theory became modified early in the present century by William Hunter and Sir William Willcox under the designation of "focal sepsis," which postulated that small localized areas of infection might exist unsuspected in certain regions of the body, notably at the roots of dead teeth and in the tonsils or prostate, and that from these sites toxins or poisons were intermittently forced into the blood stream, thus causing the disease. Belief in this possibility has, however, considerably waned of recent years.

§ "GOUTY RHEUMATISM"

The last form of arthritis to be clearly demonstrated was what we now call osteoarthritis. From Hippocratic times until the nineteenth century this disease had, presumably, been included under the all-embracing heading of gout, for we know from the evidence of numerous skeletons, not only of this period but also dating back to prehistoric times, that the disease must have been quite common then, as now. François Boissier de la Croix de Sauvages, stimulated by the example of Linnaeus in the field of botany, endeavored in 1763 to classify medical conditions in equally exhaustive fashion, and subdivided arthritis into fourteen varieties, and rheumatism into ten.

Osteoarthritis would seem to correspond with the variety which he termed *rheumatismus arthriticus*—a form of "gouty rheumatism, affecting chiefly large joints and showing no concretions." In 1801 William Heberden the Elder, who was George III's chief physician, described what are still known as "Heberden's nodes": "little hard knobs, about the size of a small pea, which are frequently seen upon the fingers, particularly a little below the top near the joint. They have no connection with the gout . . . ." Much work was also carried out on osteoarthritis by Robert Adams in Dublin and Elliot Smith in Egypt, which was summarized by the former in his book, *Treatise on rheumatic gout, or chronic rheumatic arthritis of all the joints,* published in 1857, in which he gives to osteoarthritis of the hip joint the special name of *malum coxae senilis.* Meanwhile, however, Jean-Martin Charcot, the great French clinician, was putting back the clock by teaching that both rheumatoid arthritis and osteoarthritis were variants of the same underlying pathology, which should be referred to collectively as *arthritis deformans,* a term which is, however, now obsolete. The distinction between these two diseases was only made absolute by the article on arthritis written by Sir Archibald Garrod and published in the 1907 edition of Sir Clifford Allbutt's *System of medicine,* in which he describes each type separately, each with its special pathology.

§ ANKYLOSING SPONDYLITIS

The history of ankylosing spondylitis—a condition of arthritis resembling the rheumatoid type which affects, in the first place, the spine —starts with a long, interesting, and accurate account of a post-mortem examination of a case of this disease, which was published in 1691 by Bernard Connor, an Irish doctor, who, among other positions which he held during his short but romantic life, was physician to King Sobietski of Poland and was elected an F.R.S. Hilton Fagge of Guy's Hospital described another autopsy of this condition in 1877, and in 1884 E. A. G. G. Strümpell in Germany described two clinical cases. V. M. Bechterev in Russia amplified previous accounts of the disease, and in 1898 Pierre-Marie in France named the condition *"la spondylose rhizomélique."* All this led to a somewhat confused presentation of the subject in most textbooks as "the Strümpell-Bechterev-Marie syndrome," a term not infrequently used today.

Juvenile rheumatoid arthritis was first described by Dr. (later Sir) Frederic Still, while he was still a resident at Great Ormond Street Hospital in 1897. Anatole Chauffard in Paris described it independently about the same time, and this form of disease is, therefore, frequently referred to as Still's disease or Still-Chauffard disease.†

§ SALICIN IN RHEUMATIC FEVER

The history of the treatment of these various rheumatic conditions is not a particularly interesting one until we come to modern times, unless we except the rather romantic quest of Thomas John Maclagan of Dundee, which led to his discovery of salicin as a remedy for rheumatic fever in 1876. He had noted that this disease tended to flourish best in low-lying swampy areas, and it was his firm belief that where God permitted the disease to flourish the natural remedy would be discovered not far off. Salicin is the active principle of the leaf of the willow, which he found also flourishing on his marshes.

The growth of the general ideas governing the treatment of the rheumatic diseases is part of the general history of therapeutics, and does not present any particular highlights until the year 1949. Of the exciting story of cortisone and ACTH which was opened in that year by the discovery by P. S. Hench and E. C. Kendall of the Mayo Clinic in Rochester, Minnesota, that these substances would produce a dramatic improvement in nearly every case of rheumatoid arthritis, and in some other rheumatic diseases, it is still a little early to speak with finality. Suffice it to say that this discovery has finally focused worldwide medical interest on the rheumatic diseases, and has opened out new vistas and possibilities for their treatment which were undreamed of before this discovery. Seldom has the Nobel Prize for Medicine been awarded for a discovery which is more likely to revolutionize the science and art of medicine.

† Frederick John Poynton (1869–1943) published many papers on juvenile rheumatism which were summarized in the book written jointly with Alexander Paine, entitled *Researches on rheumatism* (1913). His claim that the cause of rheumatic fever was a diplococcus of the streptococcal group was never fully accepted by the medical profession, and the controversy to which this gave rise embittered the later years of

Rheumatism

§ REFERENCES

Barlow, R., and F. Warner. (1881): "On subcutaneous nodules connected with fibrous structures, occurring in children the subjects of rheumatism and chorea." *Trans. int. med. Congr., 7* sess., *4,* pp. 116–28.

Boerhaave, H. (1724): *Aphorisms concerning the knowledge and cure of diseases.* Translated from the last edition printed in Latin at Leyden, 1722. London, W. & J. Innys.

Bouillaud, J. B. (1837): *New researches on acute articular rheumatism in general.* Translated from the French of 1836 by James Kitchen. Philadelphia, Haswell, Barrington, and Haswell.

Bouillaud, J. B. (1840): *Traité clinique du rhumatisme articulaire.* Paris, J. B. Baillière.

Copeman, W. S. C. (ed.) (1948): *Textbook of the rheumatic diseases.* Edinburgh, E. & S. Livingston. pp. 4–12.

Garrison, F. H. (1929): *An introduction to the history of medicine.* 4th ed. Philadelphia and London, W. B. Saunders.

Garrod, A. E. (1890): *A treatise on rheumatism and rheumatoid arthritis.* London, C. Griffin & Co. P. 342.

Haygarth, J. (1805): *A clinical history of the acute rheumatism.* London, Cadell & Davies.

Heberden, W. (1806): *Commentaries on the history and cure of diseases.* 3rd ed. London, T. Payne. P. 148.

Still, G. F. (1896–97): "On a form of chronic joint disease in children." *Med.-chir. Trans., 80,* 47–59.

Störck, A. (1779): *De febre continua arthritica et rheumatica.* In *Annus medicus I. Amstelodami, Sumptibus Fratrum de Tournes,* Vol. I, pp. 105–24.

Sydenham, T. (1848–50): *The works.* Translated from the Latin edition of Dr. Greenhill by R. G. Latham. 2 vols. London, Sydenham Society.

Watson, T. (1843): *Lectures on the principles and practice of physic.* London, John W. Parker. Vol. II, p. 284.

Wells, W. C. (1812): "On rheumatism of the heart." *Trans. Soc. Improve. med. and chir. Knowledge, 3,* 373–424.

---

his life spent in retirement near Bath. (See also Bate, J. G. [1952]: "Poynton and Paine." *St. Mary's Hosp. Gaz., 58,* 139–42.)

BY EDWARD F. HARTUNG
M. D.*

chapter 6 / arthritis

THIS SHORT historical sketch will stress the arthritides, but will also include some of the rheumatic disorders other than rheumatic fever, since the latter is dealt with in a separate chapter. However, it is impossible completely to isolate rheumatic fever from the rest. In the past it has been confused and entangled with the other arthritides. Even today the separation is often difficult.†

From time to time historical summaries have been written, such as those by Charles Scudamore, Sir Alfred Baring Garrod and his son, Sir Archibald Edward Garrod, R. L. J. Llewellyn, R. Stockman, Robert S. Hormell, and the excellent *Source book of orthopedics* by Edgar Milton Bick. However, medical history, like all history, could be profitably rewritten for each generation, since all history is written from the standpoint of contemporary knowledge, conceptions, aims, and even fashions of thought, and is quickly outdated. Then, too, words change their meaning and must be redefined. Nowhere are both considerations more important than in the history of arthritis. Witness, for example, the fluctuations in the meaning of the word "rheumatism" which for a millenium or so had little or nothing to do with joints; or the word "gout" 'which also at first had no exclusive

* Associate clinical professor of medicine, New York University Post Graduate Medical School, New York City, associate attending physician and chief of Arthritis Clinic, University Hospital, New York University Bellevue Medical Center; and author of several papers on arthritis.

† Editorial note: This chapter should be read in conjunction with Dr. Copeman's chapter on rheumatism. While there is some overlapping of the material treated, the approach is fundamentally different, emphasis being placed on rheumatism of the soft and of the hard tissues respectively.

relationship with joints, least of all with the disturbance of purine metabolism as we know it today.

The history of arthritis, as far as recorded history can reveal, may be divided into three phases. First there was man's attempt to explain as well as treat the heterogeneous but undifferentiated musculoskeletal and joint disorders on the basis of a unitarian theory, the most popular being the humoral theory. This unitarian theory satisfactorily rationalized all rheumatic manifestations for the medical and lay mind up to the seventeenth century. Second was man's attempt to classify these disorders into their various categories, in view of the fact that common experience showed them to fall into distinct groups, each with special characteristics. Third came man's efforts to find specific treatments for each entity.

Phase one starts with recorded history and carries through for two thousand years. Phase two—man's attempt to classify and differentiate the rheumatic disorders—is probably the most significant part of this history, starting mainly in the seventeenth century and accelerating markedly after 1800, and still more so during the last fifty years. Great strides have been made in differential diagnosis, but much still remains to be revealed in this regard. Any worker in the field is acutely conscious of the inadequacies of our present classifications. The inclusion of ankylosing spondylitis as a subheading of rheumatoid arthritis, considering its marked variations from rheumatoid arthritis, particularly its predominance in males and its localization mainly to the spine and hips, is a case in point. The very diversity of the classifications offered, the continuous controversy over terminology, and the lack of good diagnostic criteria are tokens of how much we still have to learn.

Classification, or nosology, and the differential diagnosis from which it is derived is, of course, not necessarily dependent on an understanding of etiology. Differential diagnosis is often based on purely clinical observations, at times confirmed by laboratory techniques. However, when these differentiations are supported by proven etiological concepts, the process of differentiation is complete. Concepts of etiology are at times the result of clinical observation, but often have to await advances in ancillary disciplines, such as chemistry and bacteriology. It is hardly necessary to say that this process of elucidation is still going on in arthritis and rheumatism. Only in the arthritides due to specific infections, such as tuberculosis and gonorrhea, have we arrived on firm ground concerning etiology and, fortunately, treatment as well.

Very much the same can be said about phase three. Empirical therapies we have always had. Many of our best forms of therapy, such as the use of willow bark or salicylates, the extract of the corm of *colchicum autumnale,* and physical therapy in all its forms, were and still are empirical; other more recent advances have been dependent on advances in the associated sciences, as was the case in differential diagnosis. The chemotherapeutic and antibiotic agents are outstanding examples of the latter.

At the present time a large number of classifications and terminologies are being advocated. This is not the place to present any of these. There are many "official" ones in Great Britain and in the United States of America, and these can be found in the standard textbooks. A common denominator of all of them is a group of disorders which, with some variation in terminology, can be listed as follows:

1. Arthritis due to infection
2. Rheumatic fever
3. Rheumatoid arthritis
4. Arthritis due to injury
5. Neurogenic arthropathy
6. Gout
7. Degenerative joint disease (osteoarthritis)
8. New growths
9. Hydrarthrosis, intermittent
10. Fibrositis
11. Myositis, bursitis, etc.
12. Diseases with which arthritis is frequently associated.

There is no unanimity today as to the acceptability of even these terms, least of all as to the etiology of the clinical entities they represent. That time will break each down into smaller and smaller subgroups is equally clear. The recent breakdown of category number 12 into subgroups such as lupus erythematosus, scleroderma, and the other "collagen disorders" is an example. It is also increasingly clear that most are not true arthritides, or not mainly so. Rheumatic fever is a case in point, it now being proven to be, as was surmised from very early times, a disorder of the mesenchyme, the joint manifestations being merely incidental.

§ DEFINITION OF TERMS

From Hippocrates down through the next two thousand years *arthritis* was the term of choice. What differentiation was made was on an anatomical rather than a clinical or etiological basis. Aretaeus the Cappadocian made this anatomical classification very explicit. Thus, *podagra* was arthritis of the foot, literally a seizure of the foot; *chiragra,* of the hand; *gonagra,* of the knee. The true causes of arthritis, said Aretaeus, were known only to the gods. Others such as Caelius Aurelianus were less humble and explained arthritis as "a rheumatism," that is, a flowing of a thin fluid or humor from one part of the body to another, thus producing a disproportion and congestion in the joints. Caelius Aurelianus stated that the causes and treatment were always the same, only the location varied. He used such words as *dentagra* (of the teeth) and *tenontagra* (of the tendons). He was followed closely by Galen who set the pattern for the next thousand years. Not until the writings of Conrad Victor Schneider (1614–80) did the influence of humoral pathology and theory wane, and then very slowly.

The humoral theory was based on the conception that there were four elements: earth, air, fire, and water; four qualities: dry, cold, hot, and moist; and four humors: blood, phlegm, yellow bile, and black bile. These humors flowed from one place to another, causing a disproportion in their distribution, and these arrangements in various combinations rationalized disease and indicated treatment.

The term "rheumatism" (from *rheuma,* akin to *rhein*—to flow) derives from the same humoral theory and was used, not as a term for diseases of the joints, but for "an internal defluxion of a thin humor." By this name Caelius Aurelianus, for example, understood diarrhea. The word "catarrh" is a similar concept from an identical root and was used mainly in relation to disorders of mucous membranes. The word "rheumatism" in the sense of joint disease was first used by Guillaume de Baillou (Ballonius), a Parisian physician who died in 1616.

From then on the word "rheumatism" became more or less standard nomenclature in place of the older term "acute arthritis." Hermann Boerhaave in 1728 wrote: "There is a disease ally'd to the gout, and scurvy, which is very common in England and called rheumatism." This usage continued through the nineteenth century. Thus it was used by Alfred Baring Garrod (1859) and by his son, Archibald Edward Garrod (1890) specifically for what we would call "rheumatic fever."

Parallel with this specific use of the word "rheumatism" was, and still is, the use of the term for any real or imagined, slight or severe ache or pain, the cause of which could not be diagnosed; in other words it was, and is still, often used as "a cloak of ignorance."

The word "gout" (Latin—*gutta*) again refers to a humoral concept of disease, that is, a dropping of humors from one part of the body to another, thus producing a disproportion in their distribution. The terms "rheumatism" and "catarrh" were employed by the classical authors; but the word "gout" was derived from lay use, first applied to any humoral flux, then to joint disorders in general and then as a synonym for arthritis, and gradually incorporated into medical terminology. It was first used according to Jacques-Mathieus Delpeuch in the ninth century. In the thirteenth century Ralph Bocking (Radulphus), confessor to St. Richard of Wyche, Bishop of Chichester, used the term explicitly, in a life of St. Richard, as synonymous with podagra and arthritis: *"gutta quam podagram vel arteticam vocant"* (gout which is called podagra or arthritis).

A brief outline of how we arrived at a concept of the most important of the clinical groups mentioned above will be attempted next, with particular stress on when the disease was first recognized as an entity, and an effort will be made to determine the origin of the name used to designate it today.

§ GOUT

Gout, in the modern sense of the word, appears to be the joint disease recognized and best described by the ancients. The aphorisms of Hippocrates apply mainly to true gout, referring as they do to a tendency to periodicity; to the fact that gout is more troublesome in the spring and fall; that young men are free from the disorder until after puberty; that women rarely have gout until menopause; that eunuchs

128

are not afflicted with gout; and that those with tophaceous deposits are beyond the powers of medicine. However, that he confused gout with other forms of arthritis is equally evident, some references applying to old age and to acute and chronic rheumatism.

Many statements of Celsus, Galen, Aretaeus, Caelius Aurelianus, and Alexander of Tralles are also applicable to true gout. Aretaeus, for example, says that the pain first seizes the great toe, then the rest of the foot and ankle; that friction from a new shoe, a long walk, a blow, or being trod upon, is often a precipitating factor; that sometimes the disease is confined to the feet during the patient's entire life, but that it often extends to the rest of the body; that fluid deposits are formed which are converted into hard white tophi; and that men are more frequently affected than women. The remedies are innumerable, "for the calamity renders the patients themselves expert druggists." Aretaeus also mentions that the disease is apt to recur and to become chronic, but that a gouty patient has even won the Olympic Games between attacks!

Later classical authors such as Aëtius of Amida and Paulus Aegineta also appear to be describing gout. These and the Byzantine and Arabic authors add nothing new in diagnosis and very little new in treatment, except hermodactyl or colchicum (Alexander of Tralles).

De Baillou (1642), mentioned above, was first not only to use the term "rheumatism" in the modern sense, but also clearly to draw a distinction between rheumatism and gout. General acceptance of this idea was not easy and had to await the times and writings of Thomas Sydenham (1683), who further elucidated this distinction. However, Sydenham's work was marred by his complete adherence to the humoral theory. William Cullen (1784) carried the distinction further. Others such as Thomas Willis, Friedrich Hoffmann, William Musgrave, George Cheyne, Hermann Boerhaave, Richard Mead, Gerard van Swieten, William Cadogan, Murray Forbes, and William Heberden can be only mentioned in this short sketch. By the time of Charles Scudamore (1827), the descriptions of gout have a modern tone.

In 1776 Carl Wilhelm Scheele discovered uric acid, and in 1797 William Hyde Wollaston demonstrated sodium urate in tophi. Up to this time, including Sydenham, the contents of tophi were considered to be "undigested gouty matter." A. B. Garrod completed the history in his classical book *The nature and treatment of gout and rheumatic gout* (1859), among other contributions demonstrating excess urates in the blood of the gouty (*Med.-chir. Trans.*, 1848, *31, 83–97*). Since this time we have learned very little of real value. Emil Fischer's demonstration of the relationship of purine bodies to uric acid was important. The most recent significant contributions appear to be the introduction of benemid and the demonstration of the synthesis of purine materials endogenously from simple basic elements.

It would be amusing, if space permitted, to mention countless curious epochs and items in the history of gout: its possible relation to riotous living as suggested by Seneca and others; its frequency in primitive peoples such as the Anglo-Saxons, where it was called "Fot-Adl"; its designation *morbus dominorum,* since it appeared to attack mainly the rich and well-placed; a listing of the great men past and present who have had gout; the fact that it was at times considered a blessing since at its onset other disorders ceased and it conferred on its victims considerable immunity from new infirmities. Diet was always considered of prime importance (although alcoholic spirits are not now held in such antipathy for gouty patients as in the past) up to and including the time of the elder Garrod. Social and economic position are not any longer considered important as etiological factors, but heredity appears now to be paramount as a predisposing cause.

The old ideas die hard, as witness the use of the term "rheumatic gout" by writers up to Robert Adams (1857) and A. B. Garrod (1859) to designate nongouty arthritis. Man was reluctant to give up the idea of gout as a common diathesis, causing a multiplicity of heterogeneous disorders—reluctant to accept the idea that gout is a specific separate disorder.

§ RHEUMATIC FEVER

The next entity to be segregated appears to be what we now call "rheumatic fever." This volume gives a separate detailed history of this entity, but a brief summary of certain aspects will be included here as it is an integral part of the story of how the rheumatic disorders were gradually differentiated.

Implications that nongouty acute rheumatism occurred from the earliest times are present in the writings of the ancients. De Baillou, however, more clearly defines the issues and divides the nongouty arthritides into acute and chronic forms. Thereafter, as stated above, "rheumatism" appears to be the term of choice for what we now call "rheumatic fever," and "rheumatic gout" for the large group of subacute and chronic joint disorders. Following Sydenham, Cullen (1776) and John Haygarth (1805) gave good descriptions of acute rheumatism or "rheumatic fever," the former pointing out for the first time that this form of rheumatism "almost never" terminates in suppuration. The Frenchmen, Barthez (1802), Gasc (1803), and Augustin Jacob Landré Beauvais (1800) were near to the modern viewpoint in stating that rheumatism had for its seat the structures near to and between the joints, its articular location being rather apparent than real.

It is certain that "acute rheumatism" included many other forms of arthritis, especially the infectious arthritides such as gonorrheal arthritis. Chronic rheumatism, and later the term "rheumatic gout," were scrap baskets for all the rest.

§ RHEUMATOID ARTHRITIS

The antiquity of rheumatoid arthritis is difficult to determine. Almost all the skeletal remains unearthed by archeologists, when they do reveal arthritis, undoubtedly exhibit what we now call degenerative joint disease or osteoarthritis. Cases of gout, rheumatoid arthritis, and tuberculous arthritis are described, but these are always questionable and rare. Osteoarthritis is a wearing-out of cartilage between bones, followed by spur formations at the joint margins, and is related to age and use. Thus it is an inherent eventuality in all movable joints, in man and in beast, at present and in times long antedating our records of man himself.

The existence of rheumatoid arthritis in Greek and Roman times, and in the Medieval, Byzantine, and Arabic periods, can only be surmised. Types of chronic arthritis, as distinct from acute arthritis and acute gout, are described, but their frequency and exact nature is impossible to determine. Only after the seventeenth century do we begin to get a vague, but increasingly clear picture of the existence of the entity we now call rheumatoid arthritis. We must wait till the works of Thomas Sydenham (1683) to begin to see its segregation from the great mass of arthritides. He gives an explicit description of chronic arthritis, undoubtedly rheumatoid. William Musgrave (1703), François Boissier de la Croix de Sauvages (1763), who may have coined the term "rheumatic gout," and Albrecht von Haller (1764) were more confused. Landré Beauvais (1800), although he called it asthenic gout (*"goutte asthénique primitive"*) in distinction from true gout, for the first time recognized its outstanding characteristics, calling attention to its special frequency in women, the chronic course, the destruction of cartilage, and the enlargements and deformities different from those found in true gout.

In 1801 William Heberden the Elder suggested separating what we now know as rheumatoid arthritis from other forms. He spoke of an articular disease not starting in the great toe, but preferring other joints; its clinical course so different from gout that it should be called by a distinct name, the pain being much less, but the swelling greater; and said that it causes great and lasting weakness. He described "Heberden's nodes"—the bony excrescences at the distal joints of the fingers, now considered to be osteoarthritis—but he did not separate their appearance from the syndrome of rheumatoid arthritis.

In 1805 John Haygarth gave a good description and called it "nodosity of the joints." He distinctly separated it from gout, rheumatic gout, and rheumatic fever. Kellgren (1954), however, interpreted Haygarth's description as of a form of osteoarthritis. Charles Scudamore (1827) did not think that the entity was real, that is, distinct, and one can hardly blame this excellent thinker and writer in view of the multiplicity of unrelated entities which at that time were included in this category.

Sir Benjamin Brodie (1833) made it a distinct disease. Jean Cruveilhier (1829–42) added a great deal to the understanding of its symptoms and to its anatomical characteristics. He felt the disease was separate from gout and rheumatism and "white swelling." Jean-Martin Charcot and Étienne L.-C. Trastour (1853), and J. B. E. Vidal gave excellent clinical reports. In France arthritis was considered a chronic form of rheumatism and not a specific disease.

Robert Adams's book (1857) gave good descriptions, and his engravings portraying the morbid anatomy are the foundation of our present knowledge of this phase of the subject. He advocated the term "chronic rheumatic arthritis" to distinguish it from gout.

Arthritis

Alfred Baring Garrod (1859), who contributed so much to our knowledge of gout, also coined the name "rheumatoid arthritis." He said that "although unwilling to add to the number of names I cannot help expressing a desire that one may be found for the disease under consideration, not implying any necessary relation to gout or rheumatism; perhaps rheumatoid arthritis would answer the object." His son, Archibald Edward Garrod, published a very thorough description in 1890.

Virchow offered the term *arthritis deformans* to cover all non-gouty arthritis, and most students consider that this term has markedly confused the issue.

Joel Ernest Goldthwait in 1904 offered another classification, suggesting the terms "hypertrophic" and "atrophic," and a third group called "infectious." E. H. Nichols and F. L. Richardson (1909), after an excellent study of the pathology of arthritis, offered still another classification—proliferative and degenerative: "two types of a single disease." These latter authors viewed the problem from the point of view of the soft tissue changes. Their terms are synonymous with rheumatoid and osteoarthritis respectively.

The nomenclature committee of the International League against Rheumatism, founded by Jan Frans Leonard van Breemen, considered "upward of sixty different methods of nomenclature from various countries." Van Breemen counted twenty-one names for chronic non-specific arthritis used during the nineteenth century. During the past two decades the term "rheumatoid arthritis" has gradually attained greatest popularity.

The most important subgroup of rheumatoid arthritis is rheumatoid spondylitis. It has many synonyms, including "Marie-Strümpell arthritis." It can be traced back at least to the writings of Bernard Connor (1691). Bradford reported three cases in 1883 and called it rheumatism of the spine. In 1897 E. A. G. G. Strümpell reported some cases, and in 1898 Pierre Marie described the condition well as *"la spondylose rhizomélique."* J. E. Goldthwait in 1899 wrote a comprehensive article on the subject and, although he called it osteoarthritis of the spine, distinguished it definitely from the common senile changes.

What is now considered to be rheumatoid arthritis in children was described by Frederic Still in 1897. Psoriasis in arthritis was first noted

133

by Alibert in 1872, and the term *arthropathia psoriatica* was coined by Pierre Antoine Ernest Bazin in 1860.

§ OSTEOARTHRITIS

An understanding of osteoarthritis, or degenerative joint disease, to use the designation favored by Granville A. Bennett, Hans Waine, and Walter Bauer, as we visualize it today, was difficult to achieve and can hardly be said to have been formulated before the beginning of the twentieth century. It is one of the oldest disorders, being found in the osseous remains of animals antedating man, and in man and beast at all periods of prehistory and history, but one of the most recently identified types of arthritis. At present it is considered to be an attrition and erosion of cartilage and a production of osteophytes at the chondro-osseous margins, related to use and age, but not explained completely on these factors alone. It is not merely a token of aging or merely a measure of use; it is a "senescence of joint tissues" and results from many factors, some as yet unknown. There is a generalized and a localized form.

The term "osteoarthritis" was invented by John Kent Spender (1888), not to designate this entity, but rather what was "commonly called rheumatoid arthritis." It was also adopted as the nomenclature of the Royal College of Physicians of London, but again to designate rheumatoid arthritis.

The concept of osteoarthritis was born piecemeal, as it were, item by item, as the arthritic disorders were gradually studied clinically, and eventually at autopsy. The main characteristics of the disorder were merged inextricably at first in the great group of so-called chronic arthritides, then in the category called rheumatic gout, and then as an integral part of the growing concept of rheumatoid arthritis.

Very little about the condition that we now call osteoarthritis was known or surmised until most recent times. Hippocrates noted the relationship of age to some forms of arthritis, and the joint infirmities of senescence were, of course, remarked on by countless authors, lay and medical, throughout the ages. Not until the nineteenth century, though, were specific data gradually accumulated.

In 1824 Benjamin Bell described eburnation of the femoral head. In 1835 Robert Smith proposed the term *morbus coxae senilis* and described the morbid anatomy of the condition in the hip and else-where. A. Ecker in 1843 thought this process to be senile atrophy and wear and tear on cartilage injured by previous inflammation. Anton Weichselbaum (1872–78) described the gross and microscopic changes, and the separation of rheumatoid arthritis and osteoarthritis began with his fundamental pathological studies. These were fol-lowed by the work of E. H. Nichols and F. L. Richardson (1909), R. L. J. Llewellyn (1909), H. Beitzke (1912), Gustav Adolf Pommer (1913), and Rudolph Beneke (1925). The most recent comprehen-sive study was made by Bennett, Waine, and Bauer (1942) in an ex-cellent book, *Changes in the knee joint at various ages.*

However, from a clinical point of view the old ideas died some-what more slowly. In 1802 Heberden described "Heberden's Nodes," but as a component of rheumatoid arthritis rather than of osteo-arthritis. This confusion of the two conditions carried right up and through A. E. Garrod (1890), who, although often given credit for separating rheumatoid arthritis from osteoarthritis, considerably con-fused the two. Thus he says: "All the cases . . . of rheumatoid arthritis agreed in one respect—in all there is a fibrillation and erosion of cartilage and a tendency to the formation of osteophytic growths—that the articular lesions are the sole manifestation of the disease, and are not manifestations of systemic disease but rather the result of a disturbance of nutrition similar to the arthropathies seen in locomotor ataxia." The same Garrod makes Heberden's nodes a subvariety of rheumatoid arthritis and even suspects a gouty component. The latter confusion carries through even to 1935, when J. Gutman considered osteoarthritis as due to a "faulty purine metabolism."

§ ARTHRITIS DUE TO INFECTION

The antiquity of arthritis due to infection, as we call it today (that is, arthritis due to a known microorganism), is difficult to determine. Undoubtedly acute infectious arthritis and chronic sequelae of these types were common enough, but authenticated cases, reconstructed from archeological remains or from the extant literature, are difficult to come by. Many of the acute arthritides of the past must have been of this nature; for example, some of the cases of "acute rheumatism" of de Baillou and subsequent authors.

As to tuberculous arthritis, one of the first references was that of Richard Wiseman, Surgeon General to King Charles II, who in 1672 described a specific entity, *tumor albus,* which we now recognize as tuberculosis of the joints. Gonorrheal arthritis was first described by Pierre-Martin de la Martinière (1664) in his treatise on venereal disease, by Christian Gottlieb Selle and Franz Xaver S. Swediaur at the end of the eighteenth century, and subsequently by Sir Benjamin Collins Brodie in 1818. It was referred to by A. E. Garrod (1890). However, the question he proposed was whether it was due to a metastatic infection, was of nervous origin, or was an incidental acute rheumatism brought on by the debilitating effect of the genito-urinary infection. The organism was not isolated by Albert Neisser until 1879.

J. E. Goldthwait in 1904 coined the term "infectious arthritis," as he did not feel that atrophic and hypertrophic arthritis covered all the entities he could distinguish clinically. However, his so-called infectious arthritis was, in the main, acute rheumatoid arthritis. The concept of a focal infection as a cause of arthritis was first suggested by Benjamin Rush, who in 1803 described a case of "rheumatism of the hip" cured by the removal of a painful tooth. According to Sir Humphry Rolleston this is the first authenticated case of so-called focal infection. The entire concept was formalized by F. Billings in 1912 when he described what he considered to be the relationship of focal infection to arthritis. Subsequent to this an entire generation of physicians extirpated countless teeth, tonsils, and other foci, accused of causing acute and chronic arthritis, but with equivocal results.

§ WHAT OF THE FUTURE?

A survey of what we have written above, a very cursory summary of the history of arthritis, forces one to the conclusion that we are in no sense on a pinnacle looking down and back over a laborious pathway, up which medical investigators have fought. It is rather obvious that we are now just at the foothill, just beginning to understand the joint and musculoskeletal disorders with which man may be afflicted. Undoubtedly the future is going to see a further breakdown of the above mentioned categories into other separate and etiologically distinct entities; an explanation of their causes is still to be forthcoming, and their treatment to be elucidated. It is not an exaggeration to say that only in some of the arthritides due to infection do we understand the pathogenesis and have a satisfactory and specific treatment.

§ REFERENCES

Adams, R. (1839): "Abnormal conditions of the hip joint." *Cyclopaedia of anatomy and physiology.* Edited by R. B. Todd. London, Longman. Vol. II, pp. 780–825.

Adams, R. (1857): *Treatise on rheumatic gout, or chronic rheumatic arthritis, of all the joints.* London, J. Churchill.

Aretaeus the Cappadocian (1856): *The extant works of.* Edited and translated by Francis Adams. London, Sydenham Society.

Baillou, G. de (1642): *Liber de rheumatismo et pleuritide dorsali.* Parisiis, J. Quesnel.

Barthez, P. J. (1802): *Traité des maladies goutteuses.* 2 vols. Paris, Deterville.

Bechterew, W. v. (1899): *Dtsch. Z. Nervenheilk, 15,* 37–44.

Beitzke, H. (1912): *Z.klin.Med., 74,* 215–29.

Bell, B. (1824): *Remarks on interstitial absorption of the neck of the thigh-bone.* Edinburgh, Maclachlan and Stewart.

Beneke, R. (1925): *Fortschr. Röntgenstr., 33,* 843–61.

Boerhaave, H. (1742): *Boerhaave's aphorisms concerning the knowledge and cure of diseases.* Translated from the last edition printed in Latin at Leyden, 1728. London, Innys and Hitch.

Brodie, B. C. (1814): *Med.-chir. Trans., 5,* 239–54. In (1938) *Med. Class., 2,* 919–28.

Brodie, B. C. (1818): *Pathological and surgical observations on the diseases of the joints.* London, Longman.

Canton, E. (1855): *Surgical and pathological observations.* London, Samuel Highley.

Charcot, J. M. (1853): *Thèse pour le doctorat en médecine.* Paris, Rignoux, Imprimeur de la Faculté de Médecine.

Charcot, J. M. (1867): *Leçons sur les maladies des vieillards et les maladies chroniques.* Paris, A. Delahaye.

Charcot, J. M. (1868): *Arch. Physiol. norm. path., 1,* 161–78.

Charcot, J. M. (1881): *Clinical lectures on senile and chronic diseases.* London, New Sydenham Society.

Cruveilhier, J. (1829): *Anatomie pathologique du corps humain.* Paris, J.-B. Baillière. Vol. I.

Cullen, W. (1781): *First lines of the practice of physic for the use of students in the University of Edinburgh.* 3rd edition. Edinburgh, William Creech.

Cullen, W. (1808): *A methodical system of nosology.* Translated from the Latin of Doctor W. Cullen by Eldad Lewis. Stockbridge, C. Sturtevant, Jun.

Delpeuch, A. (1900): *La goutte et le rhumatisme.* Paris. Georges Carré et C. Naud.

Ecker, A. (1843): *Arch. physiol. Heilk.*, *2*, 235–48.

Fuller, H. W. (1860): *On rheumatism, rheumatic gout, and sciatica, their pathology symptoms, and treatment.* 3rd edition. London, J. Churchill.

Garrod, Sir A. B. (1848): *Med.-chir. Trans., 31,* 83–97.

Garrod, Sir A. B. (1859): *The nature and treatment of gout and rheumatic gout.* London, Walton and Maberly.

Garrod, Sir A. B. (1866): "Rheumatoid arthritis." and "Rheumatism." In *A system of medicine.* Edited by J. Russell Reynolds. London, Macmillan & Co. Pp. 876–90, 891–919.

Garrod, A. E. (1890): *A treatise on rheumatism and rheumatoid arthritis.* London, Charles Griffin & Co.

Goldthwait, J. E. (1899): *Boston med. surg. J., 141,* 128–32

Goldthwait, J. E. (1904): *Ibid., 150,* 363–71.

Haygarth, J. (1805): *A clinical history of the acute rheumatism,* and *A clinical history of the nodosity of the joints.* London, Cadell and Davies.

Heberden, W. (1802): *Commentaries on the history and cure of diseases.* Translation into English attributed to William Heberden, Jr. London, T. Payne.

Hippocrates (1849): *The genuine works of.* Translated from the Greek, with a preliminary discourse and annotations by Francis Adams. London, Sydenham Society. Vol. I.

Hormell, R. S. (1940): *New Engl. J. Med., 223,* 754–60.

Landré-Beauvais (1800): *Doit-on admettre une nouvelle espèce de goutte, sous la dénomination de goutte asthénique primitive?* Paris. P. viii.

Llewellyn, R. L. J. (1909): *Arthritis deformans.* New York, W. Wood & Co.

Maclagan, T. J. (1881): *Rheumatism: its nature, its pathology, and its successful treatment.* London, Pickering & Co.

Marie, P. (1898): *Rev. Méd., Paris,* 18, 285–315.

Messeloff, C. R. (1930): *Med. Life, 37,* 3–56.

Musgrave, W. (1703): *Dissertatio de arthritide symptomatica.* Oxford.

Nichols, E. H., and F. L. Richardson (1909): *J. med. Res., 21,* 149–221.

Pemberton, R. (1929): *Arthritis and rheumatoid conditions: their nature and treatment.* Philadelphia, Lea and Febiger.

Pemberton, R., and R. B. Osgood (1934): *The medical and orthopaedic management of chronic arthritis.* London, Henry Kimpton.

Pommer, G. A. (1914): *Denkschr. Akad. Wiss. Wien, 89,* 65–316.

Pommer, G. A. (1915): *Virchows Arch., 219,* 261–78.

Pommer, G. A. (1918): *Über die Beziehungen der Arthritis deformans zu den Gewerbekrankheiten.* Wien, A. Hölder.

Pommer, G. A. (1920): *Arch. orthop. Unfallchir, 17,* 573–93.

Pommer, G. A.(1927): *Virchows Arch., 263,* 434–514.

Ruhmann, W. (1940): *Brit. J. Rheum., 2,* 140–62.

Rush, B. (1815): *Medical inquiries and observations.* 4 vols. 4th edition. Philadelphia, Bennet & Walton.

Sauvages, F. B. de la Croix de (1763): *Nosologia methodica, sistens morborum classes, genera et species. Amstelodami, Sumptibus Fratrum de Tournes.*

Arthritis

Schneider, C. V. (1664): *Liber de arthritide, podagra et chiragra.* Wittenberg.

Scudamore, C. (1817): *A treatise on the nature and cure of gout and rheumatism.* 2nd edition. London, Longman, Hurst, Rees, Orme, and Brown.

Scudamore, C. (1827): *A treatise on the nature and cure of rheumatism; with observations on rheumatic neuralgia, and on spasmodic neuralgia, or tic douloureux.* London, Longman, Rees, Orme, Brown and Green.

Sennert, D. (1656): "Tractatus de arthritide." In *Opera omnia.* Lugduni, J. A. Huguetan.

Spender, J. K. (1888): *Trans. med. Soc. Lond., 11,* 209–15.

Spender, J. K. (1889): *Lancet, ii,* 947–48.

Spender, J. K. (1889): *The early symptoms and the early treatment of osteoarthritis (commonly called rheumatoid arthritis) with special reference to the bath thermal waters.* London, H. K. Lewis.

Still, G. F. (1897): *Med.-chir. Trans., 80,* 47–59.

Stockman, R. (1920): *Rheumatism and arthritis.* Edinburgh, W. Green and Son.

Strümpell, A. (1897): *Dtsch. Z. Nervenheilk., 11,* 338–42.

Sydenham, T. (1683): *Tractatus de podagra et hydrope.* Londini, G. Kettilby.

Tralles, A. von (1879): *Original-Text und Übersetzung nebst einer einleitenden Abhandlung.* Ein Beitrag zur Geschichte der Medicin von Dr. Theodor Puschmann. Wien.

Vidal, J. B. E. (1855): *Thèse pour le doctorat en médecine.* Paris, Rignoux, Imprimeur de la Faculté de Médecine.

Weichselbaum, A. (1872): *Virchows Arch., 55,* 217–28.

Weichselbaum, A. (1878): *Ibid., 73,* 461–75.

Weichselbaum, A. (1877): *S. B. Akad. Wiss. Wien., 75,* 193–243.

Wiseman, R. (1719): *Eight chirurgical treatises.* 5th edition. London, B. Tooke. Vol. I.

BY TERENCE EAST

M. A., D. M., F. R. C. P.*

chapter 7 / heart disease

Until William Harvey published his *Exercitatio de motu cordis et sanguinis in animalibus* (Francofurti, Sumptibus Guilielmi Fitzeri) in 1628, no understanding of the failure of the circulation was possible. No description of the diseases of the heart and vessels was attempted. In this chapter the physiological discoveries will not find much place. Here we must confine ourselves to morbid matters. To trace the advance of the knowledge of cardiology, if we may use that word to describe the study of the diseases and derangements of functions that affect the circulation, from the time of Harvey is not easy. Sometimes a man has had an idea which led to a gain in knowledge by a new means of investigation. Sometimes it has been the correlation of observation at the bedside and in the post-mortem room. It is unsatisfactory to review the subject purely in chronological order. Rather must one in this small space pick on certain advances in some branches which have stimulated many minds and led to an extensive widening of the scope of knowledge.

§ STUDY OF THE PULSE

Physical examination must form a chief part of diagnosis, and for the cardiovascular system, and indeed the body as a whole, the study of the pulse goes back to the Ebers Papyrus of 1500 B.C. in ancient Egypt and to Chinese writers of 500 B.C. Hippocrates had little to learn from the pulse, and it was Galen at the end of the second century A.D. who made the first extensive study. As he knew nothing of the circulation,

* Senior physician and physician-in-charge, cardiological department, King's College Hospital, London; associate editor, *British Heart Journal*.

he could not get far; but his observations were acute enough and based on sound clinical facts, for he recognized the effect of emotion on the pulse and gave clear directions for its examination, as did Celsus a century earlier. Galen's writings, remarkable for their vigor, clarity, and profusion, dominated medical thought for many centuries. In 1707 Sir John Floyer, a physician in Lichfield, the family doctor of Samuel Johnson, who consulted his textbook in his last illness, published *The physician's pulse watch* (London, S. Smith and B. Walford) in two volumes. This was a great advance, for he introduced a special watch that ran for one minute (or very nearly) and used it to gauge the rate of the pulse. Perusal of these volumes is worth while, for he broke away from Galen's theory that there were pulses peculiar to diseases. He studied all possible causes of change in pulse rate with remarkable thoroughness; it is one of the first attempts at scientific clinical medicine.

When Leopold Auenbrugger published his observations in Latin on the art of percussion in 1761, *Inventum novum ex percussione thoracis humani* (Vindobonae, J. T. Trattner), the way was open for the full advance of physical examination. He was aware of the encroachment of the dullness of the heart on the resonance of the lungs when there is enlargement or when there is fluid in the pericardial sac (sections 46 and 48). The work is one of genius, remarkable for its accuracy and economy of words, but it received no recognition until it was translated into French (for the second time) by Jean-Nicolas Corvisart in 1808, one year before the author died. The translator had practiced the art for twenty years. The original, and Corvisart's shrewd and interesting comments, should be read by every young physician.

§ AUSCULTATION OF THE HEART

The link to the next great discovery, that of auscultation, is provided by Corvisart, whose pupil was René Théophile Hyacinthe Laënnec. In Corvisart's *Essai sur les maladies et les lésions organiques du coeur et des gros vaisseaux* (Paris, Méquignon-Marvis), published in 1806, there is a clear description of the thrill (*bruissement*) of mitral stenosis, in a patient who obviously had auricular fibrillation. Laënnec's *De l'auscultation médiate* appeared in 1819. That only three years elapsed between the inspiring observation of the boys playing with the log of wood and this epoch-making work is a marvel. Laënnec's attention was mainly directed to the elucidation of the signs of the lungs, but he described the murmur which accompanied the thrill felt by Corvisart. Laënnec called the thrill *"frémissement cataire,"* and he heard the systolic "bellows murmur" (*bruit de soufflet*) too. Unfortunately, he failed to grasp how the sounds of the heart were made.

Corvisart and his pupil were the first to study clinically the size and shape of the heart and were diligent in distinguishing hypertrophy and dilatation, for both followed in the path of Giovanni Battista Morgagni, who was one of the earliest to learn the "salutary lessons of the deadhouse." He had done many examinations post-mortem in his long life. He followed the earlier example of Théophile Bonet, who wrote the *Sepulchretum sive anatomia practica, ex cadaveribus morbo denatis* (Genevae, L. Chouët, 1679) and who really led the way in this study, if we exclude Antonio Benivieni, whose observations on 111 cases were published posthumously in 1507 (*De abtidis nonnulis ac mirandis morborum et sanationum causis*. Florentiae, P. Giunta). But Morgagni combined the accurate observation of the living and the dead. His volumes should have the attention of every physician. We find in them a beautiful description, written in the easy, flowing style of personal letters to a friend, of the lives and deaths of his patients. Here of interest, particularly among the famous accounts of his *De sedibus et causis morborum,* we find angina pectoris with aortic stenosis, Pick's syndrome of constrictive pericarditis, rupture of the heart, myocardial fibrosis, almost all the valve lesions, heart block, and aneurysm of the aorta. Morgagni died at the age of ninety, ten years after the publication of his work, of rupture of the heart, having greatly added to the already great fame of Padua.

He was a worthy follower of Hipólito Francesco Albertini and Antonio Maria Valsalva, who himself derived from Marcello Malpighi, and more remotely from that famous line of anatomists, Vesalius, Gabriello Fallopio, Giulio Casserio, and Adriaan van den Spieghel, all of whose names have come down to us across the years.

To Corvisart one must again refer for the accurate description of pericarditis, the valvular lesions, and some congenital defects (mentioned elsewhere). Once more the examination at autopsy was made to link up with the physical findings. So for forty years the detection of physical signs and their confirmation after death were slowly achieved. There was much more to do. In Vienna Joseph Skoda (*Abhandlung über Perkussion und Auskultation.* Wien, 1839) went on with this work, and the type of resonance he noted is still mentioned, while in England Charles J. B. Williams, who had studied under Laënnec, made clearer the method of the production of the heart sounds and murmurs by experiments under curare (Woorara) in 1828. James Hope, working at St. George's Hospital, published *A treatise on the diseases of the heart and great vessels.* (London: W. Kidd, 1831), a work on diseases of the heart and aorta far in advance of its time. Charles James Williams and Robert Bentley Todd of King's College Hospital, and J. Clendinning finally reported on "the motions and signs of the heart" (*Lond. med. Gaz.,* 1836, *19,* 360.). Hope's early death in the forties from tubercle, reminding us of the short life and the death of Laënnec, came all too soon.

During the next seventy years new and finer points of physical diagnosis were added. Jean Bouillaud described variation in the heart sounds, the *"bruit de diable"* and *"bruit de rappel"* (*J. Univ. Méd. Chir.,* Paris, 1833, *11,* 561–90; *J. Progr. Sci. Inst. Méd.,* Paris, 1834, *1,* 291;*3,* 288). His pupil, Pierre Carl Edouard Potain developed the teaching of his master in his account of gallop rhythm (*Gaz. Hôp. Paris,* 1880, *53,* 529–31)—the *"bruit de galop."*—Little could be altered in his original description, and no one has found a better name for the phenomenon, dated though it may seem to be in a mechanical age. The murmur of Austin Flint came in 1859 (*Buffalo med. J.,* 1858–59, *14,* 321; 385)—a long account of a little thing; the murmur of Paul Louis Duroziez in the arteries in cases of aortic reflux in 1881 (*Union méd. Paris,* 1881, 3. sér., *31,* 1002; 1061; 1089).

It was not until 1888 that Graham Steell described the murmur of pulmonary regurgitation (*Med. Chron.,* 1888, *8,* 89–116). The murmur of a patent *ductus arteriosus*—the last to be described—was noted by George Alexander Gibson in 1898 (*Diseases of the heart and aorta.* Edinburgh and London, G. J. Pentland). The third sound of the heart was noted by G. A. Gibson and W. S. Thayer in 1909 (*Arch. intern. Med.,* Chicago, 1909, *4,* 297–305). The study of the pulse could only distinguish those rhythms obviously abnormal in character to the educated finger. Sir Dominic John Corrigan in 1832 noted the collapsing or water-hammer type, which had already been remarked on by Raymond Vieussens. In passing one may note that the type of aortic valvular disease which gives rise to this sort of pulse is called by Corrigan's name in France to this day—distinguishing it from that due to syphilis, to which the name of Joseph Hodgson, the Birmingham surgeon, is given. Adolf Kussmaul recognized the paradoxical pulse of pericardial effusion in 1873. Thus far clinical diagnosis went with the unaided senses. The finger of Richard Bright had already suspected the increase of arterial tension in 1836 (*Guy's Hosp. Rep.*, 1836, *1*, 18–21). It was revealed later by the first practical sphygmomanometer of Riva-Rocci in 1897 (*Gaz. méd. Torino*, 1897, *48*, 161, 181).

§ DISORDERS OF RHYTHM

The disorders of rhythm had long been noted; *"pulsus irregularis perpetuus"* was continuously being referred to; but until the graphic method was developed in general practice by Sir James Mackenzie, working first with a sphygmograph of the Dudgeon type and later with his polygraph, no understanding was reached. Mackenzie's efforts culminated in the astounding feat of solving these riddles which had puzzled clinicians for generations. In *The study of the pulse, arterial, venous, and hepatic, and of the movements of the heart* (Edinburgh and London, Y. J. Pentland, 1902) he analyzed nearly all of them with a logic and clarity and economy of expression that have never been surpassed. No young physician should fail to look into this epoch-making work. The disappearance of the auricular wave in the jugular tracing, which he noted to coincide with the loss of the presystolic murmur when the pulse became completely irregular, made him think of the abolition of auricular systole. The next step, to auricular fibrillation, which Sir Thomas Lewis took (*Brit. med. J.*, 1909, *ii*, 1528) with the help of the electrocardiograph, was not a long one.

While it is true that the graphic method soon led to the solution of the arrhythmias, it must not be forgotten that the acute observations of William Stokes in Dublin, published in his book on the heart in 1854 (*The diseases of the heart and aorta*. Dublin, Hodges and Smith), recorded with absolute precision all the clinical features that can be observed in complete heart block. The account of the Cheyne-Stokes breathing in Stokes's work is unsurpassed, although Hippocrates had already noted it. The patients he studied suffered from the syncope known by his name and that of Robert Adams (*Dublin Hosp. Rep.,* 1827, *4,* 353–453). (But, of course, Morgagni had already accurately observed one case!) This period was a brilliant one in Dublin: Dominic Corrigan, John Cheyne, Robert Graves, and Francis Rynd, the surgeon who introduced hypodermic injection (*Dublin Quart. J. med. Sci.,* 1845, *13,* 167–68), were all at work there.

The part played by the electrocardiograph in the diagnosis of the arrhythmias was final. When Willem Einthoven produced a galvanometer that could record the small-voltage currents, already discovered by Augustus Désiré Waller in 1888 (*Brit. med. J.,* 1888, *ii,* 751–54), it was possible to cite the origin, time the progress, and indicate the course of the electric currents due to depolarization and repolarization in the heart muscle. Sir Thomas Lewis was the first to explore this field fully. By transferring this knowledge to the arrhythmia in question, the differentiation was easy, and with this knowledge most arrhythmias can now be diagnosed by the senses alone. Auricular flutter was first described in 1909 by A. F. Hertz and G. W. Goodhart (*Quart. J. Med.,* 1908–1909, *2,* 211–18), and in 1911 by William Thomas Ritchie and W. A. Jolly (*Heart,* 1910–11, *2,* 177–221). The clinical features of paroxysmal tachycardia had been well described by John Syer Bristowe in 1888 (*Clinical lectures and essays on diseases of the nervous system.* London, Smith Elder & Co.), and L. Bouveret in 1889 (*Rev. méd., Paris,* 1889, *9,* 753; 837). In Vienna Karel Frederik Wenckebach studied minor degrees of heart block with dropped beats and extra systoles, particularly their treatment with quinine. Max von Frey introduced quinidine for fibrillation and flutter. The character of the auricular disturbances was to some degree elucidated by the electrocardiograph, but the final understanding of them is not yet—the "circus movement" of Lewis has gone; the new work of M. Prinzmetal seems nearer the truth; high speed cinematography may give the answer.

§ INFECTIONS OF THE HEART

There are three important infections of the heart and vessels. In the past these have played a large part; in the future it seems that they will be less a menace. Syphilis of the aorta, affecting the wall, sometimes its valves and the mouths of the coronary arteries, once came first. Now it is rare. Aneurysms were beautifully described by Morgagni, but had also been noted by Vesalius, Ambroise Paré, and Giovanni Maria Lancisi. Before the return of Columbus in 1493 trauma was the usual cause. The final proof of the syphilitic origin awaited the discovery of the *treponema pallidum* by Fritz Richard Schaudinn in 1905 and the introduction of the Wassermann reaction. Good clinical accounts were given by Joseph Hodgson in 1815 (*A treatise on the diseases of the arteries and veins*. London, T. Underwood). The notable and variable physical signs were of interest to the clinicians all through the century. The introduction of X rays gave a great help to early diagnosis; there is no better account than that of Herbert Assmann of Leipzig in 1921 (*Die Roentgendiagnostik der inneren Erkrankungen*. Leipzig, F. C. W. Vogel). Treatment at this stage has never been a success. The disease will vanish when the early infection is destroyed.

Infective endocarditis in various stages was described by Bouillaud, a pupil of Corvisart, in 1835 (*Traités cliniques des maladies du coeur*). He did not clearly distinguish the rheumatic type at first. Before Louis Pasteur it was difficult to make the diagnosis. William Senhouse Kirkes of St. Bartholomew's Hospital gave an excellent account of bacterial endocarditis (*Med.-chir. Trans.*, 1852, *35*, 281–324). He understood clearly the nature of the embolic complications. Joseph Arderne Ormerod, Jean Martin Charcot, and Sir Samuel Wilks all described cases during the next few years, but Sir William Osler's Gulstonian lectures (*Brit. med. J.*, 1885, *i*, 467–70, 522–26, 577–79) gave the best account, written with all the graphic brilliance of which he was already a master. He referred again to the liability of the infection of deformed and damaged valves, first noted by James Paget in 1844. Perhaps a change in the character and incidence of the disease led to the recognition of the subacute form, *endocarditis lenta,* by Osler (*Quart. J. Med.*, 1909, *2*, 219–30) and by Horder. In this report Osler described the nodes which bear his name. Emanuel Libman in the United States described a long series of cases also.

A remarkable increase in the incidence of this disease was noted after World War I, particularly among soldiers or former soldiers whose hearts were not damaged. The diagnosis had been facilitated by the improved technique of blood culture, *streptococcus viridans* usually being found. But no treatment was of any avail; every diagnosis was a death sentence. Pencillin in the last few years has reduced mortality to 40 per cent or less. The impression is that the old malignant form is very rarely seen nowadays, and the subacute form is becoming less common. W. C. Wells of St. Thomas's Hospital gave a good account of the lesions of rheumatic carditis (*Trans. Soc. Improve. med. chir. Knowl.*, 1812, *3*, 373–424) and noted all the symptoms and signs except those that auscultation later revealed. To Bouillaud must be given credit for the first really full account of this disease (1836) (*Nouvelles recherches sur le rhumatisme articulaire.* Paris, J.-B. Baillière). He linked it with articular rheumatism, for he stated that over half of a long number of patients dated their heart disease from an acute rheumatic illness. Germain Sée introduced sodium salicylate in 1877 (*Monit. sci.*, 1877, *3*. sér., 7, 817–45), but the heart was never protected, although the joints responded. We are little better off today. But it would seem that at the present time the incidence of the acute cases, particularly in children, is becoming much less, and perhaps of the subacute, too. The crippling lesions of the mitral and aortic valves may not be so common a generation hence. Thirty years ago an attempt was made by Henry Sessions Souttar (*Brit. med. J.*, 1925, *ii*, 603–606) to relieve the constriction at the mitral valve. Now, thanks to the anesthetist and the antibiotics, the inside of the heart is relatively safe for the surgeon. Splitting of the mitral valve in carefully selected cases is now a commonplace, and the relief in disability can be remarkable; the pressure in the right ventricle and pulmonary artery, which may be thrice the normal, falls, as shown by the cardiac catheter. How much the high pressure in the pulmonary circulation is due to organic obstruction to the blood flow at the mitral valve and how much this resistance and consequent overload of the right ventricle may be aggravated by constriction of the pulmonary arterioles is a new and fascinating problem. But the riddle of rheumatic carditis seems likely to be solved on the general lines of prevention by improving health.

§ ANGINA PECTORIS

In the arterial system the great variation of structure and function of the vessels makes classification difficult. Nowhere do the effects appear more striking than in the vital vessels of the heart. The pain caused by an insufficient supply of blood to the heart muscle was first described by William Heberden in 1768 at the Royal College of Physicians of London. It was published in Latin four years later and translated by his son in 1802 (*Commentaries on the history and cure of diseases*. London, T. Payne). Under the heading *"Pectoris dolor"* Heberden described, among other pains, a very special pain, "a constrictive pain," for which he selected the rare Latin word *angina*. He was a good classical scholar. This superb account should be read by anyone who wishes to know what Heberden really had seen in his hundred cases, for his diagnosis will be greatly improved thereafter. There is little one could add to or subtract from it.

The morbid anatomy of the coronary arteries was soon noted by Allan Burns of Glasgow in his *Observations on some of the most frequent and important diseases of the heart*. (Edinburgh, Bryce & Co., 1809). Burns clearly appreciated that it was ischemia of the heart muscle which caused angina, and likened it to the pain in a limb muscle when exercised under a ligature. Over a century later Thomas Lewis proved this. About the end of the eighteenth century Edward Jenner in Gloucestershire had become interested in this disease, for his friend John Hunter in London was a victim of it. Jenner, however, did not publish much on the matter. Caleb Hillier Parry, another friend at Bath, published a paper in 1799 (*An inquiry into the symptoms and causes of the syncope anginosa commonly called angina pectoris*. London, Cadell and Davis) with some post-mortem studies that he had read eleven years before to the local medical society. The nature of symptoms and of their underlying disease would seem to have been well understood at this time in some quarters.

The treatment for the relief of angina pectoris by a vasodilator is due to Sir Thomas Lauder Brunton, later of St. Bartholomew's Hospital. When he was still a resident medical officer in Edinburgh in 1867 he realized that it lowered blood pressure; he thought a rise in blood pressure caused the pain. Various contributions were made to the knowledge of the subject in the next decade; often the addition of confusing names obscured thought, and—most important—inaccurate pathological studies gave misleading results. Perhaps the most remarkable lapse was that the infarcts, in varying stages, "myomalacia cordis" to fibrosis and aneurysm, were not associated with defects in the coronary circulation. Even the great Rudolf Virchow of Berlin called these lesions fibrous myocarditis, possibly due to syphilis, and this diagnosis stuck for seventy years; so much can the mighty mislead. So it was that the clinical diagnosis of coronary occlusion and its confirmation at autopsy was still not made. Yet Julius Cohnheim seems to have suspected that the fibrous myocarditis followed coronary disease, though he thought the coronaries were end arteries (*Virchows Arch.,* 1881, *85,* 503–37). It is clear that some of Heberden's cases were of this nature. Peter Mere Latham in *Lectures on subjects connected with clinical medicine, comprising disease of the heart* (London, 1845–46) quotes the account of a general practitioner (Dr. Bucknill) of the death of Thomas Arnold of Rugby. A more vivid and dramatic description of myocardial infarction does not exist, but the autopsy was not well done. Peter Henrik Malmsten in Sweden noted the coronary clot and the infarct in 1861. Adam Hammer in Vienna clearly diagnosed a case during life (*Wien. med. Wschr.,* 1878, *28,* 97–102), as did Carl Weigert of Silesia (*Virchows Arch.,* 1880, *79,* 390–92), and Wenser of Massachusetts in the same year. Sir William Tennant Gairdner noted "angor animi," painless cases; Latham, too, had described the sensation of dying; he clearly described rupture of an infarct of the interventricular septum. The pain of angina he thought was of the nature of muscular spasm, like cramp of the skeletal muscles. John Wickham Legg of St. Bartholomew's Hospital in 1884 described many aneurysms of the left ventricle (*Some account of cardiac aneurysms.* London, J. Churchill), but missed the coronary atheroma. He disputed Cohnheim's conclusion and showed coronary anastomoses. Henri Huchard in 1889 thought that spasm of the coronary arteries caused angina. Henri Vaquez in Paris as late as 1921 (*Maladies du coeur.* Paris, J. B. Baillière) thought it to be a neuralgia of the cardiac nerves, which certainly reflected the opinion of Laënnec a century before; even Wenckebach subscribed to this idea (*Wien. med. Wschr.,* 1924, *74,* 621, 736, 907). Mackenzie's monograph on angina (*Angina pectoris.* London, H. Frowde, 1923) contained beautifully described cases (his own is

case No. 28) and good post-mortem observations. He believed, however, that exhaustion underlay the pain, although the arterial lesions
were well understood and their relationship to those of the myocardium; of infarction he had little to say. It is curious that Sir Clifford Allbutt of Cambridge should have so long and eloquently put
forward the misleading idea that disease of the aorta caused the pain
(*Diseases of the arteries, including angina pectoris.* London, Macmillan & Co., 1915).

The very clear diagnosis of coronary thrombosis and later confirmation at autopsy by W. P. Obrastzow and Nikolaus Straschesko
(*Z. klin. Med.*, 1910, *71*, 116–32) attracted no attention. These cases
of prolonged pain had been called *status anginosus*. In 1910 (*Lancet*,
1910, *i*, 697–702, 839–44, 973–77) Osler's Lumleian lectures on angina
pectoris clearly included some of these. This review of the disease
by one who had always been interested in it is well worth reading,
as is anything he wrote. He mentioned that the frictions heard in
one case suggested the pericarditis over an infarct. He showed the
frequency of the disease among doctors—"our disease" he called it
—and the importance of family history. Yet in that day it was rare
to him, and he included some cases we would now exclude. James
Bryan Herrick in 1912 (*J. Amer. med. Ass.*, 1912, *59*, 2015) gave what
is really the first understanding account of the clinical features of
sudden obstruction of the coronary arteries. Perhaps the war in
Europe distracted attention from these discoveries. The next great
step was the association of certain abnormalities in the T wave of
the electrocardiogram with myocardial infarction. First noted by
Herrick in 1919 (*J. Amer. med. Ass.*, 1919, *72*, 387), they were described more fully by Harold E. B. Pardee (*Arch. intern. Med.*, 1920,
26, 244–57; *Amer. J. med. Sci.*, 1925, *169*, 270–83). The application
of the electrocardiogram to the detection of lesions in the myocardium,
devoted as it had been hitherto almost entirely, apart from lesions of
the conducting bundles, to disorders of rhythm, was a tremendous
advance. This came just at the moment when Lewis's magnificent
summary of electrocardiography, *The mechanism and graphic registration of the heart beat* (London, G. Shaw & Sons, 1920), had caught
the attention of the medical scientific world. Clinical and post-mortem
observations now poured out, notably those of John Parkinson and
Davis Evan Bedford in England (*Lancet*, 1928, *i*, 4), and those of

Levine and Robert Levy in the United States of America. An unmistakable clinical picture now became clear, and its recognition cleared up a host of difficulties that had caused confusion for years. The further development of the electrocardiographic technique by means of the unipolar leads of Frank Norman Wilson gives us a means of diagnosis which nowadays leaves few lesions untraced. The treatment was little more than Bucknill gave Thomas Arnold, but the introduction of anticoagulant drugs in the last few years seems to have reduced to some degree the mortality in certain cases. At the present time we are left wondering why the results of disease of the coronary arteries seem to be more common than they were fifty years ago. The solution of the riddle of atheroma and the subsequent thrombosis will one day be the next great advance.

§ HIGH BLOOD PRESSURE

Closely linked up with arterial thickening, both of the muscular middle coats and the atheromatous degeneration, is an abnormal level of the arterial blood pressure. Richard Bright recognized arterial thickening in disease of the kidneys. Frederick Akbar Mahomed also suspected that the pressure was raised. Using a sphygmomanometer invented by Samuel Siegfried Karl von Basch, Pierre Carl Edouard Potain was able in 1881 to demonstrate this increase in pressure. Ludwig Traube had suspected this in 1856 when he had published a treatise on the relationship between renal and cardiac disease (*Über den Zusammenhang von Herz- und Nieren-Krankheiten.* Berlin, A. Hirschwald, 1856). Sir William Withey Gull and Henry Gawen Sutton of Guy's Hospital produced in 1872 a remarkable work on "Arteriocapillary fibrosis" in the vascular system in cases of Bright's disease (*Med.-chir. Trans.*, 1872, 55, 273–326), and Sir George Johnson at King's College Hospital described the thickening of the small arterioles (*Lectures on Bright's disease.* London, Smith, Elder & Co., 1873). In 1877 Sir William Gowers described the thickening of the retinal arterioles seen with the ophthalmoscope in patients whose arterial tension he suspected might be high from feeling the pulse. (*Lancet*, 1877, i, 515). It was not until the portable machine of Scipione Riva-Rocci become available that Gowers' prophecy that other morbid states might be distinguished came to pass. The recognition of Allbutt of primary high blood pressure, which he called "hyperpiesia"—a better name than the hybrid "hypertension"—drew a distinction between that which arose in the course of chronic Bright's disease and the high pressure that might lead to arterial thickening and finally to granular kidney. His observations were summed up in 1915 (*Diseases of the arteries including angina pectoris*. London, Macmillan & Co., 1915). The malignant form became recognized some twenty years ago. The cause of high blood pressure still remains obscure. The experiments of Harry Goldblatt in 1934 (*J. exp. Med.*, 1934, 59, 347–79) seemed to open up a path. Treatment is still unsatisfactory in spite of the numerous drugs that can lower pressure. The familial and corporeal features of the disease are now well recognized, and its psychosomatic aspects are clearer. But the riddle of the cause of a vast amount of illness and many deaths lacks any answer as yet. Clifford Wilson's recent work seems to incriminate the suprarenal bodies.

Although before Harvey demonstrated it, the pulmonary circulation was really suspected by Michael Servetus, and by Ibñ an Nafis three hundred years earlier, little has been known about it from a clinical point of view. That it was congested in heart failure was clear to James Hope, who noted the loudness of the pulmonary second sound of the heart (*A treatise on the diseases of the heart and great vessels*. London, W. Kidd, 1831). Until the cardiac catheter became available the pressure could not be measured. It is now clear that the pulmonary circulation suffers from idiopathic high blood pressure (surmised first in 1939 and 1940). The various histological reactions of the pulmonary arterial bed to raised pressure are now becoming of great interest in chronic lung disease and mitral disease.

§ CONGENITAL HEART DISEASE

Congenital disease of the heart has always been of interest, at least to the morbid anatomist. Giovanni Battista Morgagni, of course, noted some cases. Various examples were recorded from time to time by William Hunter, Allan Burns, Matthew Baillie, and John Richard Farre. James Hope attempted a classification. The first really comprehensive account of those lesions came from Thomas Bevill Peacock (*On malformations of the human heart*. London, John Churchill & Son, 1866) of St. Thomas's Hospital. The tetrad to which the name

of Étienne Louis Arthur Fallot later became attached is clearly defined; single cases had been mentioned by some noted above, and also
by Courvoisier, who pointed out a right-sided aortic arch. Peacock's
illustrations are beautiful and his descriptions very clear. Carl Rokitansky of Vienna, where there is a fine porphyry autopsy table in-
scribed with his name, gave a masterly account of the defects of the
septa and of the complexities of transposition of great vessels. Henri
Roger predicted the lesion that goes by his name, deducing the connection between the hole at autopsy and the mid-precordial murmur
in 1879 (*Bull. Acad. Méd., Paris*, 1879, 2. sér. 8, 1074–94; 1189–91),
to be confirmed sixteen years later. Fallot's work was published in
1888 (*Marseille-méd.*, 1888, 25, 77–93; 138–58; 207–23; 270–86; 341–
54; 403–20). Victor Eisenmenger described his cases of large pulmonary artery and patent interventricular septum in 1897 (*Z. klin.
Med.*, 1897, 32, suppl. 1–28). Sir Arthur Keith described the importance of the absorption of the bulbus cordis in causing an infundibular
type of pulmonary stenosis.

The really great comprehensive treatise of Maude Abbott, based
on one thousand cases, came out in 1936 (*Atlas of congenital cardiac
disease*. New York, American Heart Association, 1936). An earlier
series had appeared in 1908 (In *Modern Medicine* [Osler], 1908, 4,
323–425). Owing to the possibility of surgical treatment interest in
these lesions is now great. By the angiogram the shadows of the cham-
bers and vessels can be outlined, and by the cardiac catheter (André
Cournand and Hilmert A. Ranges) the pressure and the oxygen
content of the blood within them measured (*Proc. Soc. exp. Biol.,
N.Y.*, 1941, 46, 462–66). Diagnosis can now reach a remarkable degree of precision. Pulmonary stenosis can be evaded by short-circuit
implantation of a convenient artery (Blalock-Taussig) (*J. Amer.
med. Ass.*, 1945, 128, 189–202), or relieved by dilatation (Brock)
(*Brit. med. J.*, 1948, i, 1121–26). The aortic valves and the defects of
the cardiac septa are now already under attack. Ligation of the patent
ductus, first done by Robert E. Gross in the United States of America
(*Ann. Surg.*, 1939, 110, 321–56), is now a commonplace. Excision of
the coarctation in the aorta, first done by Clarence Crafoord in Sweden (1945) (*J. thorac. Surg.*, 1945, 14, 347–61), is often performed.
The future history of these treated cases will be interesting reading.

Fluid in the pericardial sac was first detected clinically by Auenbrugger, and the signs of active pericarditis were fully described by Laënnec. In the post-mortem room the diseases of the pericardium had already been described and to some extent linked with certain clinical phenomena. Morgagni noted several types of pericarditis and described the results of pericardial constriction. Raymond Vieussens, and later, Lancisi and Jean Baptiste Senac had all been impressed by their possible importance; until the time of Sir William Broadbent (1898) more was laid to their account than was really true (*Trans. med. Soc., Lond.,* 1898, *21,* 109–22); now only the constrictive adhesions are blamed. They can now be released by the brilliant operation devised by Paul Dudley White and Edward D. Churchill in the United States of America (*Arch. Surg.,* 1929, *19,* 1457–69), and the venous and hepatic congestion, so well described by Norman Chevers of Guy's Hospital in 1842 (*Guy's Hosp. Rep.,* 1842, *7,* 387–439), relieved and certain death avoided.

§ THE FAILING HEART

The idea of failure of the heart and circulation grew very slowly. It is true that James Hope in 1831 gave a very clear account of the effects of various lesions of the heart on the circulation; but before this Jean Nicholas Corvisart understood that accumulation of blood in the lungs causes cardiac dyspnea. Hope put forward the "back pressure" theory of heart failure to explain the signs of congestion. But there had been a forerunner in Raymond Vieussens of Montpellier, who in a case of mitral stenosis seems to have glimpsed the whole picture and integrated the findings at autopsy with the clinical (*Traité nouveau de la structure et des causes du mouvement naturel du coeur.* Toulouse, Jean Guillemette, 1715). This was only one case, but he made a departure from the old idea that once was expressed, that the heart could not be diseased. (The pulse of aortic incompetence astonished him, "the like of which I had never seen before, and do not wish to see again.") Lancisi, who wrote on sudden death at the request of the Pope (*De subitaneis mortibus.* Romae, J. F. Buagni, 1707), also led the way in proving that disease of the heart caused failure. A little later (1749) the treatise of Jean Baptiste Senac was one of the first devoted solely to heart disease and its symptoms (*Traité de la structure du coeur, de son action, et de ses maladies*). The post-mortem observations are good here. The alternative possibility, "forward failure," was noted by Julius Cohnheim and based on experimental work in 1889. Sir James Mackenzie was entirely in support of the "forward" theory (*Diseases of the heart*. 3rd ed. London, Oxford University Press, 1913), but he always stressed the importance of the efficiency of the myocardium and did much to correct the undue emphasis on auscultatory findings (which had grown during the century) when no general textbook put forward the idea of failing muscle. Lewis, too, was a supporter of the "forward failure" theory. In France the idea of separate failure of either ventricle was an important conception that has gained general support in the last twenty-five years.

The vast amount of information gained by accurate studies of the output of the heart with the help of the cardiac catheter, by the estimation of the circulatory rate, of the blood volume, and of the venous pressure, and of the earlier studies of Fraser on the oxygen content of the blood, are not yet co-ordinated. One thing seems certain: the law of the heart laid down by Ernest Henry Starling (*The Linacre lecture on the law of the heart, given at Cambridge in 1915*. London, Longman, Green & Co., 1918) is a sound physiological basis on which the final understanding will be established. Except for management on general lines, failure of the heart once had little to expect. William Withering, whose great botanical knowledge enabled him to pick on digitalis as the important ingredient in the mixture of simple herbs of a countrywoman's remedy for dropsy, in a remarkable work, perfect in form, statement, and clarity, brought in the first really effective drug (*An account of the fox-glove* .... Birmingham, G. G. & J. Robinson, 1785). Squill had already been in use for ages and had won the approval of Samuel Johnson. Nothing can really be added to Withering's superb monograph, yet the proper use of digitalis was lost until Mackenzie revived it. The discovery of digoxin was an important addition for intravenous use, for which strophanthus, popular on the continent of Europe, was never very satisfactory. In recent years the introduction of an efficient diuretic, an organic preparation of mercury (Saxe and Heilig, 1920), first with a view to treating syphilis, was an enormous benefit. Venesection, once the vogue for everything, still retains a place of life-saving value in suitable cases when the venous pressure, which Sir Thomas Lewis has shown can be so easily estimated, is too high. Oxygen can now be given really effectively and may provide great help. Morphine has long been a stand-by; as a cardiac sedative, quinine was recommended by Senac; and its isomer, quinidine, came to the fore in 1918 (von Frey). Recently the part played by the retention of sodium has led to an important line of treatment for persistent edema whereby the substance is strictly reduced and fluids are freely taken—ion-exchange resins helping to limit the absorption of sodium.

It will be seen from this survey that knowledge has progressed by fits and starts. First came clinical observation and then post-mortem confirmation. Then the introduction of technique: percussion and auscultation. Then years of painstaking description and correlation. Then the extension of the senses by the X rays and the graphic methods, and the further application of the understanding of the electrical phenomena of the heart. Later, methods for recording pressure anywhere in the vascular system and for sampling the blood, and for accurately gauging the work of the heart. All these give possibilities for a remarkable degree of accuracy in diagnosis. The more elaborate methods have often confirmed the clinical diagnosis given, and what was uncertain became sure, and the complicated way could be dropped. Although any real control of the causes of heart disease is still very weak, the possibilities of treatment of its effects based on accurate and early diagnosis are now strong. The quotation from Vergil—*"Haeret lateri lethalis harundo"*—that Corvisart put in his book, and which Walshe already thought less opportune in 1862, is to us, nearly one hundred years later, of still less sinister import.

BY RALPH H. MAJOR

M. D.*

chapter 8 / BRIght's disease

THE EARLY HISTORY of nephritis is shrouded in the same obscurity that surrounds the early history of most diseases. The ancient Egyptians, whom Herodotus praised as the greatest physicians of antiquity, have left no accounts of nephritis that have come down to us. Indeed, we are not sure that they had a word for kidney. James H. Breasted suggests that the word *phd.w* in the Ebers Papyrus means "kidneys," although B. Ebbell gives it the meaning of "buttocks." Sir Alan Gardiner's dictionary does not include an Egyptian equivalent for kidney. In spite of this silence, however, we can scarcely doubt that the Egyptians, who prepared countless bodies for embalming so well that their mummies have lasted several millenia, saw and recognized such obvious organs as the kidneys. It should also be noted that a passage in the Ebers Papyrus, composed *circa* 1500 B.C., the translation of which has not been questioned, states: "There are two vessels to the bladder; it is they which give urine."

Hippocrates, whom every generation of physicians has honored for two thousand years, while extolled as a great master of clinical observation, is admitted by his most doughty champions to have been a bit weak on anatomy. In the Hippocratic fragment Περι Ανατομης he notes: "The kidneys have the same shape, the color of them resembles that of apples: from each kidney comes an oblique duct which goes to the top of the bladder."

Hippocrates, however, studied the urine with great care. A firm believer in the humoral theory of disease, that recovery from disease was produced by coction or pepsis—a kind of cooking whereby the excess humor was discarded and excreted as a waste product—it was

* Professor of medical history, University of Kansas.

but natural that he should study the urine in which this waste product was excreted. Hippocrates (in E. Littré's translation) refers to the characteristics of the urine in disease 188 times. He describes the urine in various diseases as thin, watery, black, purulent, pale, fatty, and bloody, and mentions suppression of urine with convulsions. The thirty-fourth aphorism of Hippocrates states: "When bubbles settle on the surface of the urine, they indicate disease of the kidneys and that the complaint will be protracted." Francis Adams, the learned translator of Hippocrates, comments on this passage thus: "It can scarcely admit of a doubt, that our author here refers to *albuminous* urine, which it is well known is also *frothy,* and is now generally admitted to be connected with disease of the kidneys."

All the disciples and followers of Hippocrates refer to the urine, but their observations add little to those of Hippocrates. The great encyclopedist, Aurelius Cornelius Celsus, in his *De medicina,* which was written at the beginning of the Christian era, reviews in great detail the opinions of the Greek physicians on disease from the time of Hippocrates to his own era. While he adds nothing original to their descriptions, he does note that the Greeks described a disease they called *hydrops* (ὕδρωψ), and distinguished three varieties: *tympanites* (τυμπανίτης), *hyposarka* (ὑπὸσάρκα), and *ascites* (ἀσκίτης). He discussed diuretics at length and makes the sage observation: "Nor is it a bad plan to measure his drink and urine; for, when the quantity of execreted fluid exceeds that which is ingested, then, at last, there is some hope of recovery."

While Gulielmus de Saliceto (1476) has been credited with being the first medical writer to have definitely associated dropsy with contracted kidneys, Rhouphos (or Rufus) of Ephesus, who lived about A.D. 100, describes sclerosis of the kidneys with dropsy. This account appears in a fragment preserved by Oribasius, and is entitled περὶ σκληρίας νεφρῶν ("Concerning sclerosis of the kidneys, nephrosclerosis"). It is as follows:

Sclerosis which develops in the kidneys causes no pain, but it seems to the patients as if a weight were hanging from their body in the region of the flanks; they note a numbness about the hips, weakness of the legs, scanty urination, the condition of the body resembling most closely a dropsy. In this condition one should soften the kidneys with cataplasms

158

and massage, administer substances which increase the urine and soften the abdomen with enemata.

Aëtios of Amida, the earliest Greek physician of note who was thought to have been a Christian, lived from A.D. 502–575 and practiced in Constantinople. The Latin edition (1534) of his *Six books on medicine* contains the following description in Chapter XVII, *De duricie renum:*

> When sclerosis arises about the kidneys, it does not cause pain but it seems to the patient as if something hung from around the stomach, numbness attacks the hips, there is weakness of the legs and they urinate little, the rest of the body appears much like in those suffering from water in the skin. Further, in time they develop obvious hydrops as if spreading from the other hardened viscera.

The preceding chapter, *De renum inflammatione,* carries the notation that it is copied from Rhouphos. It seems safe, therefore, to assume that Aëtios knew the writings of Rhouphos.

Paul of Aegina, who lived from A.D. 625–690 and practiced in Alexandria, wrote on *Hardness of the kidneys.* He says:

> When hardness occurs in the kidneys, it does not occasion pains, but they seem, as it were, to hang from the loins, and the haunches are torpid, and the limbs lose their strength, little urine is passed, and the whole habit resembles that of dropsical persons.

Here again, paraphrasing a well-known passage in the Old Testament, the hands were the hands of Paul, but the voice was the voice of Rhouphos.

Arabian physicians greatly admired both Paul and Rhouphos. The surgical works of Paul formed the basis for the seventh book of Rhazes' *Liber ad Almansorem* and for the well-known surgical treatise of Albucasis. Rhouphos was called by Ibn abī Uṣaibi'a, the historian of Arabian medicine, in his *Lives of the physicians,* "the great Rhouphos" and "the first physician of his time," and he is quoted many times in the works of Serapion, Mesuë, Rhazes, and Ibn Baitar. Rhazes (A.D. 850–923) in his *Liber ad Almansorem* writes:

When an apostem in the kidney does not produce pus, it on the contrary becomes sclerotic (*transit in duritiem*) and progresses with heaviness in the kidneys without fever . . . and, if the urine is seen to be diminished, stimulants are given, not in small amounts because this condition leads to dropsy.

Avicenna (A.D. 980–1037), the "Prince of Physicians," states that in hardening of the kidneys there is "great heaviness but no pain . . . numbness of both legs, numbness of the hips . . . the lower extremities become thin, the urine is small in quantity . . . swellings like that in cachexia . . . and very often dropsy."

These brief extracts have been quoted in order to show that by the year A.D. 1000 at least five physicians, Rhouphos, Aëtios, Paul of Aegina, Rhazes, and Avicenna, were familiar with sclerosis of the kidneys and described as its characteristic signs weakness, absence of pain, scanty urination, and dropsy. It also seems evident that all these descriptions stem from the original account of Rhouphos. The descriptions of Aëtios, Paul, Rhazes, and Avicenna not only stress the same symptoms, but they employ almost identical language.

Gulielmus de Saliceto, who was professor at Bologna from 1269 to 1274, wrote his well-known description of *durities in renibus,* first published in his *Liber . . . in scientia medicinali* (1476): "The signs of hardness in the kidneys are that the quantity of urine is diminished, there is heaviness in the kidneys and of the spine with some pain: and the belly begins to swell up after a time and dropsy is produced." Though his description was written more than a thousand years after that of Rhouphos, once more the old similarity is apparent.

The Middle Ages added little to our knowledge of kidney disease. The Arabians, undisputed leaders of science during this period, studied the urine, but did not go beyond their Greek masters. The latter part of the Middle Ages witnessed the phenomenal rise of the uroscopists, who claimed to be able to make diagnoses solely by examination of the urine. This pseudo science seized the medical profession and the laity as astrology had once seized them. The physician was identified in art and in the popular imagination by his urine glass, just as the bishop was by his crozier and the pope by triple tiara. One interesting illustration of this period portrays Jesus as the Great Physician, holding up a urine glass.

The uroscopists of this period, however, failed to advance our knowledge of nephritis. They attempted too much diagnosis with too little knowledge. The famous poem of Gilles de Corbeil (Aegidius Corboliensis), who died about 1220, on the urine, *Carmina de urinarum judiciis,* for long remained the authoritative treatise on the subject. The first part describes the colors of the urine: black, gray, white, pale blue, pale, milky, lemon, red, green, and various combinations. The second part deals with the things contained within the urine: the circles it makes, the bubbles, grains, clouds, foam, pus, fat, chyme, blood, sand, hair, and scurf. This poem had a great vogue and summarized the existing knowledge of uroscopy. Its author recognizes that pus in the urine indicates ulceration of the kidneys or of the bladder; that blood indicates disease of the kidneys and of the bladder; and that sand indicates a kidney or a bladder stone. Nevertheless, the poem does not aid us in the diagnosis of chronic nephritis.

Nicolaus Cusanus (1401–64), as Henry Viets has pointed out, in his *De staticis experimentis* offered some interesting suggestions "in regard to the value of comparing the weights of equal volumes of the blood or urine of a healthy man and of a weak one." This suggestion, however, along with many others, as Viets notes, "fell on deaf ears." Jan Baptista van Helmont (1577–1644), the founder of the iatrochemical school, appears to have been the first to carry out this procedure. In his *Oriatrike* (1662) he describes the experiments in which he compared the weights of equal quantities of water and of urine from patients—the first recorded gravimetric examinations of the urine. He also examined the bodies of patients who had died of dropsy and, finding the liver normal in appearance, attacked the ancient doctrine that dropsy was caused by disease of the liver. He found the kidneys diseased in some patients and described one patient whose kidney was "scarce of the bigness of a Filburd-nut [filbert]." Dropsy, he writes in his characteristic mystical jargon, is caused by a fury, or indignation, of the Archeus of the kidneys since "the Kidney hath received the dominion of the water."

The systematic and scientific study of the urine, according to Camille Vieillard, began with the observations of Lorenzo Bellini (1643–1704) and of Hermann Boerhaave (1668–1738). Abandoning the ancient concept of the uroscopists who studied only the appearance of the urine, Bellini and Boerhaave stressed the importance of investigating the composition of the urine, the former emphasizing its physical examination, the latter its chemical. Boerhaave, harking back to van Helmont, introduced the routine determination of the weight of urine as compared with water—the estimation of the specific gravity.

Meanwhile, Frederik Dekkers (1648–1720), who was a colleague of Boerhaave's, demonstrated for the first time the presence of albumin in the urine, first boiling the urine and then adding "a drop or so of acetic acid." His observation (1694) was made on a patient with phthisis. Domenico Cotugno in 1764 showed that the urine of a dropsical patient when partially evaporated showed "a white mass already loosely coagulated like egg albumen." In 1811 William Charles Wells read a paper before the Society for the Improvement of Medical and Chirurgical Knowledge in which he described tests on the urine of 130 dropsical patients, in 78 of whom he found albumin. He also described the kidneys in two dropsical patients: in one the "kidneys were much harder than they usually are and their cortical part was thickened and changed in its structure"; in the other, the "kidneys were larger and softer than if in a healthy state, and on the outside of both were several vesicles, partly imbedded in their cortical substance." In 1818 John Blackall in his book, *Observations on the nature and cure of dropsies,* describes the urine in dropsy as being coagulable by heat, and notes that in two cases "the kidneys were firmer than ordinary, in one of them very strikingly so, approaching to scirrhus."

To recapitulate—by 1818 it was known that in many cases of dropsy the urine was scanty and contained albumin, and that certain of these patients had small hardened kidneys. However, no one as yet had stressed the association of albuminous urine, sclerosis of the kidneys, and dropsy, grouped them together as a clinical entity, or pointed out the frequency of this syndrome. This was the great achievement of Richard Bright (1789–1858).

§ RICHARD BRIGHT

Richard Bright was born in Bristol in 1789, the third son of an influential banker and prominent citizen who resided at Ham Green House (now one of the city's isolation hospitals). He was educated at Dr. Estlin's School in Bristol and subsequently at Edinburgh University and at Guy's Hospital, London. He took the degree of M.D. at Edinburgh in 1813 and in 1820 was appointed assistant physician at Guy's, becoming in due course physician. He was twice married; the eldest son of the second marriage was the famous historian who became Master of University College, Oxford. Illness caused Richard Bright to retire from the active staff of Guy's in 1843 at the early age of fifty-four. His remaining years were devoted to consulting practice, to travel, and to his many artistic interests. In spite of ill health, his practice, which had been slow in coming, grew to be perhaps the largest in London. The announcement of the discovery of "Bright's Disease" was made in 1827, when the first volume was published of his *Reports of medical cases selected with a view of illustrating the symptoms and cure of diseases by a reference to morbid anatomy*. The completeness of Bright's account of those forms of renal disease associated with his name will be realized from the fact that he described the uremic symptoms, cerebral hemorrhage, loss of sight, hard pulse, edema, pleural, pericardial, and peritoneal effusions, bronchitis, cardiac hypertrophy, and the enteritis which may attend the disease. But even if he had not discovered the disease which bears his name, he would still have been one of the greatest of English physicians. His powers of observation were marvelous; none of his observations have been shown to be incorrect. According to Sir Samuel Wilks, he could not theorize but he could *see,* and he could also write well. Sir William Hale-White said in the account of his life, which he contributed to the *Guy's Hospital Reports* in 1921: "Many modern textbooks would be vastly improved if some of their pages were deleted to make room for Bright's descriptions." Bright was an artist, too; no medical work has more beautiful pictures than are to be found in his *Reports of medical cases.*

In the words of William Sydney Thayer's address delivered at Guy's Hospital on July 8, 1927: "Happy in his birth and the surroundings and conditions of his early life, cultivated by travel and society, an artist, a linguist, a man of scholarly tastes, Bright made full use of his opportunities." He died after a short illness on December 14, 1858.

Bright's *Reports of medical cases* state in the introduction that he first observed "the altered structure of the kidney in a patient who had died dropsical" nearly twelve years before. His *Reports* consist of twenty-three cases with clinical histories and autopsy records, together with some beautiful illustrations of the pathological lesions. He describes three forms of the disease. In the first "a state of degeneracy seems to exist, which from its appearance might be regarded as marking little more than simple debility of the organ. In this case the kidney loses its usual firmness, becomes of a yellow mottled appearance externally." The second form "is one in which the whole cortical part is converted into a granular texture, and where there appears to be a copious morbid interstitial deposit of an opake white substance." The third form is "where the kidney is quite rough and scabrous to the touch externally . . . the feel is hard, and on making an incision, the texture is found approaching to semi-cartilaginous firmness, giving great resistance to the knife." Bright adds: "Although I hazard a conjecture as to the existence of these three different forms of disease, I am by no means confident of the correctness of this view." He thinks it possible that the second and third forms may be "more or less advanced states of one and the same disease."

According to Hale-White, Bright in 1842 studied the microscopical appearances of diseased kidneys, but so far as we know, these results were never published. The first careful microscopical studies of the kidney were those of Jacob Henle in 1841 and 1847, who, impressed by the increase in connective tissue, writes: "This alteration may be called cirrhosis of the kidneys, in so far as this term means not the original idea of color, but a decrease in the size of the organs caused by a new growth of contractile fibers."

In his paper in the first volume of *Guy's Hospital Reports* (1836), entitled "Tabular view of the morbid appearances occurring in one hundred cases in connexion with albuminous urine," Bright notes the great frequency of cardiac hypertrophy in these patients and observes: "The hypertrophy of the heart seems, in some degree, to have kept pace with the advance of disease in the kidneys." He further notes that as the disease progresses the amount of urea in the urine diminishes, while the amount in the blood increases.

The masterly description of the new syndrome by Bright made a deep impression on his contemporaries, and the term *Morbus Brightii* soon appeared in the British and French medical literature and somewhat later in the German. The kidneys of these patients were carefully examined, both grossly and microscopically, and the urine was studied chemically and microscopically. Urinary casts were described by Franz Simon and by Christian Friedrich Nasse in 1843, and in 1844 by Henle in sections of kidney tissue. In 1858 Siegmund Rosenstein found casts in normal urine—an observation which has been repeatedly confirmed in recent years.

Bright and his co-workers, particularly John Bostock, also found that the urine of normal persons at times contained albumin. Their usual method of examination was "the application of heat, by taking a small quantity of the urine in a spoon and holding it over the flame of a lamp or candle. In healthy urine, no change follows from this exposure to heat." However, when they tested normal urine with bichloride of mercury or with ferroprussiate of potash, a trace of albumin was frequently present.

Bright and his associates had no method available of estimating the blood pressure, but in their clinical notes the pulse of the patient is often described as being full and hard. In discussing the causes of cardiac hypertrophy, Bright speaks of an "altered quality of the blood . . . that so affects the minute and capillary circulation, as to render greater action necessary to force the blood through the distant subdivisions of the vascular system." This thought was carried further by George Johnson, who advanced the theory that impurities which should have been eliminated by the kidneys are retained and cause constriction of the arterioles, a rise in blood pressure, and cardiac hypertrophy. This view was attacked by William Withey Gull and Henry Gawen Sutton, who maintained that the increased blood pressure was due, not to arteriolar contraction, but to arteriocapillary fibrosis, or a hyaline fibroid change in the capillaries and arterioles.

Karl Vierordt, who made the first instrument for estimating the blood pressure in man, in 1855 reported several cases of Bright's disease which showed high blood pressure. Samuel Siegfried von Basch, who constructed the first practical sphygmomanometer in 1881, made similar observations, but the estimation of the blood pressure became a routine procedure in Bright's disease only after the introduction of Scipione Riva-Rocci's well-known instrument in 1896. Sir William Henry Broadbent, in his classic book, *The pulse* (1890), devotes a chapter to kidney disease and stresses the importance of high blood pressure. He makes no mention, however, of instrumental determination of blood pressure, although he shows sphygmographic tracings of high tension pulses. He used his fingers to diagnose increased arterial tension.

William Senhouse Kirkes in 1855 connected cerebral hemorrhage with renal disease. By this time clinical instruments of precision were being invented so that Friedrich Moritz Heymann of Dresden in 1856, employing the ophthalmoscope, first observed the occurrence of albuminuric retinitis, and Clifford Allbutt made the ophthalmoscope an indispensable instrument for physicians. Hermann Senator, by means of von Basch's sphygomomanometer, recorded the systolic arterial blood pressure and found it raised in kidney disease.

Bright's teaching was bitterly opposed, especially in London, where, it will be recalled, Lister's discoveries were even less readily accepted. It was very largely due to Pierre-François-Olive Rayer that Bright's views generally gained ground. Rayer's classic work, *Traité des maladies des reins. . . .* (Paris, 1839–41), was the first systematic treatise on the diseases of the kidneys, and it confirmed Bright's observations. In England this book was followed by George Johnson's *On the diseases of the kidneys. . . .* (London, 1852). Julius Vogel made known the new work to German readers in his article, "Krankheiten der harnbereitenden Organe," contributed to Volume VI of Virchow's *Handbuch der speciellen Pathologie.* (Erlangen, 1856–65). Ludwig Traube separated several individual diseases which had previously been included under the term "Bright's disease," distinguishing renal congestion, contracted kidney, and amyloid disease. Christian August Bartels showed interstitial nephritis to be distinct from chronic parenchymatous, which was a tubular or glomerulotubular form.

Albumosuria associated with myeloma was described by Henry Bence Jones in 1848, and true albumosuria by Hermann Senator in 1882.

Since Bright's original classification of albuminuria many reclassifications have been suggested, one of the most important being the recognition of physiological or orthostatic albuminuria in contrast to pathological. The modern classification we owe chiefly to Franz Volhard and Theodor Fahr in 1914:

1. Glomerulonephritis, the clinical counterpart of a kidney showing inflammatory glomerular destruction.

2. Nephrosclerosis associated with thickening of the small renal arteries.

3. Nephrosis, which is a degenerative process affecting most markedly the tubules.

Hemoglobinuria was first distinguished from hematuria by H. O. Dressler in 1854.

In recent years much attention has been paid to the pathological physiology as contrasted with the pathological anatomy of the kidney in disease. Leonard G. Rowntree and John T. Geraghty in 1910 introduced the phenolsulphonephthalein tests for renal function, which has stood the test of forty years. Thomas Addis, in a series of observations extending over several years, has pointed out the importance of the qualitative and quantitative examination of the urinary sediment.

As we look back over the history of nephritis, the figure of Richard Bright towers in the field like that of Vesalius in the history of anatomy. Thomas Addis remarks: "It is often said, and with some justification, that we have made no real advance in this field since the time of Richard Bright." While this may be an overstatement, it emphasizes the pre-eminence of that great old physician of Guy's Hospital.

§ REFERENCES

Addis, T. (1948): *Glomerular nephritis: diagnosis and treatment.* New York, Macmillan.

Avicenna (1562): *Liber canonis.* Venice, Giunta. P. 359.

Blackall, J. (1818): *Observations on the nature and cure of dropsies.* 3rd ed. London, Longman.

Breasted, J. H. (1930): *The Edwin Smith surgical papyrus.* Chicago, University of Chicago Press. P. 111.

Bright, R. (1827): *Reports of medical cases selected with a view of illustrating the symptoms and cure of diseases by a reference to morbid anatomy.* 2 vols. London, Longman.

Broadbent, W. H. (1890): *The pulse.* London, Cassell & Co.

Celsus, A. (1831): *De medicina.* Translated by G. F. Collier. London, Simpkin and Marshall. P. 108.

Cotugno, D. (1775): *De ischiade nervosa commentarius.* Naples and Bologna, St. Thomas Aquina. P. 27.

Dekkers, F. (1695): *Exercitationes practicae circa medendi methodum.* Leyden, Bontesteyn. P. 338.

Dressler, H. O. (1854): *"Ein Fall von intermittirender Albuminurie und Chromaturie."* Virchows Arch., 6, 264.

Ebbell, B. (1937): *The papyrus Ebers.* Copenhagen, Levin and Munksgaard; London, Oxford University Press. P. 116.

Falck, C. P. (1848): *"Die Geschichte der Brigt'schen Krankheit vom Jahre 1827 bis zum Jahre 1847."* Janus, 3, 133-53, 456-94.

Galen (1916): *On the natural faculties.* Translated by A. J. Brock. New York, G. P. Putnam. P. 51.

Gardiner, Sir A. H. (1950): *Egyptian grammar: being an introduction to the study of hieroglyphs.* London, Oxford University Press.

Helmont, J. B. van (1662): *Oriatrike or physick refined.* London, Lodowick Loyd. Pp. 507, 1056.

Hippocrates (1839-61): *Oeuvres complètes. Traduction nouvelle avec le texte grec en regard, . . . Par É Littré.* 10 vols. Paris, J. B. Baillière.

Johnson, G. (1852): *On the diseases of the kidney.* London, Parker.

Jones, H. Bence (1848): "On a new substance occurring in the urine of a patient with millities ossium." *Phil. Trans., 138,* 55-62.

Major, R. H. (1930): "The history of taking the blood pressure." *Ann. med. Hist., N. S. 2,* 47.

Major, R. H. (1949): "Notes on the history of nephritis." *Bull. Hist. Med., 23,* 453-60.

Nixon, J. A. (1934): "Bright's Disease." In *A short history of some common diseases.* Edited by W. R. Bett. London, Oxford University Press. P. 101-107.

Paul of Aegina (1844): *The seven books of.* Translated from the Greek by Francis Adams. London, Sydenham Society. Vol. I., p. 546.

Rayer, P. (1839-41): *Traité des maladies des reins et des altérations de la sécrétion urinaire. . . .* 3 vols. Paris, J. B. Baillière.

Rhazes (1480): *Liber nonus ad Almansorem cum expositione Joannis Arculani.* Padua, Petrus Maufer.

Rosenstein, S. (1858): *"Beitrag zur Aetiologie der parenchymatösen Nephritis."* Virchows Arch., 14, 110.

Rosenstein, S. (1894): *Die Pathologie und Therapie der Nierenkrankheiten.* Berlin, Hirschwald.

Rowntree, L. G., and J. T. Geraghty (1910): "An experimental and clinical study of the functional activity of the kidneys by means of phenolsulphonephthalein." *J. Pharmacol, 1,* 579-661.

Rufus of Ephesus (1873): In *Oeuvres d'Oribase. Traduit par U. C. Bussemaker et C. Daremberg.* Paris, L'Imprimerie Nationale. Vol. V, p. 514.

Senator, H. (1902): *Die Erkrankungen der Nieren.* Vienna, Hölder.

Simon, F. (1843): *"Über eigenthümliche Formen im Harnsediment bei Morbus Brightii."* Arch. Anat. Physiol., Lpz., 28.

Vieillard, C. (1903): *L'urologie et les médecins urologues.* Paris, F.-R. de Rudeval.

Vierordt, K. (1855): *Die Lehre vom Arterienpuls in gesunden und kranken Zustanden.* Braunschweig.

Wells, W. C. (1812): "On the presence of red matter and serum of blood in the urine of dropsy which has not originated from scarlet fever." *Trans. Soc. Improve. med. and chir. Knowledge, 3,* 194.

BY R. SCOTT STEVENSON
M. D., F. R. C. S. Ed.*

chapter 9 / tonsils and adenoids

THE RISE in the incidence of the operation for the removal of tonsils
and adenoids is one of the major phenomena of modern surgery, for
it has been estimated that some two hundred thousand of these operations are performed annually in Great Britain and that they form
one-third of the number of operations performed under general
anesthesia in the United States of America. Tonsillotomy, or cutting
off part of the tonsil, is one of the most ancient of surgical procedures,
though tonsillectomy, or removal of the whole tonsil, is a concept of
quite recent surgery. As for adenoids, they were discovered for the
first time in 1868.

Hippocrates, the "Father of Medicine," who flourished about 400
B.C., does not mention tonsillotomy, but describes tonsillitis accurately
and vividly and advises that a swollen tonsil should be opened up.
He writes:

> When the tonsils become diseased, there forms on the jaw on both sides
> a swelling; it is hard to the touch, the uvula is inflamed. When this hap-
> pens, introduce the finger and push aside the tonsils; rub the uvula with
> dry flowers of copper; give warm gargles, externally apply warm plaster
> of barley-flour cooked in wine and oil. When the swellings appear soft
> touched from inside, open them with a bistoury. Some heal spontaneously.

According to T. A. Wise, the historian of Indian medicine, the
treatment of enlarged tonsils was considered and the operation of
tonsillotomy practiced by early Hindu surgeons round about 1000
B.C., long before the time of Hippocrates. "The tonsils are to be
seized," he quotes, "between the blades of a forceps and drawn for-

* Surgeon to the Metropolitan Ear, Nose and Throat Hospital, London.

ward, and with a semicircular knife one-third of the swelled part is to be removed. If all be removed, so much blood may be discharged as will destroy the individual. If too little is removed, it will produce an increase in the swelling with fainting."

§ FIRST DESCRIPTION OF TONSILLOTOMY

The earliest description of tonsillotomy (or it may even have been tonsillectomy) is given by Celsus, a Roman nobleman who did not practice medicine but wrote an extensive medical encyclopedia in eight books, *De medicina*. Although this was written in the first century A.D., it was apparently overlooked and virtually lost until 1478, when it was found in the Vatican library and was one of the first medical works to be printed. Celsus describes the operation as follows:

Tonsils that are indurated should be disengaged all round by the finger and pulled out. If they are not separated by this method, it is necessary to take hold of them with a small hook and cut them out with a knife: then to wash the ulcer with vinegar and rub the wound with a styptic medicine.

Galen, the Greek dictator of medicine for a thousand years, was born at Pergamos in Asia Minor in A.D. 131, became surgeon to the gladiators of his native city, and was drawn by ambition to Rome, where he attended the Emperor Marcus Aurelius. He was a good anatomist, and classified inflammation of the throat as five varieties. He advised the use of a snare in amputating enlarged tonsils—the first mention of this method: *"Adenas excedentes naturam in tonsillis adversis plagis amputamus,"* which sounds as if it were quite a common practice in those days.

§ EARLY ACCOUNTS OF TONSILLOTOMY

Oribasius (born A.D. 326), one of the so-called Byzantine compilers who kept medical learning alive in the Dark Ages, describes tonsillotomy in the medical section of his vast general encyclopedia: the tonsil was to be pulled forwards by a hook and the projecting part cut off with a knife, but the incision had to include only the prominent portion, as there was danger of hemorrhage if the gland were incised too deeply.

Paul of Aegina, another Byzantine writer, born in A.D. 607, in the seventh book of his great work on medicine has a chapter on the surgery of tonsils. He writes:

Place the patient in the sunlight and let him open his mouth while an assistant holds his head with one hand and presses down the tongue by means of a spatula with the other; take a hook, stick it into the tonsil gland and drag it as far as possible upwards, without dragging out the membranes as well; then cut it completely away by means of a curved knife. There are two such instruments with opposite curves. Then remove the other tonsil in the same way. After operation the patient gargles with cold water . . . if there is severe bleeding he gargles with other decoctions, such as the juice of plantain or comfrey.

For centuries the methods employed for incision of the tonsil showed little or no change. Jan Yperman, the "Father of Dutch Surgery," wrote in 1350:

Direct your attention to tonsils, for they are the true seat of the disease. For that purpose you will have with you, if you are practiced in the art, a hook made of copper or iron. Pull the tonsil forward with this and incise with a "vhem" or some other knife made for this purpose. Then make the patient gargle.

The great French surgeon Ambroise Paré (1510–90) described inflammations of the tonsils and incised a quinsy with a knife, but did not describe tonsillotomy. Most surgeons of the time feared to excise tonsils because of hemorrhage and contented themselves by removing portions with cautery or ligature.

Peter Lowe of Glasgow, who flourished around 1600, in his *A discourse on the whole art of chirurgerie* writes that some remove swollen tonsils by means of the snare, others use a cautery, and others again "pull them away with crossets and other instruments either all whole or by pieces." Richard Wiseman, surgeon to King Charles II, writes in his *Severall chirurgicall treatises* (5th ed., 1719): This way of excision is by making a ligature about the basis of them and snipping them close off with a pair of crooked probe-scissors." He also

172

frequently used escharotics and the actual cautery when he had reason to fear hemorrhage or when the tonsils was very adherent.

The French surgeon Pierre Joseph Desault, born 1744, seems to have been the first to use a special instrument for the removal of the tonsils. It was a modification of an instrument known as the cysto-tome or "kiotome," which was used for dividing cysts of the bladder. It consisted of a metallic sheath cut into the shape of a half-moon at one end and with two rings at the proximal extremity by which it could be held. A knife blade was arranged so as to pass through the sheath across the half-moon notch after the latter had been adjusted to the tonsil, which was drawn into it by means of a hook. But Desault's instrument was not generally adopted and eventually lapsed into desuetude. Desault was also accustomed to make use of a ligature around the tonsil, which he tightened daily for a day or two until the tonsil fell off.

Samuel Sharp of Guy's Hospital, in his book *A critical enquiry into the present state of surgery* (1750) writes: "The extirpation of Scirrhous Tonsils by Ligature seems to be a practice as yet almost entirely confined to England, though for no other reason as I imagine, but because it generally requires some time for the propagation of an improvement."

The eighteenth-century surgeons, as well as the modern, had a wholesome respect for the dangers of hemorrhage in operations on the tonsils. Lorenz Heister in Germany in 1743 differentiated the following methods of operating: (1) application of corrosives; (2) abscission according to the methods of the ancients; (3) ligation, using the apparatus of Hildanus for the uvula. A method attributed to William Cheselden was to pierce the tonsil with a double-threaded needle and tie off each half of the tonsil in a ligature. Benjamin Bell in 1784 employed his double cannula snare, previously used for nasal polypi, for ligation of the tonsils.

§ THE FIRST TONSIL GUILLOTINE

The first tonsil guillotine or tonsillotome was designed by Philip Syng Physick of Philadelphia (a graduate of Edinburgh) in 1828, modified from the uvulatome in use at the end of the eighteenth century. Physick's tonsillotome had two plates with a knife sliding between them; a strip of waxed linen was passed round the posterior semi-circumference of the aperture, so as to obviate not cutting clean through the tissues, the waxed linen supporting and holding them. By increasing the size of the aperture in the guillotine he found that he could adapt it to the removal of the tonsils. Physick wrote of the operation that it is "easy to cut off the whole or any portion that may be necessary of the enlarged tonsil in this manner. The operation can be finished in a moment of time. The pain is very little, and the haemorrhage so moderate that it has not required any attention in four cases in which the doctor has lately performed it." Physick's method was eagerly taken up by many of his American colleagues, several of whom devised modifications of his instrument. William B. Fahnestock of Lancaster, Pennsylvania, introduced a guillotine with a prong or fork to catch the tonsil, which, somewhat modified, became known in France as "Mathieu's guillotine" and maintained its popularity up to the first years of the present century. But Morell Mackenzie of London in the sixties should be regarded as the true founder of the modern tonsil guillotine operation. His guillotine was a modification of that devised by Physick, but with many improvements, and in his skillful hands the technique of the operation was greatly improved. He did much to popularize the operation by the excellent results achieved by his methods; indeed, until the early years of the twentieth century the guillotine remained the favorite instrument for the removal of the tonsils throughout the world.

James Yearsley of London, however, in the eighteen thirties was still skillfully dissecting out tonsils with a curved bistoury after seizing them with a tenaculum; in the third edition of his book *On throat ailments* (1850), he mentions that he had operated thus upon 1,400 patients. But the pioneer of the modern operation of complete tonsil dissection was George E. Waugh of Great Ormond Street Hospital, London, who published in 1909 his method of simple, methodical dissection, using dissecting forceps and snare, and tying off bleeding points. Waugh had observed that the results of the tonsil operations of his day were poor, particularly in relation to the incidence of tuberculous glands in the neck, and he taught that in order to control infection reaching the cervical glands from the pharynx the entire tonsil must be dissected out.

The principle thus laid down marks a definite period in the history of the tonsil and adenoid operation. It is true that there was for some years a recrudesence of the popularity of the guillotine operation through the writings of Samuel S. Whillis and Frederick C. Pybus of Newcastle-on-Tyne and of Greenfield Sluder of St. Louis, but they accepted Waugh's principle of complete removal. When Whillis and Pybus in 1910 revolutionized guillotine tonsillectomy by employing the reverse method, pressing the tonsil outwards and into the aperture of the guillotine by pressure on the anterior pillar of the fauces with the finger, in their first series of two hundred cases they made the modest claim that they were able to enucleate 42 per cent of the tonsils complete in their capsule in one piece; in a later series of one hundred cases they were able to claim 74 per cent of the tonsils complete in one piece. Greenfield Sluder in 1912 published a paper (originally read before the American Medical Association in 1910) claiming 99.6 per cent of completely successful results in tonsillectomy by using a guillotine in a somewhat similar manner—dislocating the tonsil forwards with the guillotine on to the mandibular eminence at the posterior end of the mylohyoid ridge, which forces it through the ring. Practice in this method no doubt has increased the percentage of complete results in skillful hands, but it is improbable that the average operator with the guillotine achieves anything near 100 per cent of complete tonsillectomies, as complete dissection undoubtedly does.

Diathermy, radium, and X rays have all been recommended in the treatment of unhealthy tonsils, but none of them are satisfactory methods; with diathermy the danger of secondary hemorrhage is considerable, and in many cases the removal is incomplete. Radium and X rays cause fibrosis or even destroy the lymphoid tissue of the tonsils, but have no effect on the crypts and their infected contents. The application of radium, for a brief period and under a radiologist's supervision, to shrivel adenoid remains has, however, apparently proved effective.

The gross anatomy of the faucial tonsils had been studied and described from the earliest times, but Albert von Kölliker in 1852 was the first to study their structure with the microscope. He described the follicles in their walls and the epithelium, and believed them to be part of the lymphatic system and related to the Malpighian corpuscles of the spleen. The finer structure of their lymphatic network was more precisely investigated by Wilhelm His of Basel in

1862; in 1884 H. W. G. Waldeyer of Berlin pointed out the still imperfectly understood arrangement of lymphoid tissue around the intersection of the air and food passages.

§ ADENOIDS

Kölliker, in describing the faucial tonsils, mentioned the existence of similar tissue in the nasopharynx; Jacob Henle in 1866 insisted that the "pharyngeal bursa" was a normal structure; and Hubert von Luschka in 1868 fully described the median and lateral recesses of the pharyngeal tonsil. James Yearsley of London in 1842 removed mucous membrane from behind the uvula to improve the hearing, and Johann Nepomuk Czermak and F. E. R. Voltolini introduced posterior rhinoscopy about 1860; but it was Hans Wilhelm Meyer of Copenhagen who in 1868 first described adenoids. Mayer's paper "On adenoid vegetations in the nasopharyngeal cavity" appeared in several languages, first in the Danish *Hospitalstidende,* and in *Medico-Chirurgical Transactions* in London in 1870. In the course of examining a young patient for a possible cause of deafness associated with nasal obstruction, Meyer pushed his finger up into the nasopharyngeal space and became aware of the presence there of an abnormal growth. Once his attention had been drawn to it, he recognized the condition as so common that he found it present in 102 cases during the next eighteen months. He described the signs and symptoms of adenoids so fully that any doctor, however inexperienced in rhinoscopy, was able to suspect and detect their presence at once. He described his first case as follows:

I had cleared the obstructed passage through the nose, removed the enlarged tonsils and the swelling of the throat and soft palate, but the manner of speaking remained as deficient as ever. The patient, a young lady, now underwent a regular course of training in pronunciation, but with no better result. She then came to me again. Having found rhinoscopy impracticable, I now passed my forefinger behind the soft palate up into the so-called "naso-pharyngeal cavity," and was very much astonished to find this almost entirely filled up by *soft masses,* which, giving way to the finger, felt very much like a bunch of earthworms, and hanging down from the roof of the pharynx, completely closed up the posterior nares. There was rather free bleeding during and for some minutes after this digital examination. These growths were quite new to me then, and I found no allusion made to them in any of the ancient or modern works on Surgery and Morbid Anatomy which I consulted.

Ambroise-Arnold-Guillaume Guye of Amsterdam in 1884 emphasized the influence of adenoids in retarding the development of a child's mentality, giving this symptom the name of "aprosexia." Meyer was accustomed to remove adenoids with the aid of a ring-knife, others employed the index finger with a "steel nail" upon it; but later Karl Stoerk's choanal forceps and (in 1885) Jacob Gottstein's curette came into use and have since been modified in design by various surgeons. The operation was at first performed without any anesthetic, but in the early nineties it began to be realized that general anesthesia was beneficial to patient and surgeon alike.

§ REFERENCES

Celsus (1935–38): *De medicina.* With an English translation by W. G. Spencer. 3 vols. London, William Heinemann.

Guye, A. A. G. (1889): "On aprosexia, being the inability to fix the attention and other allied troubles in the cerebral functions caused by nasal disorders." *Brit. med. J., ii,* 709–11.

Hippocrates (1923): *Works of.* With an English translation by W. H. S. Jones. London, William Heinemann.

Mackenzie, M. (1880): *A manual of diseases of the throat and nose.* Philadelphia, P. Blakiston. Vol. I, p. 10.

Meyer, W. (1870): "On adenoid vegetations in the naso-pharyngeal cavity." *Med.-chir. Trans., 53,* 191–215.

Mollison, W. M. (1928): "The work of Samuel Sharp and his predecessors on the functions and surgery of the tonsils." *Guy's Hosp. Rep., 78,* 93–103.

Moore, I. (1928): *The tonsils and adenoids and their diseases including the part they play in systematic diseases.* St. Louis, C. V. Mosby.

Physick, P. S. (1828): "Description of a forceps employed to facilitate the extirpation of the tonsil and invented by P. S. Physick." *Amer. J. med. Sci., 2,* 116–17.

Sluder, G. (1923): *Tonsillectomy by means of the alveolar eminence of the mandible and a guillotine.* St. Louis, C. V. Mosby.

Waugh, G. E. (1909): "A simple operation for the complete removal of tonsils." *Lancet, i,* 1314.

Whillis, S. S., and F. C. Pybus (1910): "The enucleation of tonsils with the guillotine." *Lancet, ii,* 875.

Wise, T. A. (1845): *Commentary on the Hindu system of Medicine.* Calcutta, Thacker.

BY DOUGLAS J. CAMPBELL
T. D., F. R. C. P., D. P. H.*

chapter 10 / the venereal diseases

THE VENEREAL DISEASES, so called because they are in the main acquired during sexual intercourse, have provided the most conflicting of all medicosocial problems throughout the history of man. Since scientific understanding and evaluation only reached rational levels in the twentieth century, their history is chaotic and full of glaring contradictions. Until 1905 diagnosis depended on clinical observations alone, and a cure was equally assessed by appearances, unsupported by laboratory confirmation. Once the specific microorganisms were demonstrated and their predilection for warmth, moisture, partial anaerobic conditions, and in some, particular body structures realized, the mode of spread by venery became more understandable.

Three main diseases have been recognized in the past. Gonorrhea or clap resulted in sterility and stricture from chronic inflammatory changes and, in the new-born, blindness from infection of the eyes resulting in ophthalmia neonatorum. Soft sore or chancroid (the latter name given by Freeman Bumstead of New York in 1861), long associated with poor personal hygiene and filth, led to destructive ulceration of the genitals and buboes in the groin. Syphilis or the great pox is a disease of many stages, the first being a hard ulcer or chancre, ultimately destroying health and efficiency, especially of the cardiovascular and central nervous systems, usually at a time of life when the individual should be at his best and able to make the greatest contribution to family and social life. Being passed *in utero* to the developing child, it causes a high fetal mortality or the birth of congenitally infected children, who may suffer deformities, impaired vision, mental disease, and the like.

* Consultant venereologist, Sheffield (England) area.

178

The Venereal Diseases

All three infections may occur together, hence the centuries-long confusion of diagnosis and treatment. In more recent times other venereal diseases have become widely known, some of which are found mainly in far off countries, such as *lymphogranuloma venereum* and *granuloma inguinale*. Many infections of the urethra, grouped under nongonococcal or nonspecific urethritis, and Reiter's syndrome, present a new formidable clinical picture. A world-wide problem resulting from treponematoses includes yaws, found in the tropics, bejel, found in Arabia, and pinta in Mexico. They have long been endemic in close communities, but may alter in character as a result of the wider and more rapid contact of modern life and travel. These diseases are apparently nonvenereal in spread, but in all bacteriological and clinical respects are similar to syphilis.

§ HISTORY

Medical historians are agreed that gonorrhea and soft sore existed from Biblical times. In Leviticus, chapters 12 and 15, the advice on ablution after copulation must have been intended to prevent or cure diseases acquired during sexual intercourse. In Proverbs, Wisdom advises her pupil to avoid strange women lest his flesh and body be consumed. Gonorrhea, called an "issue," is often mentioned, and Moses warned the Israelites against "carnal knowledge of strange women," while the "visitations of the Lord" probably allude to epidemics of venereal disease amongst the promiscuous and nomadic peoples. The practice of circumcision was probably an hygienic measure against venereal infections, and diseases which were described as passing "to the third and fourth generation" in the Bible might suggest acquired and congenital syphilis. However, many cemeteries examined by the survey department of the Egyptian Government, the burials ranging over a period of five thousand years, failed to show unmistakable signs of syphilis in the bones. Singularly, in view of the looseness of morals in the Greek and Roman era, no reference is made to the disfiguring effects associated with syphilis in classical literature. Hippocrates and Celsus describe soft sore. Celsus in his account of phimosis (Book vi, ch. 18, sect. 2) says:

The foreskin should be drawn back when ulcers will be found on the glans or body of the penis itself, either clean and dry, or moist and purulent. The pus in the latter case may be abundant and smell offensively. The ulceration may become deep and extensive and may even cause so much damage beneath the foreskin that the glans is destroyed and may slough off. The patient in such cases should be circumcised, and there is some danger of the urethra becoming closed.

While the satyric poets hint at the existence of what might be gonorrhea, the condition was not described fully until the twelfth century when *"chaude pisse"* was widely recognized by such men as Henri de Mondeville and John Arderne. Gonorrhea and soft sore dominated the picture until the end of the fifteenth century and remained unchanged as grave problems until the advent of the sulphonamides in 1937.

In 1493, as described by Ruy Diaz de Isla, a surgeon in practice at Barcelona, "a disease previously unknown, unseen and undescribed, first appeared in that City...and spread thence throughout the world." This new disease was syphilis, brought to Europe from the new-found America by Columbus and his crews. That it existed in America is apparently established by the finding of bony syphilis in the skeletons of Indians dating back to the year A.D. 1000. Had the disease in fact never been in Europe before? Could leprosy, so long recognized, not have included syphilis? Might not the disease have reduced in morbidity through the centuries and so gone unrecognized? Was the infection brought by Columbus a new and virulent strain introduced to a nonimmune community and rapidly disseminated by the mercenary armies of Charles VIII of France when Italy was invaded and Naples occupied for a long period, or by the hordes of persecuted Jews expelled from Spain at that time and forced to migrate all over central Europe in search of new homes, or by the era of greater travel associated with Columbus, Vasco da Gama, and the like? This is the great controversy. Is there any conclusive evidence on either side? Many quotations suggest that syphilis did exist in Europe before 1493. Some historians hold that the descriptions from the fifth century might well be early syphilis, while others are equally dogmatic that they refer to other venereal diseases. In the fifth century diseases of the genitals were considered a judgment of Heaven on promiscuity. In the twelfth century were described "hot humours from foul women," and later leprosy again enters the lists. Gulielmus de Saliceto of Placenza in 1270 spoke of "cold and hot humours which proceed from the liver and cause a bubo in the groin after lying with an unclean woman." In 1290 Theodoric Borgognoni said: "Whoever converses with a woman who has lain with a Leper shall catch the distemper," and Lanfranchi of Milan described chancres of the penis after foul women. In 1398 Trevisa quotes Bartholomew de Glanville (*De proprietatibus rerum.* Translated by John of Trevisa, 1398) as describing a disease which arises from adultery or is passed from "fader or moder" or "when a chylde is fedde with corrupte mylke of a Leprouse nourryce," in which the nose is stopped up, the voice is altered, and the hair falls. In 1752 Antonio Nuñez Ribeiro Sanchez in his *Origine de la malade vénérienne* decided that the disease existed before the supposed introduction by Columbus. Whatever the truth, a great scourge quickly spread all over Europe from 1493. It was severe in Naples following the occupation by Charles's army. In 1497 it had spread to England, and the town councils of Aberdeen and Edinburgh tried to arrest it by segregating sufferers on islands off the coast of Scotland. Foul and destructive lesions of the skin, especially of the face, pains in bones and joints, involvement of the lungs, and other gross manifestations which we now recognize as secondary lesions, were the main symptoms, and, in contrast to the present day, when such manifestations are much less fulminating, death frequently occurred during these early stages.

The foulness of the lesions and the knowledge that they followed promiscuous intercourse gave rise to that abhorrence which exists in the public mind to this day. The scourge baffled the physicians for the next four centuries and provoked voluminous writings and theories, coinciding as it did with the introduction of printing and wood block illustration. At first it was named after the peoples who were supposed to have spread it, thus "Neapolitan disease," "French disease," and "Spanish disease." In 1527 Jacques de Bethencourt of Rouen called it "venereal" from Venus, the goddess of love. The fatal influence of the stars, especially Venus, Mars, and Jupiter, were expounded by Gasparo Torella and Fracastoro. In 1530 Girolamo Fracastoro of Verona, humanist, poet, geologist, and physicist, wrote *Syphilis sive morbus gallicus,* and from the hero of this poem came the word which now designates the disease. For the next three hundred and fifty years another great controversy was the cause of syphilis and whether syphilis and gonorrhea were but different phases of a common infection. Reputation and friendships amongst medical men suffered and conflicted. Jean François Fernel (1497–1558) said that it was due to an "occult and poisonous quality contracted by contagion and inherent in some matter or humour which serves as a vehicle and carries it into the economy." In 1736 Jean Astruc, physician to Louis XV of France, wrote a treatise on venereal disease, dividing it into two parts, the first describing the early affection of the genitals such as is seen in syphilis and gonorrhea, the second describing what we would recognize now as late or tertiary syphilis. In 1793 Benjamin Bell argued that syphilis and gonorrhea were different, and his views were also subscribed to by Jean François Hernandez of Toulon in 1812. John Hunter described a virus which affected the system, primarily or locally and secondarily or constitutionally. He thought that the point of inoculation decided the type of disease, thus, via the mucous membrane, gonorrhea; via the skin, chancres. To prove his theory he inoculated himself in May, 1767, with matter from a patient with gonorrhea. It now appears that this patient also had syphilis, for Hunter developed signs of both diseases. Thus this famous and courageous surgeon, after whom the initial syphilitic lesion was called the Hunterian chancre, ruined his own life and retarded science for many years.

François Joseph Victor Broussais and his pupils rejected Hunter's virus theory and fell back on "irritation" as the cause. In 1838 Philippe Ricord tabulated the disease as "syphiloid" and "syphilis." Later he repeated Hunter's experiment of inoculation and showed that gonorrhea was distinct from syphilis. P. I. A. Léon Bassereau in 1852 and François Félix Clerc in 1854 taught that soft sores were not caused by the same poison as syphilis, nor did the cause of the difference lie within the constitution, age, sex, or tissues affected, but that a different virus was responsible. Eventually a bacteriologist settled the issue; in 1879 Albert Neisser of Breslau identified the gonococcus. In 1889 Auguste Ducrey discovered the bacillus in the pus of buboes associated with chancroids, and Paul Gerson Unna found it in the walls of the ulcers themselves. In 1905 Fritz Schaudinn, a protozoologist at the Berlin Health Institute, working on trepanosomes and spirochetes, demonstrated a spirillum in the exudate from a syphilitic chancre to Paul

The Venereal Diseases

Erich Hoffmann. It was named *Treponema pallidum* or *Spirochaeta pallida* after its shape and characteristic pallor as viewed with a dark ground microscope. Further experiments at the Pasteur Institute in Paris proved it to be the causative organism which physicians had sought for centuries. Laboratory research has still been retarded because the *Spirochaeta pallida* does not affect animals other than man, higher apes, and rabbits, and the last named do not develop the generalized manifestations of the former two. The stimulus of the new discovery soon led pathologists to establish the spirochete as the cause of aortic disease, while Hideyo Noguchi found the organism in the brains of general paralytics.

In 1906 August von Wassermann, Albert Neisser, and Carl Bruck evolved the complement fixation test we now know as the Wassermann, based on the Bordet-Gengou complement fixation phenomenon. The antigen first used was considered "specific," being made from fetal syphilitic liver. Later, extract of beef heart was found effective—a fortuitous result, considering the modern preventive measures make syphilitic fetal liver a rarity. This test is still a basic one despite modifications. An era of cardiolipin antigens is upon us, promising greater specificity and fewer false results. From 1917 a group of flocculation tests—the Meinicke, Kahn, Sachs-Georgi, Eagle, Hinton, and others, named after their respective originators—have rivaled, but not ousted, the Wassermann. The latest serological test in our diagnostic armamentarium is the Nelson treponemal immobilization test. The serological tests, while confirming the syphilitic nature of active lesions, also revealed that a latent syphilis could be present in an individual, though not showing active lesions at the time. They also explain Colles's law of 1837 which expounded that a mother, due to the pregnant state, was immune to syphilis herself, but could give birth to a congenital syphilitic child, infected by the paternal route. We realize now that the mother herself was already infected, but in a latent phase of the disease. Of other diagnostic aids, X rays have proved of considerable help. Thus we now know that each venereal disease has its own causative organism, but we have not reached finality, for nonspecific urethritis viruses, pleuropneumonia-like organisms, and inclusion bodies constitute the present-day controversy, while the behavior of the spirochete in its long periods of inactivity or latency may one day be explained by such contrivances as the electron microscope.

§ TREATMENT

Since the identification of the causative organisms of venereal disease is so recent, treatment was for centuries entirely empirical, and in their hopelessness the victims often turned from the physician to the quack.

In gonorrhea, treatment until 1937 consisted of trying to heal the affected mucous membranes by instillations and irrigations with antiseptic lotions. Numerous concoctions from herbs were often palliative. Attempts to stimulate specific antibody reaction by vaccines, injections of milk, etc., proved ineffective in the main, and the condition became recognized as "self-limiting." In 1937 the sulphonamides brought a cure in some five days to a condition which had previously taken many months or years of tedious practices. This happy state continued until 1943, when, in German-occupied Europe, the writer discovered sulphonamide-resistant gonorrhea—a condition which occurred all over the world in the succeeding months, reducing the disease to the hopelessness of the past. Fortunately, another ally was at hand in penicillin, and so far the gonococcus has not become resistant, but who knows what the promiscuous use of the antibiotic for so many conditions may ultimately produce?

Similarly, chancroid had no specific cure, not even in a vaccine prepared from the causative organism, until the sulphonamides provided a rapid cure. This position is still maintained, and throughout the world chancroid is a rapidly disappearing problem, partly due to the better hygiene of all peoples.

The history of the treatment of syphilis begins with the traditional treatment by bleeding, as practiced generally by physicians and surgeons at the time of Columbus. In the past the Arabs had used mercury for the treatment of the filthy sores which we know included chancroids, and in the early days following the scourge of 1493 *unguentum Saracenicum* was much in use. This ointment, containing mercury, was a particularly fortunate choice, for of all drugs then known mercury was to prove the most effective against syphilis. It was not without danger, because it was believed that it had to be pushed to the stage of copious salivation or "fluxing," which brought pains in the belly, foul ulceration of the mouth, and loosening of the teeth. Its toxicity was so great that in 1517 guaiacum, which had been used in the West Indies for the treatment of the established endemic syphilis, was introduced into Europe. It proved less toxic than mercury, but gave rise to more relapses. This in turn was replaced by sarsaparilla, which remained popular until the present century, at least as a "blood purifier" and was sold in tumblerfuls from a cart in Broad Sanctuary, opposite Westminster Abbey, and within a few yards of Westminster Hospital, as related by Sir D'Arcy Power and J. Johnston Abraham. The relapses following guaiacum and sarsaparilla brought mercury back into favor. Fumigation replaced inunction in its application, but mercury poisoning proved worse than the disease, and the accounts of the so-called hospitals in which the sufferers collected with their foul syphilis and still more foul mercurialism, nursed by the lowest prostitutes, make harrowing reading. In 1836 William Wallace of Dublin introduced potassium iodide, which was much more moderate in its effects than mercury, but not so specific. In 1853, as a result of work on vaccination by Jenner, attempts were made to produce natural immunity by "syphilization," which was inoculating the pus from a soft sore, as this was thought to be an attenuated form of syphilis. In 1861 Jonathan Hutchinson and Jean Alfred Fournier returned to mercury given over long periods and always short of salivation. In 1868 G. Lewin of Breslau introduced intramuscular injections, which were effective but painful. Thus, from a pharmaceutical mist in which it was believed that through a Divine Providence there was a curative herb for each disease, mercury's popularity ebbed and flowed throughout the centuries. Following Schaudinn's discovery of the spirochete in 1905, Paul Ehrlich, working in his laboratory in Frankfort, experimented to find a drug which would destroy the spirochete without being harmful to the host. In 1909, on his "606th" experiment, he produced an organic compound of arsenic which promised these requirements. Thus Salvarsan opened up the era of arsenotherapy. As with iodides nearly a century before, the great cure had arrived! One injection seemed to suffice, but the drug was highly toxic, and relapses did occur even when the number of injections were increased, so experiments were continued. Silver-Salvarsan was produced in 1912, and as the result of the 914th experiment neo-salvarsan was discovered. This trivalent arsenical proved highly successful and is still firmly approved by many venereologists today. Experience showed that pro-

185

longed courses of weekly injections up to two years or longer in duration were necessary. Bismuth, which has high spirocheticidal properties and lower toxicity than mercury, was advocated by Félix Balzer in 1889, but was not universally accepted. In 1921 R. Sazerac and Constantin Levaditi revived its popularity, and since that date it has replaced mercury and was given in conjunction with arsenic until 1943. A pentavalent arsenical (tryparsamide) has been considered particularly selective in neurosyphilis, but is thought to increase the danger of optic atrophy, while the addition of quinine and iodine to bismuth has also had a vogue in the treatment of this group. Ever straining at short courses for patients who have a high default rate, researchers produced arsenoxide at the end of the nineteen thirties, but again toxicity was high. Other adjuvant therapy has been heat in the form of malaria or artificial methods using hypertherms, particularly for neurosyphilis, following the work of Julius Wagner von Jauregg in 1917. Sir Alexander Fleming's discovery of penicillin has opened yet another era in the treatment of syphilis, for this antibiotic seems to achieve in days what took arsenic and bismuth months. It combines speed and low toxicity. The number of courses advocated and the voluminous literature on the subject in the last ten years make it apparent that we have certainly not yet reached finality. Arising from the problem of large masses of native peoples throughout the world suffering from treponematosis, experiments with "one shot" penicillin therapy are being carried out under the auspices of the World Health Organization. Parallel with this is a marked improvement in general health standards in such peoples, with a much higher expectation of life. May not the failures from such rapid therapy cause a marked increase in late manifestations similar to those occurring among more civilized races?

In England the medicosocial aspect was finally tackled following the Royal Commission of 1916, which established adequate, well-staffed and equipped treatment centers at which patients could obtain free treatment and, above all, outlawed the quack.

Venereal diseases are as old as man. Their severity gradually diminishes the longer they are present in any race, even under the influence of inadequate treatment, but fresh contacts bring at least temporary exacerbations and renewed severity, as was seen in the United Kingdom early in World War II when Allied and colonial soldiers served in that country. Promiscuity increases with travel, absence from home, war, famine, and other economic upsets, and while the prostitute is still universally indicted, her amateur sister is not blameless. From time to time great hopes of final eradication have surged through the picture. Disappointment has always followed. Today the newly infected are rendered noncontagious faster than ever before, established cases are cured or patients are enabled to enjoy longer lives because of penicillin. While the organism as yet shows no resistance, there is a marked increase in intolerance of the drug by human beings, and none of the other antibiotics seem to hold such promise. Might the historian of the future describe this era as yet another in the long list of disappointments?

§ REFERENCES

Astruc, J. (1736): *De morbis venereis libri sex.* Lutetiae Parisiorum, G. Cavelier.

Bell, B. (1793): *A treatise on gonorrhoea virulenta, and lues venerea.* 2 vols. Edinburgh, J. Watson and G. Mudie.

Colles, A. (1837): *Practical observations on the venereal disease, and on the use of mercury.* London, Sherwood, Gilbert and Piper.

Diaz de Isla, R. (1539): *Tractado cótra el mal serpentino.* Sevilla, D. de Robertis.

Ehrlich, P., and S. Hata (1910): *Die experimentelle Chemotherapie der Spirillosen (Syphilis, Rückfallfieber, Hühnerspirillose, Frambösie).* Berlin, J. Springer.

Ehrlich, P. (1912): *"Über Laboratoriumsversuche und Klinische Erprobung von Heilstoffen."* Chemiker Zeitung, Köthen, *36,* 637–38.

Fracastoro, G. (1530): *Syphilis, sive morbus gallicus.* Veronae.

Hernandez, J. F. (1812): *Essai analytique sur la non-identité des virus gonorrhoïque et syphilitique.* Toulon.

Hunter, J. (1786): *A treatise on the venereal disease.* London.

Neisser, A. (1879): *"Über eine der Gonorrhoe eigenthümliche Micrococcusform."* Zbl. med. Wiss., *17,* 497–500.

Ricord, P. (1838): *Traité pratique des maladies vénériennes.* Paris, De Just Rouvier and E. Le Bouvier.

Sanchez, A. N. R. (1752): *Dissertation sur l'origine de la maladie vénérienne.* Paris, Durand and Pissot.

Sazerac, R., and C. Levaditi (1921): *"Traitement de la syphilis par le bismuth."* C. R. Acad. Sci., Paris, *173,* 338–40.

Schaudinn, F., and E. Hoffman (1905): *"Vorläufiger Bericht über das Vorkommen von Spirochaeten in syphilitischen Krankheitsprodukten und bei Papillomen."* Arb. GesundhAmt., Berlin, *22,* 527–34.

Wassermann, A., A. Neisser, and C. Bruch (1906): *"Eine serodiagnostische Reaktion bei Syphilis."* Dtsch. med. Wschr., *32,* 745–46.

§ FURTHER READING

Bloch, I. (1901 and 1911): *Der Ursprung der Syphilis.* Jena, G. Fischer. Pt. 1 (1901), pt. 2 (1911).

Jeanselme, E., *et al.* (1931): *"Histoire de la syphilis."* In *Traité de la syphilis.* Edited by E. Jeanselme and E. Schulmann. Paris, G. Doin. Tome I.

Pusey, W. A. (1933): *The history and epidemiology of syphilis.* Springfield, Illinois, C. C. Thomas.

Sudhoff, K. F. J. (1912): *Aus der Frühgeschichte der Syphilis.* Leipzig, J. A. Barth.

Sudhoff, K. (1925): *The earliest printed literature on syphilis. Being ten tractates from the years 1495–98.* . . . Adapted by Charles Singer. Florence, R. Lier & Co.

BY A. WHITE FRANKLIN
M. B., B. Ch., F. R. C. P.*

chapter 11 / Rickets

THE HISTORY of rickets is the history of the rise and fall of a disease. Rickets is now rare, but it was once common, and by its presence hundreds of thousands of children grew up damaged and deformed. In prehistoric and classical times there is little trace of it. From the seventeenth to the mid-nineteenth centuries, doctors, struck by its increasing frequency, described it well, while treating it badly. In the last one hundred years the experimental method let men learn the causes and contrive the cure through studies which taught and spread important new ideas in human and animal nutrition. But the same complex social organization, with whose growth rickets increased, is needed to prevent it. With social breakdown rickets would return. Henry E. Sigerist writes: "There is very little evidence for the occurrence of the disease in prehistoric and early historic times." Sir Grafton Elliot Smith has shown that "clear, unmistakable evidence of rickets has not been found in human bones in any cemetery in Egypt or Nubia." But Carl Fürst did find traces in neolithic bones in Denmark and Norway. These results of research into paleopathology cause no surprise. Nudity, sunlight, and the South would always discourage what Sigerist calls a disease of city slums and of the North, but what is also a disease of darkness, ignorance, and poor hygiene.

Soranus of Ephesus described the many deformed children found in the great city of Rome in the second century A.D. In the *Treatise on diseases of women* he compares Roman children and their mothers unfavorably with the Greeks. A few years later Galen gives a similar description in *De morborum causis* of deformities that might have been due to rickets:

* Physician to the children's department, St. Bartholomew's Hospital, London.

The bodies of new-born infants, being soft and almost flexible are easily distorted .... The natural shape of the limbs can be altered and distorted ... if the infants are wrongly handled. And indeed, in the whole of the subsequent rearing many limbs suffer distortion, partly by immoderate feeding or by incorrect movements—being permitted to stand or to walk too soon—or by too violent exercise .... The legs, from the weight of the body, are distorted either outwardly or inwardly according to the propensity of the tibiae. For those whose legs are altogether straighter than is natural become knock-kneed, while those who have curved legs become bandy. Many parts of the thorax are also deformed.

The belief that sitting too early and too long bends the spine and that standing or walking too early bends the thighs recurs through the ages in accounts of deformed children. It survives now, particularly in the minds of old nurses and grandmothers, and may no more have referred to rickets in the past than it does today.

The evidence of rickets in the Middle Ages is weak. The court jester, like Thersites in Homer, has been accused of rickets, and John A. Foote (1927), discussing rickets in medieval art, reproduces a Nativity by the Swabian Master of Augsburg to show rickety cherubs. In the picture the Virgin and Joseph share with the cherubs a large square forehead and a large skull, so that the artist appears to have painted the members of one family, if indeed he painted from life at all. Even in modern times many conditions where deformity complicates dwarfism, have been called rickets. No doubt medieval rickets included gargoylism, achondroplasia, osteogenesis imperfecta, osteochondrodystrophies of varies kinds, and even cleidocranial dysostosis.

Theodosius of Bologna in the sixteenth century recorded a pale seventeen-month-old infant with a lower dorsal curvature of the spine, who could neither move nor sit. In the first half of the seventeenth century Ambroïse Paré described valgus and varus deformities of the legs, so rickets was probably active in France at the time.

George Frederic Still follows earlier historians in quoting a Basel thesis of 1582, *De tabe pectorea,* in which a certain Jerome Reusner is said to have given the first modern account of rickets. The description was quoted by Giovanni Verardi Zeviani in a treatise on the cure of rickets in 1761 to show that the condition had been described in the sixteenth century, one hundred years before Francis Glisson.

No copy of Reusner's thesis can be traced. The second period of the history of rickets must date from the mid-seventeenth century clinical descriptions.

§ WHISTLER, BOOT, GLISSON, AND MAYOW

Four medical works on rickets were published within the space of twenty-five years. In 1645 Daniel Whistler presented for his M.D. thesis at Leyden *De morbo puerili Anglorum quem patrio idiomate indigenae vocant the Rickets;* four years later a Dutchman, Arnold Boot, included a description of rickets in his work *Observationes medicae de affectibus omissis* (London, 1649); and in 1650 appeared the most important work of all, *De rachitide sive morbo puerili, qui vulgo The Rickets dicitur,* published by Francis Glisson; translated, it appeared in 1651 as the first account of the disease in the English tongue. In 1668 John Mayow, writing in more philosophical vein, discusses the problem in *De rachitide,* one of his *Tractatus duo.* This was revised and enlarged to form the fifth part of *Tractatus quinque* in 1674.

Rickets must have been a striking disease at this time, and nothing suggests that Whistler, Boot, or Glisson had any knowledge of each other's work. All three were engaged with the disease at the same time, but the credit for the first published description of what we know as rickets today belongs to Daniel Whistler. "Some twenty-six years ago," he writes in 1645, "the disease was first observed in our country and is said to have acquired its name 'The Rickets' from the surname of some quack who was the first to treat it." Others traced it to the Dorset dialect "to rucket," meaning to be short of breath. Whistler lists seventeen diagnostic symptoms including abdominal enlargement, enlarged bony epiphyses, swelling of the costochondral junctions, bending of the long bones and of the back, a large skull, flabby soft tissues, late eruption of teeth and caries, and narrowness and deformities of the chest. He blames a fault of proportion in the clot-forming part of the blood, the spreading of the serous portion into the whole system causing softness and swelling. The author thought well of his thesis and justly so, and he republished it in 1684 when he was president of the College of Physicians of London.

Arnold Boot (Bootius), born in Holland in 1606, includes his account in a book of overlooked affections. He prefers the name *tabes pectorea,* the name used by Reusner in Basel. Boot blamed enlargement of the liver, which he had always found in the many postmortem examinations of children who had died of the disease. The chest deformity and bending of the ribs were later accompanied by enlargement of the head, weakness and wasting of limbs, inability to stand, and curving of the spine. Boot spent some time in Ireland as chief of the medical staff to the Viceroy; and in *Ireland's Naturall History* (1652) his brother Gerald (Boate) described rickets as one of the reigning diseases there. Arnold moved in 1644 to Paris, where he found various children "labouring with the disease."

The first book in any language devoted entirely to rickets is the famous *De rachitide* of Francis Glisson. A. F. Hess calls it "the mature and well-balanced product of a master" and adds that "it is one of the first English monographs treating of a single disease . . . leaving . . . little to the future clinician or pathological anatomist." Glisson regarded rickets as "absolutely a new disease" and, like Whistler, pointed to its appearance in Dorset in 1620. His book includes accounts of post-mortem findings, of symptoms (adding little to what Whistler had already described), more on physiology within the framework of the ancient humoral theory, and all that could be conceived at the time about treatment—from issues through blisters, leeches, splints, and simples to the control of the diet.

In one respect Glisson and the seven other Fellows of the College of Physicians, who contributed their own observations to him, were in error. They found the affected bones hard rather than soft, and they blamed the bending on the unequal growth of the two sides. Mayow in his tract relies largely on Glisson's clinical description, but "deduces the symptoms of the disease from obstruction of the spinal marrow." Because the cure of obstruction is catharsis, he catalogues under treatment: enemata, emetics, cathartics, bloodletting, issues, blisters, cupping, diaphoretics, and even the warm springs of Bath—a choice of formidable therapy for the feeble, debilitated infant patient.

§ A NEW DISEASE?

Is it possible that rickets really was a new disease? Rickets certainly appears for the first time and as the cause of fourteen deaths in the bills of mortality in 1634; and a contemporary, Captain John Graunt, the pioneer with Sir William Petty of medical statistics, himself argued the point, believing the disease to be new. Dr. Henry Power wrote from Halifax in August, 1649 to Sir Thomas Browne:

> There is only one inbred & late disease amongst us (The Ricketts) wch puzles mee in the cure: for I know not well what ℞'s are pat for that purpose. Neither can I be relieved by any Authour, it being of so late a standing that none I know of have attempted to write thereon.

This is the year before Glisson published his work. Sir Jack Drummond and Anne Wilbraham in their study of *The Englishman's food* felt certain that rickets had existed in earlier periods of dearth, but blamed the terrible depression and poverty in the last decade or two of the Tudors for a noticeable increase in southern England, where "white meats," especially milk, became dear and scarce, reducing the daily calcium and phosphorus intake as well as that of the anti-rachitic vitamin D.

Whatever doubts arise about the origin of rickets, its frequency increased mightily during the next two centuries. Glisson observed that the "disease doth more frequently invade the cradles of the rich than afflict poor men's children." Samuel Gee also noted that while the severer forms might be peculiar to the poor, "slight or even considerable rickets is really common in the children of the comparatively rich." At this time, in 1867, he wrote of his Great Ormond Street Hospital experiences: "30.3 per cent of sick children under two years of age are rickety." This figure was universal in the big cities of Europe at that time.

For Gee, rickets existed in all possible gradations between "simple genuine debility and the special form called rickets." He recognized the condition by delayed dentition and walking, separation of cranial sutures, the large head, craniotabes (discovered in clinic and post-mortem room and christened by C. L. Elsässer in 1843), thoracic deformities, beading of the ribs with a transverse depression at the level of the xiphoid articulation (now known as Harrison's sulcus), absence of fever, and a spasmodic disposition (laryngismus and carpopedal spasms), to which Sir William Jenner had drawn attention in lectures in 1859. Gee writes that a "child not idiotic or weakened by some recent acute disease, not walking at eighteen months, is rickety or paralysed." He describes as a symptom of rickets the "agony when he is lifted," which is typical of scurvy; he was writing ten years before W. B. Cheadle drew attention to infant scurvy and fifteen years before Sir Thomas Barlow's classical paper (1883) separating scurvy from rickets. Glisson's description of scurvy complicating rickets, causing lassitude, pain in the joints, and swelling of the gums, had remained unnoticed through the centuries. There is no mention of the sweating described by Mayow.

Gee wrote with sarcasm of the idea that rickets was due to lack of earthy phosphates in the bones—rickets was really due to a debility —and here the great clinician exposes his Achilles' heel to posterity. In 1838 J. Guerin had already reproduced in dogs the rickety swelling of epiphyses and the bending of bones by feeding a diet deficient in lime. In 1842 Chossat described soft bones in pigeons fed on a low calcium diet. The chemists were already invading medicine, and all Gee's sarcasm would not stop them.

§ PRE- AND POST- POMMER

There was still some descriptive work to be done. Clinical criteria are not enough for the experimental method. It was Gustav Pommer in 1885 who first established the specific histological picture of the bones in rickets and osteomalacia—two diseases whose essential identity had already been proved by Armand Trousseau and C. Lasègue (1849). The children's diseases section of the London International Medical Congress of 1881 had listened at length to J. M. J. Parrot on the syphilitic nature of rickets. Such absurdities would hereafter be impossible. Leonard Findlay wrote that the history of rickets is divided into the pre-Pommer and the post-Pommer periods and that "Pommer did in the pathological field what Whistler and Glisson had done in the clinical." Pommer showed that the bone lesion of rickets consisted in a great and irregular overgrowth of cartilage with deficient calcification and the formation of osteoid issue. Such change could not be produced by a calcium-poor diet alone.

From Whistler to Pommer was two hundred and forty years; forty years after Pommer, A. F. Hess and H. Steenbock had shown the antirachitic activity of irradiated oils.

Rickets

The history of rickets now leaves the ward and the outpatient department and moves into the laboratory and into realms presently to be administered by the adepts of social medicine. A survey prompted by the Medical Congress of 1884 showed that the distribution of rickets in Great Britain coincided with the industrial population. In Clydeside every child examined was found to be affected. In India, William Huntly, a medical missionary, was struck by the absence of rickets. He had learned from Cheadle the idea that absence of animal fat was the chief cause of the disease. This could not apply to India where the diet of the masses was eminently poor in fat. Huntly, comparing climatic conditions in India and Glasgow, concluded that although diet might play some part in rickets, "the absence of open-air exercise and sunlight appear as the main factors in accentuating the tendency to its production." The publication of these observations in 1889 led T. A. Palm to make a geographical survey of the distribution of rickets, finding it prevalent where sunshine was scarce, and rare when sunshine was abundant.

As usual in medicine, the discovery of new facts in one field is applied to others in the hope of lighting up dark places. The dawn of endocrinology in the late years of the century led some to wonder whether the glands of internal secretion held the clue. In 1894 O. Lanz claimed good results with thyroid gland treatment, and in 1900 W. Stoeltzner recorded benefit from the use of adrenalin. Karl Basch in 1906 described the onset of rickets in a dog, following removal of that most deceitful of all glands, the thymus, and in 1911 J. Erdheim believed that he had produced rickets in the rat by parathyroidectomy. None of these results was later confirmed.

During this same period the question was discussed whether rickets was an infection. Parrot was convinced that it was due to syphilis. Clemens von Pirquet as late as 1919 held the view "that it was an infectious disease . . . comparable to some extent with tuberculosis." B. Morpurgo in 1900 supposed that he had found in the feces of rats suffering from epidemic rickets a diplococcus with which he could reproduce rickets in other animals. Over the next decade several other workers reported producing the disease in fowls inoculated with bacteria (A. Iovane, G. Moussou, and Josef Koch). These curious reports bear witness to the difficulties of the experimental method.

Meanwhile, the main stream of research led along two channels—the place of the external environment and the importance of diet in the production of the disease. By the turn of the century it had become clear that rickets favored civilized countries and the cities; that primitive races escaped under natural conditions, but were exceedingly susceptible when living in the white man's habitations; and that animals, never affected while in a state of nature, succumbed when reared in captivity. These facts led D. Hansemann in 1906 to formulate the opinion that the cause of the disease was to be found in domestication, which for him meant everything that made civilization contrast with nature. Two years later (1908) Leonard Findlay recorded that he had successfully caused rickets in dogs simply by confining them in cages.

At this time work on the vitamins was in its infancy, and the need to take stock of other factors in the diet than the proximate principles and salts was not appreciated. It had long been recognized that scurvy was due to the absence of something present in fresh fruit and vegetables, but all ideas on the subject were rather nebulous. In 1881 N. Lunin had discovered that mice fed on a synthesized diet composed of protein, fat, carbohydrate, and salts could not live and that something else in addition had to be present if life were to be preserved, and in 1897 C. Eijkman had demonstrated that fowls fed on polished rice developed neuritis which could be cured by feeding on an extract of the polishings. It was the work and writings of Casimir Funk, F. Gowland Hopkins, and Lafayette B. Mendel and T. B. Osborne which brought this aspect of dietary studies into prominence and revealed the necessity for a revaluation of all previous experimental work on rickets. In 1906 Hopkins, while discussing the far-reaching importance to nutrition of qualitative differences in the composition of the protein molecule, remarked that rickets and scurvy were almost certainly due to dietetic errors "which comprise these minimal qualitative factors" and for which in 1912 Funk devised the name "vitamine."[†] In 1913 E. V. McCollum and M. Davis, and Mendel and Osborne almost simultaneously identified one of these minimal qualitative factors which was essential for growth, and because it was associated

† Funk thought that they were amines. When this was found untrue, Drummond suggested the name without the terminal "e."

with the fat, it was called the fat-soluble A vitamin or accessory food factor. It was shortly after this that Edward Mellanby, by careful dietary studies, began the investigation of the disease in the dog, and in 1918 he stated that rickets was a "deficiency disease due to the absence of an accessory food factor related to the growth promoting factor," although he admitted with Findlay that confinement did play a part. At this time Mellanby did not consider the antirachitic substance identical with the growth-promoting factor, "since the disease is most prominent in quickly growing animals," but in 1921, when he published his complete study, he concluded that the potent agent was probably the fat-soluble A vitamin.

In spite of all the experimental work detailed above, there still prevailed the greatest uncertainty regarding the cause of the disease. Indeed, it might almost be said that, instead of helping towards the solution of the problem, this work had rather increased the confusion, for it seemed quite impossible to reconcile the various findings. But in 1919 Kurt Huldschinsky, by means of a clinical experiment, reported an observation which was destined to clarify the whole position. Huldschinsky had no clear conception of the cause of the disease and, like other clinicians, employed a multitude of therapeutic measures. Because of the economic conditions in Germany after the war, the high cost of cod-liver oil, and the scarcity of fresh fruit and vegetables, Huldschinsky, by exposure of the children to artificial sunlight, endeavored to obtain the well-known benefits of residence in the country during the summer and found that within a period of two to three months they were completely healed, clinically and radiologically.

§ DIET VERSUS ENVIRONMENT

The last two paragraphs are taken almost verbatim from Findlay's essay in the original edition of this book. Findlay was brought up by Noël Paton in the environmentalist camp and fails to do justice to the work of Mellanby. At the very same time that Mellanby was producing rickets in growing dogs by feeding them on a diet deficient in an accessory food factor, Paton and A. Watson, and Findlay himself, were doing their best to prove him wrong by devising experiments to support the importance of environmental hygiene as an opposing theory. As Findlay wrote: "These observations at first increased the controversy of 'diet versus environment' as the cause of the disease"; but the quarrel was shortly to be resolved. E. V. McCollum has told (in the *Festschrift* in honor of Dr. Edwards A. Park) how he set up a rat colony in the School of Hygiene and Public Health at the Johns Hopkins University in 1917 and how with his associates he was able regularly to produce rickets in rats by variations in the diet, especially with an abnormal ratio of calcium to phosphorus. The identity of the rickets was clearly established by Park's careful studies of the histology of the bones, which showed the characteristic changes described by G. Schmorl in 1909 in the human. The next step was to prevent those changes by a small addition of cod-liver oil or a large addition of butter fat, or by regular daily exposure to sunlight. Cod-liver oil remained effective even after being treated to destroy the vitamin A property. As this treated cod-liver oil lacked the vitamin A property of preventing and curing xerophthalmia, clearly a second vitamin was responsible and this was named vitamin D.

§ COD-LIVER OIL

The value of regular cod-liver oil in preventing rickets in Negroes in New York had been shown by A. F. Hess and Lester J. Unger in 1917, and its curative value in the dispensary was shown by Edwards A. Park and J. Howland in 1921 in a series of observations well controlled by X-ray photographs of bones. Despite the carefulness with which all this work was done and the consistency of the results, many doubters remained. In 1919 the Medical Research Council and the Lister Institute sent to post-war Vienna, where rickets was reported to be rampant, a team under the direction of Dr. Harriette Chick, with the task of confirming or disproving Mellanby's work on dogs. It was these *Studies of rickets in Vienna 1919–1922*, published in 1923, which finally convinced the world that the chief cause of rickets had been found and that a method of its cure and its prevention had been discovered.

The curative power of cod-liver oil could no longer be denied. Indeed, its antirachitic activity could now be measured by its effect in healing experimentally produced rickets in rats, using the delicate line test of McCollum and his associates (1922). Two hundred and fifty years earlier (1668–69) Sir Thomas Browne had written to Dr. Christopher Merrett about the birds of Norfolk: "Many [rooks] are killd for their Livers in order to the cure of the Rickets." Perhaps some devotee will one day assay the vitamin D content of this material.

Fish-liver oil, extracted by heat or pressure, had been used for centuries in the fishing villages of Iceland and the Northern European coastline. Large quantities were sold in the markets of Bergen and Hamburg for the purpose of tanning hides, lighting lamps, and rubbing painful joints and limbs. The first record of its use in medicine is found in a letter from Dr. Robert Darbey to Dr. Percival (February 12, 1782) about the treatment of patients with chronic rheumatism attending the Manchester Infirmary, to whom a total of a hogshead was prescribed annually. *Oleum jecoris aselli* or cod-liver oil first appeared in the *Pharmacopoeia* in 1771. In 1807 Samuel Argent Bardsley, also of Manchester, found the oil, given in warm table-beer, valuable in the treatment of women who had repeated attacks of rheumatism after childbirth and who were possibly suffering from osteomalacia. The next British publication was John Hughes Bennett's *Treatise on the oleum jecoris aselli* (1841), and curiously enough he learned of its virtues for rheumatism and rickets in Germany. It seems that a professor in Marburg had adopted its use from experience during a visit to England. A Dutch pupil Scherer or Schenck, wrote about it in 1822 and published in 1826 an account of three infants cured of rickets by the oil. D. Schütte in 1824 claimed to have used cod-liver oil as a specific remedy for rickets and osteomalacia for twenty-five years in Germany, and he makes the remarkable suggestion that its value might lie in the presence of imponderable amounts of substances which produce marked changes in the body but cannot be determined by the chemist.

Through Bennett in Edinburgh, cod-liver oil once more found popularity in Great Britain. The pharmacy accounts (*l*, p. 584) of St. Bartholomew's Hospital show that the oil was first purchased there in 1847.

1847.					
April 29	3 lb.	4 oz.	... 3/6	....	11s. 5d.
May 14	9 lb.	10 oz.	... 2/6	....£1.	4s. 1d.
June 21	6 lb.	4 oz.	... 2/6	....	15s. 8d.
June 25	5 galls		... 7/–	from Duncan, Flockhard, Edinburgh	
Nov. 9	10 galls		... 7/–	from Duncan, Flockhard, Edinburgh	

The purchase for 1848 was 20 gallons; 1849, 134 gallons; 1850, 214 gallons; and by 1877, 811 gallons at five shillings. Dr. Gee, whose account of rickets in the *St. Bartholomew's Hospital Reports* (1868) has already been quoted, wrote: "In cod liver oil we possess a pharmaceutical agent worthy of a place beside iron, Peruvian bark and mercury."

But once again the oil lost favor, possibly because of adulteration or substitution. By 1912 Still could write in his textbook that cod-liver oil was no better than olive oil, pilchard, or cottonseed oils. The seventh edition of Cushny's *Pharmacology* in 1918 was no more complimentary, regarding it as a food, but as having no place in pharmacology—a statement which did not prevent him from writing in the next edition (1924): "The value of cod-liver oil in malnutrition in the young and in rickets has long been recognised."

The discovery that cod-liver oil contained vitamin D, which protected rats, dogs, and babies from rickets, put an end to all doubts, but at once led to experiments to find alternative vehicles for the vitamin. The value of sunlight and of ultraviolet radiation in curing and preventing rickets both in children and in experimental animals had been established by Huldschinsky, McCollum, and others. In 1924 H. Steenbock showed that irradiation of the ricket-producing diet prevented the development of rat rickets, and Hess proved that antirachitic power could be imparted to naturally inactive oils like cottonseed or linseed oils by exposure to the mercury-vapor lamp. The next years saw many attempts to identify the chemical nature of the antirachitic agent, culminating in the preparation of pure crystalline vitamin D (calciferol) by the vacuum distillation of the products of irradiation of ergosterol by Bourdillon and his co-workers (F. A. Askew, *et al.,* 1932). Steenbock (1932), working at the University of Wisconsin, showed that, judged by the effects on chickens, the vitamin of irradiated ergosterol was different from that found in cod-liver oil (7-dehydro-cholesterol); the former remains the main source of manufactured vitamin D for human beings.

A wartime survey in 1943 of 3,328 children aged three to twelve months living in Great Britain gave an incidence of rickets of 4 per cent in the first year of life—in Newcastle-on-Tyne, Manchester, Leeds, and Sheffield 10 to 12 per cent, in Dublin 8 per cent, in Belfast higher—but in no other area more than 3 per cent. Florid deforming of the skeleton and stunting of growth were seldom found. The diagnosis depended on the beading of the ribs, the bowing and bending of the limbs described by Whistler in 1645, on craniotabes described by Elsässer (1843), and on radiological signs such as had been recognized since H. Gocht published his textbook on X-ray examination (1898) three years after Roentgen's first paper. Some attention was paid to the blood phosphatase levels. Clinical rickets, radiological rickets, and chemical rickets were all found, but not all three always in the same patient.

Many mysteries remain—among them the site of action of vitamin D, the nature of vitamin D poisoning, the subtleties of calcium and phosphorus inter-relations and metabolism in the processes of bone growth, and the factor of heredity in rickets. But men do know that rickets can be prevented. Yet in 1952, deaths from rickets were still recorded in England and Wales as 3 per 100,000 inhabitants. To feed a nation (or a world) too large for its own food supply, each family must be able to secure the minimum quantity of food and vitamins essential for health and must have the knowledge and the wit to give its ration to each member. This is much to ask of the human race, both governors and governed. It is, nevertheless, only this that will drive rickets from the world.

§ REFERENCES

Any one now writing on the history of rickets is under a debt of gratitude to A. F. Hess's book on *Rickets, including osteomalacia and tetany* (Philadelphia, Lea and Febiger, 1929), and to Leonard Findlay's chapter in the original edition of this book. For an intellectual treat the medical reader should follow the exciting story of "The etiology of rickets" told by Professor Park in *Physiological Reviews,* 1923, *3,* 106.

Askew, F. A., *et al.* (1932): *Proc. roy. Soc. B., 109,* 488–506.
Bardsley, S. A. (1807): *Medical reports of cases and experiments.* London, R. Bickerstaff.
Barlow, T. (1883): *Med.-chir. Trans., 66,* 159–220.
Basch, K. (1906): *Jb. Kinderheilk., N. F. 64,* 285–335.
Bennett, J. H. (1841): *Treatise on the oleum jecoris aselli, or cod liver oil.* Edinburgh, Maclachlan, Stewart & Co.

Boot, A. (1649): *Observationes medicae de affectibus omissis*. London, T. Whitaker.

Browne, Sir T. (1931): *The works of*. Edited by Geoffrey Keynes. London, Faber and Faber. Vol. 5, p. 385; Vol. 6, p. 287.

Chossat (1842): *C. R. Acad. Sci., Paris, 14*, 451–54.

Cushny, A. R. (1918): *A text-book of pharmacology and therapeutics*. 7th ed.; (1924) 8th ed. London, J. and A. Churchill.

Drummond, J. C., and A. Wilbraham (1939): *The Englishman's food*. London.

Eijkman, C. (1897): *Virchows Arch., 148*, 523–32.

Elsässer, C. L. (1843): *Der weiche Hinterkopf*. Stuttgart and Tübingen, J. G. Cotta.

Erdheim, J. (1911): *S. B. Akad. Wiss., Wien, 96*, abt. 3.

Findlay, L. (1908): *Brit. med. J., ii*, 13–17.

Foote, J. A. (1927): *Amer. J. Dis. Child., 34*, 443–52.

Funk, C. (1912): *J. State Med., 20*, 341.

Fürst, C.: *See* Sigerist, H. P. 47.

Gee, S. (1868): *St. Bart's Hosp. Rep., 4*, 69–80.

Glisson, F. (1650): *De rachitide sive morbo puerili, qui vulgo The Rickets dicitur*. Londini, typ. G. Du-gardi.

Gocht, H. (1898): *Lehrbuch der Röntgen-Untersuchung zum Gebrauche für Mediciner*. Stuttgart, F. Enke.

Greenwood, M. (1948): *Medical statistics from Graunt to Farr*. Cambridge, Cambridge University Press. P. 29.

Guerin, J. (1838): *Gaz. méd. Paris, 6*, 332.

Hansemann, D. von (1906): *Berl. klin. Wschr., 43*, 249–54; 629–31; 670–73.

Hess, A. F. (1924): *Amer. J. Dis. Child., 28*, 517–20.

Hess, A. F. (1929): *Rickets, including osteomalacia and tetany*. Philadelphia, Lea and Febiger.

Hess, A. F., and L. J. Unger (1917): *J. Amer. med. Ass., 69*, 1583–86.

Hopkins, F. G. (1906): *Analyst, 31*, 385–404.

Huldschinsky, K. (1919): *Dtsch. med. Wschr., 45*, 712–13.

Huntly, W. (1889): *Investigation into the habits and diet of the natives of Rajputana with reference to the etiology and treatment of rickets*. Ajmere, Rajputana Mission Press. P. 23.

Iovane, A., and S. Forte (1907): *Pediatria, Napoli, 2., sér. 5*, 641–70.

Koch, J. (1911): *Z. Hyg. InfektKr., 69*, 436–62.

Lanz, O. (1894): *Samml. klin. Vortr., N. F.* No. 98, 29–62.

Lunin, N. (1881): *Hoppe-Seyl. Z., 5*, 31–39.

Mayow, J. (1907): *Medico-physical works, 1674*. London, Simpkin, Marshall, Hamilton, Kent & Co.

McCollum, E. V. (1952): *J. Pediat., 41*, 646–50.

McCollum, E. V., and M. Davis (1913): *J. biol. Chem., 15*, 167–75.

McCollum, E. V., et al. (1921): *J. biol. Chem., 45*, 333; (1922) *Ibid., 50*, 5–29; *51*, 41.

Rickets

Mellanby, E. (1918): *J. Physiol.*, *52*, xi–xii, liii-liv.

Mellanby, E. (1921): *Spec. Rep. Ser. med. Res. Coun., Lond.*, No. 61.

Morpurgo, B. (1900): *Beitr. path. Anat.*, *28*, 620–26.

Moussou, G. (1903): *Bull. Soc. cent. Méd. vét.*, *21.*, 303–309.

Osborne, T. B., and L. B. Mendel (1913): *J. biol. Chem.*, *15*, 311–26.

Palm, T. A. (1890): *Practitioner*, *45*, 270, 321.

Paré, A. (1649): *The workes of.* Translated out of Latin and compared with the French by Tho. Johnson. London, Richard Cotes and Willi Du-gard. P. 584.

Park, E. A., and J. Howland (1921): *Bull. Johns Hopk. Hosp.*, *32*, 341–44.

Percival, T. (1783): *Lond. med. J.*, *3*, 392–401. In *Essays medical, philosophical, and experimental.* 4th ed., 1789. Vol. II.

Pirquet, C. (1923): See Preface to *Spec. Rep. Ser. med. Res. Coun., Lond.* No. 77.

Pommer, G. (1885): *Untersuchungen über Osteomalacie und Rachitis.* Leipzig, F. C. W. Vogel.

"Report on the incidence of rickets in war-time." (1944) *Minist. Hlth Rep. publ. Hlth med. Subj.*, No. 92.

Reusner, J. (1582): *See* Still, G. F. (1931).

Scherer: See Hess, A. F. (1929).

Schmorl, G. (1909):*Ergebn. inn. Med. Kinderheilk.*, *4*, 403–54.

Schütte, D. (1824): *Arch.med. Erfahrung*, *2*, 79–92.

Sigerist, H. (1951): *A history of medicine.* New York, Oxford University Press. Vol. I, p. 47.

Steenbock, H., and M. T. Nelson (1924): *J. biol. Chem.*, *62*, 209–16.

Steenbock, H., and S. W. F. Kletzien (1932): *J. biol. Chem.*, *97*, 249–64.

Still, G. F. (1912): *Common disorders and diseases of childhood.* 2nd ed. London, Henry Frowde and Hodder and Stoughton.

Still, G. F. (1931): *The history of paediatrics.* London, Oxford University Press.

Stoeltzner, W. (1900): *Jb. Kinderheilk.*, *51*, 73–98, 199–221.

"Studies of rickets in Vienna 1919–1922." (1923): *Spec. Rep. Ser. med. Res. Coun., Lond.*, No. 77.

Theodosius, J. B. (1553): *Medicinales epistolae.* Basileae, N. Episcopium.

Trousseau, A., and C. Lasègue (1849): *Arch. gén. Méd.*, 4. sér., t. *19*, 257–87.

Whistler, D. (1645): *De morbo puerili Anglorum quem patrio idiomate indigenae vocant the Rickets.* Lugduni Batavorum, Wilhelmi Christiani Boxii.

Zeviani, G. V. (1761): *Della cura de' bambini attaccati dalla rachitide.* Verona.

BY A. P. CAWADIAS
O. B. E., M. D., F. R. C. P.*

chapter 12 / Diseases of the
endocrine glands

THE FACT that certain organs—glands—of the body secrete into the
bloodstream chemical substances necessary for life was first established through the pioneer work and thought of Thomas Willis in
the seventeenth century, Théophile de Bordeu in the eighteenth century, and J. J. C. Legallois (1801), Thomas Wilkinson King (1836),
and George Gulliver (1840) in the nineteenth century. It was only
in the middle of the nineteenth century, however, that this conception was definitely proved. Arnold Adolph Berthold, completing the
work of John Hunter and giving the experimental stamp to the in-
tuitions of Thomas Willis, in 1849 showed the presence in the testis
of a substance acting on the body as a whole. In 1855 Claude Bernard
also established experimentally the doctrine of internal secretion, and
in the same year—the peak of the history of endocrinology—Thomas
Addison published his great work, *On the constitutional and local
effects of disease of the supra-renal capsules,* and in 1856 C. E. Brown-
Séquard made the first experiment of adrenalectomy. Since then endocrine physiology has made steady progress.

Knowledge of the existence of such glands of internal secretion
allows for the understanding that there are diseases predominantly
due to disturbances of these glands, and the mid-nineteenth century
marks the beginning of endocrine nosology. Diseases which were
isolated and described before the knowledge of internal secretion—
eunuchism, eunuchoidism, cretinism, gigantism, dwarfism, Graves'

* Professor Emeritus of Medicine, Athens University; former endocrinologist of
the Order of St. John Clinic.

disease—were subsequently demonstrated as based on endocrine disturbances, and other diseases are isolated and described as based on such disturbances. There is a tendency, however, among many contemporary endocrinologists to enlarge the physiopathology of these diseases, because the endocrine glands have been demonstrated through recent physiological work to form a part of a large system of metabolic, or constitutional, regulation and integration—a system composed of the cerebral psycho-associational cortex, of the neurovegetative system, of the endocrine system, and of the nuclear genes. Thus, the "diseases of the endocrine glands" of even a few years ago are now considered as constitutional diseases with, however, a more or less important endocrine factor.

From the numerous endocrine diseases described in our textbooks a few will be chosen to show the mode of progress of endocrine nosology and physiopathology.

It is important in each disease to consider: (A) Its natural history, its clinical, anatomical, and laboratory features; its mode of onset, course, and termination. This is the basis of nosology. (B) Its physiopathology and etiology. The disturbance of the function of the organism (the *pathos* of the Greeks), which is manifested as "disease" (the *nosos* of the Greeks), and the etiological conditions which have determined this disturbance. (C) Its treatment.

This division has to be particularly kept in mind in endocrinology because there has been too great a tendency to make clinical medicine (a separate science, the true clinical science) the servant of physiology and pathology; in other words, to recognize clinical pictures in so far as they reflect physiological laws, and to read them in the light of temporary—and often distorted—physiological conceptions.

§ THYROID DISEASES

Graves' Disease. Three clinical scientists dominate the introduction of this disease into nosology. Caleb Hillier Parry of Bath gave the first description in 1825; Robert James Graves of Dublin studied it more completely in 1835; Carl Adolph von Basedow of Merseburg rounded off the work of Graves by adding various symptoms, particularly regarding the eyes, in 1840. The central position occupied by Graves in the history of this disease justifies the eponym "Graves' disease" given by Armand Trousseau in 1860.

Since Basedow's time, highlights in the natural-historical study of this condition are the investigation of the histological features of the thyroid of such patients by William Smith Greenfield (1893), the demonstration of increased basal metabolism by Adolf Magnus-Levy (1895), the account of incomplete (*fruste*) forms by Trousseau in 1860, and later by Pierre Marie and by Jean Martin Charcot, and the differentiation between real Graves' disease and toxic adenoma, mainly by Henry Stanley Plummer in 1913. Contemporary research has enriched the natural history of Graves' disease with various laboratory features, in particular the increase of protein-bound iodine in the blood and the demonstration of the avidity of the thyroid of patients with this disease for iodine (work with iodine isotopes).

From the physiopathological point of view the condition was first considered as a neurosis similar to hysteria, and it was later attributed to a disturbance of the sympathetic nervous system, but in 1886 Paul Julius Möbius ascribed it to abnormal thyroid activity. Recent work has united the nervous and the thyroid conception and it is accepted that Graves' disease is hyperthyroidism due to an abnormal function of the diencephalopituitary system. The causes of this physiopathological disturbance are not as yet well understood, but a certain importance is attached to psychological factors.

From a therapeutic point of view the first methods employed were the general constitutional procedures of good nutrition and hygiene, mental and physical rest, climatotherapy, hydrotherapy, and psychotherapy. Later, iodine was applied, at first sporadically and with a certain hesitation (William Stokes, 1854; Trousseau, 1860), but since David Marine (1912), H. Weller (1914), and principally, H. S. Plummer (1923), more systematically. The more active thiouracil series was introduced by E. B. Astwood in 1943. Radioactive iodine is the latest arrival of these active medicines.

While medical treatment was thus developing, surgery entered into the arena. Partial thyroidectomy was first performed by Sir Patrick Heron Watson in 1874, but it is to William Stewart Halsted since 1907 and to Sir Thomas Peel Dunhill since 1908 that the more general application of this procedure is due. The first interventions were fraught with heavy mortality, but with the perfectioning of anesthetic technique and of pre-operative treatment with the general constitutional methods, iodine, and the thiouracil series, these operations have become very safe. Most clinicians now prefer surgical treatment complemented by medical treatment in the majority of cases, but there are many advocates of an exclusive medical treatment. The recent trend—as in clinical medicine in general—is to consider each case individually. X-ray treatment directed to the thyroid was introduced in 1902 by F. H. Williams of Boston. Deep X-ray treatment directed to the pituitary was first attempted by G. Étienne and P. L. Drouet, but these methods have not found great favor. Radioactive iodine is, in fact, a mode of irradiation, but the results are not yet definite.

Myxedema. This disease was first described in its congenital form by Charles Hilton Fagge in 1871 as "sporadic cretinism," and in the adult form by Sir William Withey Gull in 1874 as "a cretinoid state supervening in adult life in women." The term "myxedema," based on the much discussed and inconstant excess of mucin in the skin of such patients, was coined by William Miller Ord in 1878. Subsequent clinical work resulted in the description of other forms: postoperative myxedema by Jacques Louis Reverdin (1882) and Theodor Kocher (1883), the important *formes frustes* by E. Hertoghe and Léopold Lévi and Henri de Rothschild in the nineties, and, in the last twenty years, the "secondary hypothyroidisms" due to a pituitary lesion or a tumor pressing on the hypothalamus. Important biochemical features were added, beginning with the hypometabolism discovered by Magnus-Levy in 1895.

A certain confusion was introduced in the eighties by the unification—on the basis of the highly simplified physiological conceptions of those days—of myxedema and cretinism. Clinically, cretinism is a different endemic disease, and the application by certain authors of the term "sporadic cretinism" to congenital hypothyroidism is no longer justified.

Effective treatment began with the work of George Redmayne Murray, who in 1891 treated myxedema by subcutaneous injection of a glycerin extract of sheep thyroid, thus initiating one of the greatest discoveries in endocrinotherapy. In the following year H. W. G. Mackenzie used fresh thyroid gland by the mouth. Since then thyroid powder has been used, but recently synthetic thyroxine has been proposed, although its advantages have not been demonstrated.

The Goiters. Goiter was described as bronchocele by the Greeks, translated as struma in Latin, but this term included many other tumors
of the neck, mainly of the lymphatic glands. The isolation from these
bronchoceles of a swelling of the thyroid, thus of a real goiter, is
ascribed to Guilielmus Fabricius in 1617, and since then goiter has
been dismembered into various diseases: goitrous cretinism (Paracelsus), endemic goiter (allied to cretinism), simple sporadic goiter,
the goiter of Graves's disease, and—more recently—cancer of the
thyroid, and certain forms of chronic thyroiditis such as Hashimoto's
disease and Riedel's disease.

The physiopathology of goiter has recently been attributed to an
excess of thyrotropic hormone due to inability of the thyroid to produce thyroid hormone. The causes of this physiopathological disturbance have been studied particularly for endemic goiter, and a
leading role has been attributed, since the work of A. Chatin during
a number of years after 1850, to iodine deficiency, mainly in drinking
water. Recently, various other goitrogens have been described, and
as a development of K. H. Bauer's conception (1926) genetic factors
have been accepted.

Preventive treatment of endemic goiter is based on the iodine
deficiency conception. Important public health measures consisting
of the administration of iodized salt have been instituted in Switzerland, and in the United States of America prophylactic use of iodine
is applied according to the method of D. Marine and O. P. Kimball.

Treatment of the goiter itself with iodine dates from Roger of
Palermo, a surgeon of the school of Salerno in the twelfth century,
who advocated burnt sponge and seaweed, but the treatment was
principally introduced by Jean François Coindet of Geneva in 1820.
This method, however, has been shown to be dangerous in certain
cases, mainly by Kocher in 1910, and is, on the whole, not applied in
simple sporadic or endemic goiters. Surgical treatment was probably
applied in ancient Greek times, if we are to believe Celsus, but its
real introduction was made by the Swiss surgeons Kocher and Reverdin, and developed by William Stewart Halsted of Baltimore and
Sir James Berry of London.

Diseases of the Endocrine Glands

§ DISEASES OF THE ADRENALS

Addison's Disease. This disease was first isolated and described by Thomas Addison in his famous monograph, *On the constitutional and local effects of disease of the supra-renal capsules* (first published in *Lond. med. Gaz.,* 1849, *43,* 517–18), and the eponym "Addison's Disease" for this condition was given by Trousseau in 1856. Addison completely described the clinical features, the anatomical lesions, and tuberculosis and cancer (now considered rare) of the suprarenals. Subsequent work on various biochemical signs and physiological tests enlarged the clinical picture and added adrenal atrophy to the anatomical features. Since the nineties, through the work of Émile Sergent and Léon Bernard, knowledge of other forms of this disease —mainly *formes frustes*—has progressed.

In his original work Addison accepted adrenal disturbance as the physiopathological basis of this disease. Many subsequent authors attributed a greater role to the abdominal sympathetic. However, progress in knowledge of adrenal physiology again directed attention to an adrenal mechanism, which is accepted as consisting mainly in deficiency of the adrenal cortex. The cause of this physiopathological disturbance has been considered for a long time chiefly as a tuberculous infection, but more complete research discovered other etiological factors such as neoplasm—otherwise rare—and, principally, certain obscure factors leading to adrenocortical atrophy.

Treatment has for long been concentrated on the general constitutional methods which have lately been developed parallel with more specific procedures. Adequate nutrition and treatment of digestive disturbances have been recognized from the beginning. Since the work of Jacques Loeb in 1901 the importance of salt has been demonstrated, and since Albert Szent-György's investigations in 1928 vitamin C has been applied. Low potassium diet was advised in 1936 by R. L. Zwemer and R. Truszkowski, but its indications are limited. Specific treatment began with the isolation of active adrenocortical extracts. In 1928 F. A. Hartman applied cortin experimentally, and in 1930 Wilbur Willis Swingle and Joseph John Pfiffner prepared another potent extract, which was successfully applied clinically by Julius Moses Rogoff and George Neil Stewart (1929). The isolation of special adrenocortical steroids such as desoxycorticosterone marks a notable practical advance, but it is the isolation of cortisone which seems to reveal new horizons.

Adrenal Female Intersexuality. Female *pubertas praecox* with masculinization was described long ago. Recognition of a special form connected with adrenocortical hyperplasia or tumor dates from the observation of William Cooke in 1811, followed by other isolated cases, but principally from the work of William Bulloch and James Harry Sequeira in 1905. This last contribution established the adrenocortical physiopathological mechanism, and determined that this condition is due to an hypersecretion of adrenocortical sexual steroids from the tumor or the hyperplasic cortex, occurring after birth but before puberty. Treatment is mainly surgical and consists in the removal of the tumor, or in adrenalectomy developed in England by Lennox Ross Broster. The first successful operations were those of A. Riche in 1907 and H. Gaudier in 1908. Estrogens have been used as palliatives in mild cases, and L. Wilkins has applied cortisone with success (*Arch. Neurol. Paris,* 1907, *3 sér.,* t. 2, 185.).

Female pseudohermaphroditism (genital gynanadroidism) was also known of old. The special form connected with adrenocortical lesion was first described by A. W. Otto in 1816 and principally by Luigi de Crecchio in 1865. Following the memoirs of Bulloch and Sequeira the physiopathological mechanism has been accepted as consisting of adrenal sexual steroids hypersecretion occuring before birth. Palliative treatment has been described by Hugh Hampton Young of Johns Hopkins University.

Virilism also was known of old. The connection between virilism and adrenocortical lesions, dating from the memoirs of Bulloch and Sequeira, is accepted as being determined by hypersecretion of adrenocortical sexual steroids occurring after puberty. Estrogens have been used in mild cases. Adrenalectomy has been developed by Broster.

Cushing's Disease. In 1932 Harvey Cushing isolated from the various constitutional syndromes the disease that bears his name and completely described its clinical features and a basophil adenoma of the pituitary as an anatomical feature. Subsequent authors reported other lesions in cases showing Cushing's symptom complex—principally adrenocortical tumors or hyperplasia. P. Heinbecker (1944) described hypothalamic lesions, and A. C. Crooke (1935) a special pituitary lesion independent of basophile adenoma.

The physiopathological mechanism accepted through this recent work is one of hypersecretion of adrenocortical steroids either primarily or following abnormal hypersecretion of pituitary adrenocorticotropin (ACTH). In fact, cortisone and ACTH in humans have produced Cushing's disease.

Therapeutically, Cushing applied X rays to the pituitary. Other clinicians used estrogens, and F. Albright (1941) used testosterone. Adrenalectomy was applied in cases with adrenal tumor.

Phaeochromocytoma. Ernest Marcel Labbé, Jules Tinel, and E. Doumer first described the anatomical (adrenal medullary tumor) and clinical (paroxysmal hypertension) features of this disease in 1922. During these last years the clinico-anatomical picture was completed by the description of a form with chronic hyperpiesia and the addition of biochemical signs and certain physiological tests (benzodioxane). Surgical treatment has been applied since 1929 (Maurice C. Pincoffs).

§ DISEASES OF THE PITUITARY

Acromegaly. This disease was first isolated and described by Pierre Marie in 1886. His first description was purely clinical, but in 1891 with G. Marinesco he added the pituitary lesion. C. Benda in 1900 developed the anatomical features by showing microscopic increase in eosinophile cells. Recent work has added biochemical features— mainly an increase in inorganic phosphorus.

Oscar Minkowski in 1887 accepted a pituitary dysfunction as a physiopathological basis of this condition, a conception which was upheld and elaborated by Pierre Marie himself. R. Massalongo in 1892 accepted this dysfunction as hyperpituitarism, and Dean Lewis accepted it in 1905 as eosinophile hyperpituitarism. The discovery of the growth hormone and the experimental work of Harvey Cushing demonstrated that the ultimate mechanism was hypersecretion of growth hormone.

Therapeutically, F. T. Paul applied decompression in 1893. J. Hochenegg in 1909 performed the first operation for the removal of

211

the causal eosinophile tumor, and this procedure was followed on a large scale by Cushing. Radiological treatment was introduced simultaneously in 1909 by A. Gramegna of Turin and A. Béclère of Paris. Recently, estrogens and testosterone have been applied as palliatives.

Adiposogenital Dystrophy (Babinski-Fröhlich Disease). This disease was first described by Joseph Babinski of Paris in June, 1900. In June, 1901, Alfred Fröhlich described the same disease, curiously without any reference to Babinski's description, which, however, was more complete. Babinski, and later Fröhlich, connected the clinical picture with a tumor of the pituitary. Later, postencephalitic and functional adiposogenital dystrophies (that is, without any pituitary lesions) were reported.

Babinski and Fröhlich first accepted a pituitary dysfunction as the basic physiopathological mechanism. The work of Gustave Roussy and his pupils, however, showed that the basic mechanism was hypothalamic dysfunction, the pituitary tumor pressing on the hypothalamus.

Simmonds' Disease (Pituitary Cachexia). This disease was described by Morris Simmonds of Hamburg in 1914, although the Pole, L. K. Glinski, may be considered as the precursor according to Douglas Robertson. Simmonds described the clinical and anatomical features and insisted on cachexia as a prominent symptom.

Anatomically, he described pituitary necrosis following septic embolus and pituitary tumor. H. L. Sheehan in 1939 reported in detail a special form of this disease connected with postpartum necrosis, in which cachexia does not seem a leading symptom. Subsequent work showed the existence of a general atrophy or sclerosis of nearly all the endocrine glands—easily understood on account of the prominent role of the anterior pituitary in the endocrine system—and thus included in this disease the "pluriglandular insufficiency" of H. Claude and H. Gougerot. Various biochemical symptoms were added recently.

An attempt has been made to consider anorexia nervosa as a special form of Simmonds' disease, but from the point of view of natural history it is a separate disease. "Functional" forms, that is, without pituitary lesions, and *formes frustes* (G. von Bergmann's (1934) "pituitary leanness") have been described.

212

From a physiopathological point of view, this condition has been considered as based on a failure of all pituitary hormones, a failure due to hemorrhage, necrosis, sepsis, trauma of the pituitary, or to a diencephalic infection.

Active treatment began with the discovery of the first potent anterior pituitary preparation, the prolan of Hermann Zondek. Later, testosterone, growth hormone, and adrenocortical preparations were added and proved more effective. Pituitary grafts have been attempted (E. W. V. Kylin).

§ DISEASES OF THE PANCREAS

Diabetes Mellitus. As with so many diseases, knowledge of diabetes is of great antiquity; it was probably known in ancient Egypt and ancient India, but the first scientific isolation and description of this disease dates from Aretaeus of Cappadocia in the first century A.D. His description was clinical, and he insisted on the polyuria—hence the name "diabetes," which he adopted—and the emaciation.

Suśruta, the Indian, in the fifth century A.D. and Avicenna in the eleventh century noted the sweet taste of the urine in Aretaeus's disease, and this was confirmed by Thomas Willis in 1674. In 1776 Matthew Dobson of Liverpool proved that the sweet taste was due to sugar, and this enabled Johann Peter Frank in 1794 to separate from Aretaeus's disease—known from that time as *diabetes mellitus* or *verus*—the spurious or "insipid" diabetes. The next milestones in the natural history of diabetes were the description of diabetic coma by William Prout (1840), of diabetic acidosis in general by Bernard Naunyn in 1906, and the differentiation between fat and lean diabetes by Étienne Lancereaux in 1880. Recent work has added important biochemical signs. For a long time anatomical features were not characteristic, but in 1778 Thomas Cawley described pancreatic calculi in one of his cases, and towards the middle and end of the nineteenth century Lancereaux, Richard Bright, and F. T. Frerichs reported pancreatic lesions.

The physiopathology of diabetes was centered, according to Lancereaux, in the pancreas (at least for thin diabetics), and this was confirmed by the famous experiment of pancreatectomy of Joseph von Mering and Oscar Minkowski in 1889. As E. Laguesse of Lille and E. Hédon of Montpellier in 1893 ascribed an endocrine function to the islands of Langerhans of the pancreas, this disease became an endocrine disease of pancreatic origin, and the discovery of insulin by Sir Frederick Grant Banting and Charles Herbert Best in 1921—one of the greatest discoveries in medicine—crowned this conception.

However, things were not so simple. The carbohydrate metabolism, the disturbance of which makes diabetes, is controlled not only by insulin, but by other hormones—principally by the diabetogenic factor of the anterior pituitary—as shown by the work of B. A. Houssay and F. G. Young (1937), and thus diabetes is considered to be determined by the upsetting of the balance between insulin and contra-insulin hormones.

Treatment of diabetes before the discovery of insulin was focused on diet and was not very successful. Apollinaire Bouchardat's method of carbohydrate restriction was popular in the last half of the nineteenth century. Since the work of Guillaume Guelpa (1910), total restriction of food was adopted and was codified by Frederick M. Allen in 1914. With the advent of insulin, diet became more rational, and with the help of this hormone diabetics can now live and work.

Hypoglycemia. The existence of this disease—the converse of diabetes —was postulated in 1924 by Seale Harris, but it was not until 1927 that this condition was introduced into nosology through the work of R. M. Wilder and his associates, who described hypoglycemia as being connected with a pancreatic tumor originating in the islands of Langerhans. Later, other hypoglycemias unconnected with pancreatic tumor were reported, the most interesting being the "functional hypoglycemias" of neurogenic origin. Hyperinsulinism was considered the physiopathological basis of the pancreatic neoplastic form of hypoglycemia. The first successful result through removal of the pancreatic tumor was accomplished by E. Mathias in 1928.

§ DISEASES OF THE GONADS

Eunuchoidism. Male eunuchoidism was first mentioned by Hippocrates, but a more complete description is to be found in the work of Théophile de Bordeu in the eighteenth century. French and Italian clinicians of the nineteenth century completed the clinical picture, and modern research has added biochemical and, principally, hormonic features. The similarity of the symptoms of this condition to the symptoms found in eunuchs centered the physiopathological mechanism on testicular endocrine deficiency of primary or pituitary origin.

Female eunuchoidism was first described by Bordeu under the term of "the Female Eunuch."

Climacteric Disease. Female climacteric disease was described in olden times, but its modern knowledge dates from the work of Gregorio Maranon (1929). Unfortunately, too many dissimilar conditions have been dumped into this syndrome, and a clearer study is awaited. The physiopathological mechanism is centered on the involutional hypoovarism, but recent work has demonstrated the great role of psychological factors. The use of estrogens and a rational psychotherapy have greatly improved the prognosis of this condition.

Male climacteric disease also has been the dumping ground for many morbid conditions of middle age and has been completely dismissed on the basis of lack of definite laboratory features. Sir Henry Halford described this condition in 1831, and clinicians recognize the accurateness of his description.

§ DISEASES OF THE PARATHYROIDS

Hypoparathyroidism. The natural history of hypoparathyroidism began with the discovery by Giulio Vassale and F. Generali in 1896 of the connection of certain tetanies with a parathyroid lesion. The next important step was the finding in these cases of a diminution of calcium in the blood (William George MacCallum and Carl Voegtlin, 1908). Many other clinical and laboratory features were added later. John Abercrombie (1880) and František Chvostek (1876) directed attention to the facial irritability elicited by tapping the facial nerve.

The first cases described were those following strumectomy (i.e., parathyroidectomy). Later, "idiopathic" forms were considered, and F. Albright recently described the "pseudohypoparathyroidism," in which hormonic secretion of the parathyroids is normal, but sensitiveness of the target cells to this hormone is deficient.

The hypoparathyroidean physiopathological basis of this condition developed slowly, but progress of knowledge of the function of the parathyroids was crowned by James Bertram Collip's discovery of parathormone in 1925.

The outstanding therapeutic agent for this condition, calcium administration, was introduced through the work of W. M. Boothby in 1930.

Hyperparathyroidism. The natural history of this disease began with the discovery by J. Erdheim in 1907 of the connection between osteitis fibrosa cystica (described by Friedrich Daniel von Recklinghausen in 1891) and parathyroid lesion, and was crowned by the therapeutical result of parathyroidectomy (Felix Mandl, 1926). Recent work has completed the clinical picture and has added the important renal syndrome. The basic parathyroid lesion first considered was neoplasm (adenoma and more rarely carcinoma), but lately the presence of hyperplasia has been demonstrated.

§ PINEAL AND THYMUS

Pineal Pubertas Praecox. Pubertas praecox—principally male— associated with a pineal tumor, usually a teratoma, was described in 1899 by O. Heubner. There is some discussion regarding its physiopathology, as some authors consider that the sexual precocity and the macrogenitosomia in general is due to a hormone secreted by the tumor, and others hold that it is determined by the pressure of the tumor on the hypothalamic centers of the endocrine system. These tumors are highly radiosensitive, and X-ray treatment is usually applied. Pinealectomy was first performed by Walter Edward Dandy in 1921, but it is a very dangerous operation.

Status Thymicolymphaticus. The clinical and anatomical features of this condition were described in 1889 by A. Paltauf, and the physiopathological basis was considered as centered in a disturbance of the thymus. However, as this physiopathological mechanism was not demonstrated, the passing of this disease was announced. In fact, status thymicolymphaticus exists as a clinico-anatomical entity. Only its original thymic conception has passed and is being replaced by an adrenal deficiency conception introduced by David Marine in 1926,

216

and even this present-day physiopathological conception may be replaced tomorrow by yet another.

The history of our knowledge of status thymicolymphaticus is one more illustration of the necessity for separating clinical science (the nosology of the Greeks)—the science of disease as manifested to us —from physiopathology (the pathology of the Greeks)—the science of morbid processes. It shows, also, that clinical pictures remain, while pathological conceptions are ever changing.

§ REFERENCES

Abercrombie, J. (1880): *On tetany in young children.* London, Baillière, Tindall and Cox.

Addison, T. (1855): *On the constitutional and local effects of disease of the supra-renal capsules.* London, Samuel Highley.

Albright, F., *et al.* (1942): *Endocrinology, 30,* 922–32.

Albright, F., W.Parson, and E.Bloomberg (1941): *J. clin. Endocrinol., 1,* 375–84.

Allen, F. M. (1914): *J. Amer. med. Ass., 63,* 939–43.

Aretaeus the Cappadocian (1856): *The extant works of.* Edited and translated by Francis Adams. London, Sydenham Society. P. 338.

Babinski, J. (1900): *Rev. neurol., 8,* 531–33.

Basedow, C. A. von (1840): *Wschr. ges. Heilk., 6,* 197–220.

Béclère, A. (1909): *Bull. Soc. méd. Hôp. Paris, 3 sér., 26,* 274–93.

Benda, C. (1900): *Berl. klin. Wschr., 37,* 1205–10.

Bernard, C. (1855): *Leçons de physiologie expérimentale appliquée à la médecine.* Paris, J.-B. Baillière. P. 100.

Berthold, A. A. (1849): *Arch. Anat. Physiol. wiss. Med., 42,* 6.

Bordeu, T. (1818): *Oeuvres complètes.* Paris, Caille and Ravier. Vol. II, p. 492.

Broster, L. R., and H. W. C. Vines (1933): *The adrenal cortex.* London, H. K. Lewis.

Bulloch, W., and J. H. Sequeira (1905). *Trans. path. Soc. Lond., 56,* 189–208.

Caton, R., and F. T. Paul (1893): *Brit. med. J., ii,* 1421–23.

Cawley, T. (1788): *Lond. med. J., 9,* 286–308.

Chvostek, F. (1876): *Wien. med. Pr., 17,* 1201, 1226, 1314.

Collip, J. B. (1925): *J. biol. Chem., 63,* 395–438.

Cooke, W. (1809): *Med.-chir. Trans., 2,* 17–23.

Creccio, L. de (1865): *Sopra un caso di apparenze virile in una donna.* Napoli, F. Vitale.

Crooke, A. C. (1935): *J. Path. Bact., 41,* 339–49.

Cushing, H. (1932): *Bull. Johns Hopk. Hosp., 50,* 137–95.

Dobson, M. (1776): *Medical observations and inquiries by a society of physicians, 5,* 298–316.

Erdheim, J. (1906): *Mitt. Grenzgeb. Med. Chir., 16,* 632–744.

Fagge, C. H. (1871): *Med.-chir. Trans., 54*, 155–70.

Fröhlich, A. (1901): *Wien. klin. Rdsch., 15*, 883, 906.

Gaudier, M. (1908): *Bull. Soc. Chir. Paris, N. S. 34*, 712–14.

Graves, R. J. (1835): *Lond. med. surg. J.* (Renshaw), 7, 516–17.

Greenfield, W. S. (1893): *Lancet, ii*, 1493–97, 1553–55.

Guelpa, G. (1910): *Brit. med. J., ii*, 1050–51.

Gull, Sir W. W. (1874): *Trans. clin. Soc. Lond.*, 7, 180–85.

Halsted, W. S. (1907): *Amer. J. med. Sci., 134*, 1–12.

Hartman, F. A., *et al.* (1928): *Amer. J. Physiol., 86*, 353–59.

Hédon, E. (1893): *Arch. Physiol. norm. path. Paris*, 5, sér., t. 5, 154–63.

Heinbecker, P. (1944): *Medicine, Baltimore, 23*, 225–47.

Hochenegg, J. (1909): *Dtsch. Z. Chir., 100*, 317–26.

Houssay, B. A., and M. A. Magenta (1924): *Rev. Asoc. méd. argent., 37*, 389–406.

Kussmaul, A. (1874): *Dtsch. Arch. klin. Med., 14*, 1–46.

Kylin, E. (1937): *Acta med. scand., 91*, 428–34.

Labbé, M., J. Tinel, and Doumer (1922): *Bull. Soc. méd. Hóp. Paris, 3 sér., 46*, 982–90.

Laguesse, E. (1893): *C. R. Soc. Biol. Paris, 45*, 819–20.

Lancereaux, E. (1877): *Bull. Acad. Méd. Paris*, 2, ser., t. 6, 1215–40.

Lewis, D. D. (1905): *Bull. Johns Hopk. Hosp., 16*, 157–64.

Loeb, R. F. (1932): *Science, 76*, 420–21.

MacCallum, W. G., and C. Voegtlin (1909): *J. exp. Med., 11*, 118–51.

Mackenzie, H. W. G. (1892): *Brit. med. J., ii*, 940–41.

Magnus-Levy, A. (1895): *Berl. klin. Wsch., 32*, 650–52.

Mandl, F. (1926): *Arch. klin. Chir., 143*, 245–84.

Maranon, G. (1929): *The climacteric*. London, Henry Kimpton.

Marie, P. (1889): *Progr. méd., Paris*, 2 sér., 9, 189–92.

Marie, P. (1886): *Rev. Méd.*, 6, 297–333.

Marie, P., and G. Marinesco (1891): *Arch. Méd. exp.*, 3, 539–65.

Marine, D. (1912): Quoted in L. M. Warfield (1924): *Trans. Ass. Amer. Phys., 39*, 179.

Marine, D. (1926): *Arch. Path. (Lab. Med.)*, 1, 175–79.

Massalongo, R. (1892): *Rif. med.*, 8, 74, 87.

Mathias (1928): *Med. Klinik, 24*, 1814. Quoted in K. A. Meyer, L. Amtman, and L. Perlman (1941): *J. Amer. med. Ass., 117*, 16–20.

Mayo, C. H. (1927): *J. Amer. med. Ass.*, 89, 1047–50.

Mering, J. von, and O. Minkowski (1889): *Arch. exp. Path. Pharmak., 26*, 371–87.

Minkowski, O. (1887): *Berl. klin. Wschr., 24*, 371–74.

Möbius, P. J. (1896): In *Nothnagel's Spezielle Pathologie und Therapie*. Vienna, A. Hölder. Band 20.

Murray, G. R. (1891): *Brit. med. J., ii*, 796–97.

Naunyn, B. (1898): *Der Diabetes melitus*. Vienna, A. Hölder.

Otto (1816): Quoted in Bulloch and Sequeira.

Diseases of the Endocrine Glands

Paltauf, A. (1889): *Wien. klin. Wschr.*, 2, 877–81.

Papaspyros, N. S. (1952): *The history of diabetes mellitus.* London.

Parry, C. H. (1825): *Collections from the unpublished medical writings.* London, Underwoods. Vol. II, pp. 111–29.

Prout, W. (1840): Quoted in H. Rolleston (1936): *The endocrine organs in health and disease.* London, Oxford University Press.

Recklinghausen, F. v. (1891): In Rudolf Virchow's *Festschrift.* Berlin, Georg Reimer.

Riche, A. (1907): *Thèse.* Lille.

Robertson, D. J. (1951): *Brit. med. J.,* i, 921–23.

Rogoff, J. M., and G. N. Stewart (1929): *J. Amer. med. Ass.,* 92, 1569–71.

Sheehan, H. L. (1939): *Quart. J. Med.,* N. S. 8, 277–309.

Simmonds, M. (1914): *Dtsch. med. Wschr.,* 40, 322–23.

Swingle, W. W., and J. J. Pfiffner (1930): *Science,* 71, 321.

Vassale, G., and F. Generali (1896): *Riv. Patol. nerv. ment.,* 1, 95–99.

Watson, P. H. (1873): *Edinb. med. J.,* 19, 252–55.

Williams, F. H. (1902): *The roentgen rays in medicine and surgery.* 2nd. ed. New York, Macmillan. P. 679.

Willis, T. (1674): *Pharmaceutice rationalis.* Oxoniae, E. Theatro Sheldoniano. Sect. IV. Cap. III.

Young, F. G. (1937): *Lancet,* ii, 372–74.

Young, H. H. (1937): *Genital abnormalities.* Baltimore, Williams and Wilkins.

Cortisone

Hench, P. S., E. C. Kendall, *et al.* (1949): *Ann. rheum. Dis.,* 8, 97.

Kendall, E. C., *et al.* (1934): *Trans. Ass. Amer. Phys.,* 49, 147.

Proc. Mayo Clin., 1935, 10, 245.

Wintersteiner, O., and J. J. Pfiffner (1935): *J. biol. Chem.,* 109, C.

Only a few of the more important references from an historical point of view can be given. More detailed references will be found in:

Rolleston, Sir H. D. (1936): *The endocrine organs in health and disease with an historical review.* London, Oxford University Press.

Cawadias, A. P. (1947): *Clinical endocrinology and constitutional medicine.* London, Frederick Muller.

BY DONALD C. BALFOUR

M. D., LL. D., D. Sc., F. R. C. S. Eng.*

chapteR 13 / Gallstones

THE HISTORY of gallstones was so concisely summarized by the late Sir David Wilkie† in the first edition of this book that any revision of his article becomes not only unnecessary but would detract from the orderly presentation of the significant contributions which have led to our present concept of this disease. For this reason it seems appropriate to preserve Sir David's chapter as it was written, with the addition of a brief summary of the further advances which have been made since his death in 1938.

Sir David divided this subject roughly into three periods: (1) an early period when the presence of gallstones was noted in bodies dissected or embalmed; (2) a period when the structure and composition of gallstones were investigated and when the clinical significance of their presence in the gall bladder or ducts was appreciated and the complications to which they give rise described; and (3) a modern period, the outstanding feature of which has been the development of the surgical treatment of the condition.

In ancient medical records there is a curious and possibly significant absence of any mention of gallstones. Greek writers are silent on this subject, and the suggestion has been advanced that the athletic life and simple fare of the Greeks rendered them relatively immune to biliary trouble. Although Trallianus in the sixth century is often credited with the first definite reference to gallstones, we find that Galen in the second century was familiar with them and considered

---

* Chief, surgery division, Mayo Foundation, Rochester, Minnesota.

† Sir David Percival Dalbreck Wilkie (1882–1938), professor of surgery, University of Edinburgh (1924–38).

that they were due to coagulation of the bile. Haly Abbas, a Persian physician of the tenth century, recorded the presence of calculi in the liver, and Gentile da Foligno in the fourteenth century described gallstones found by him in a body which he was embalming. Vesalius (1543) and Fallopius both described the presence of gallstones in dissected bodies, and Johann Kentmann (1665) gave illustrations of gallstones of various shapes and sizes and noted that the more numerous they were the more angular were their shapes.

That gallstones occur in lower animals was recognized by the Jews, as shown by reference to Joseph Caro's sixteenth-century *Shulhan 'Aruch,* the final and authoritative codification of the Talmudic law. After mentioning certain abnormalities of the gall bladder, some of which were held to render the carcase either fit to be eaten (*kosher*) or unfit for food (*terefah*) it continues: "If hard things are found in the gall-bladder, which are like the pits of dates, without sharp edges, the animal is *kosher:* but if the edges are sharp, as in the pits of olives, the animal is *terefah*."

§ THE STRUCTURE AND FORMATION OF GALLSTONES

Jean François Fernel (1554) made important observations, notably that gallstones will float in water and that occlusion of the cystic duct was often present when gallstones were found in the gall bladder. He considered, therefore, that stasis of the bile was an important factor in determining their formation. Paracelsus (1616) in his doctrine of "Tartarus," expressed the belief that this noxious matter could be formed from the nourishment taken and from the destruction of tissues, and that this impure material might precipitate in the biliary passages, bile being a coagulant of "tartarus." He may therefore be described as the founder of the metabolic theory of gallstone formation, a theory of which Aschoff is the modern protagonist.

Morgagni (1767) discovered the presence of glands in the wall of the gall bladder. He emphasized the importance of age, sedentary habits, and irritation or inflammation of the glands in the gall bladder wall as factors in gallstone formation. He may therefore be regarded as the father of the inflammatory theory of gallstone formation.

The isolation of cholesterol by Pouilletier de la Salle in 1740 gave a new impetus to the study of gallstones, and Vicq d'Azyr a few years later described the two types of gallstone, those composed of cholesterol and those containing, in addition, bile pigment.

Meckel von Hemsbach (1856) made many important observations on both the origin and structure of gallstones. He supported strongly the view of Morgagni that a catarrh of the mucous membrane of the gall bladder was a leading factor in gallstone formation. In later years the name of Bernard Naunyn has been associated with this theory. Meckel was a geologist, and he studied particularly the secondary changes which occur in gallstones. He pointed out how, by the recrystallization of cholesterol, the structure of a gallstone may be slowly changed and noted the tendency for cholesterol crystals to assume a radiate arrangement.

The discovery of Antonio Vallisnieri (1730) that gallstones were soluble in turpentine led to the use of this drug, both as a preventive measure and as a means of dissolving gallstones—a practice which persisted for many years.

§ THE CLINICAL RECOGNITION OF GALLSTONE DISEASE

Antonio Benivieni and Jean François Fernel in the sixteenth century gave graphic descriptions of biliary colic, and Fernel made the important observation that the presence of jaundice and clay-colored stools was associated with the arrest of a stone in the common bile duct. Francis Glisson (1597–1677) was himself a sufferer from gallstones and recorded his own symptoms in an attack of colic, mentioning the peculiar pain radiating to the right shoulder and the clavicular region and the jaundice which followed the pain. Friedrich Hoffmann (1733) first identified the phrenic nerve as the link between the abdominal and shoulder tip pains of biliary colic.

Many discriminating and important observations were made by Michael Ettmüller (1708), and his conclusions in the correlation of symptoms with the underlying pathology have stood the test of time. He argued that since Teckof, a student in Leyden, had removed the gall bladder in dogs without causing jaundice, stones may be present in the gall bladder and may give rise to pain without jaundice. He made particular note of the nausea, precordial pain, and catch in the breathing which accompany some gallstone attacks and the jaundice and pale stools which follow in certain cases.

Alexis Pujol (1823) made an important observation, namely the sensation of extreme epigastric tension in a gallstone attack, a sensation accentuated when pressure is made by the hand over the gall bladder. He was the first to record the correct explanation of many attacks of biliary colic, namely that a stone becomes impacted in the cystic duct, and that the subsidence of the colic is due either to the cessation of contraction of the gall bladder wall or to the stone disengaging and dropping back into the lumen of the gall bladder.

Attacks of acute obstructive cholecystitis were described by many medical writers, but perhaps the most graphic descriptions were the following from the letters of Sir Walter Scott, who suffered from recurring attacks at the time of his greatest literary activity. To J. B. S. Morritt he wrote in March 1817:

I have been plagued all through this winter with cramp in my stomach which I endured as a man of mould might, and endeavoured to combat them by drinking scalding water and so forth. On the 5th I had a most violent attack which broke up a small party at my house and sent me to bed, roaring like a bull-calf, and all sorts of remedies were applied, as in the case of Gil Blas' pretended colic, but such was the pain of the real disorder that it out-devilled the doctor hollow. Even heated salt, which was applied in such a state that it burned my shirt to rags, I hardly felt when clapped on my stomach. At length the symptoms became inflammatory, and dangerously so, the seat being the diaphragm.

Again he wrote to Miss Clephane:

The cause was a cramp in my stomach which, after various painful visits, as if it had been sent by Prospero and had mistaken me for Caliban, at length chose to conclude by setting fire to its lodging like the Frenchmen as they retreated through Russia, and placed me in a proper state of inflammation.

The syndrome associated with the presence of stones in the common bile duct was described by many early writers, but the classical picture of the intermittent colic, with rigors and fever, followed by jaundice and associated with loss of weight, was given by Jean-Martin Charcot in 1877.

Ludwig George Courvoisier (1890) remarked that in cases of obstructive jaundice, due to causes other than stone, the gall bladder was distended; when due to stone in the duct the gall bladder was usually contracted from preceding inflammation. This observation, which has come to be known as "Courvoisier's law," is found to hold good in over 80 per cent of cases.

§ THE SURGICAL TREATMENT OF GALLSTONES

While the surgery of the biliary passages is mainly a development of the post-Listerian period, there are many isolated records of operations for gallstones during the two preceding centuries. The first recorded operation is of doubtful authenticity—that of Johann Georg Fabricius (1618). The patient certainly did not survive the operation, which was possibly a post-mortem one. There are several records of what may be termed accidental gallstone operations, e. g. Cornelius S. Stalpart van der Wiel (1687) and Amyord (1738) recorded the removal of gallstones after opening abscesses which were pointing in the upper part of the abdomen.

The founder of the surgery of the gall bladder was unquestionably Jean Louis Petit. In 1733 this surgeon suggested that when the diagnosis of a large and inflamed gall bladder adherent to the anterior abdominal wall was made it should be cut down on and the pus and gallstones evacuated. In 1743 he carried out such an operation with success, puncturing the gall bladder, passing in a probe to detect the stone, and then enlarging the opening and removing the stone. His advocacy of this operation fell on deaf ears, as the fear of opening the peritoneal cavity possessed the minds of all the surgeons of his day.

Guilielmus Michael Richter (1798) suggested that adhesion of the gall bladder to the abdominal wall was not an essential preliminary to operation.

During the first half of the nineteenth century several writers, among whom may be mentioned Sebastian (1828), Robert James Graves of Dublin shortly afterwards, and Johann Ludwig Wilhelm Thudichum (1859), advocated a two-stage operation for gallstones. At the first operation the fundus of the gall bladder was exposed and an endeavor made to produce adhesions to the anterior abdominal wall by packing down to it or by stitching it to the wall (Thudichum).

John Stough Bobbs of Indianapolis is frequently referred to as the pioneer of modern gall bladder surgery. His first recorded case (1867) was one of an abdominal tumor of unknown origin. He exposed a large cyst, opened it, and evacuated much clear fluid and several gallstones. He then closed the dilated gall bladder and returned it to the abdomen. The patient made a good recovery.

With the adoption of the Listerian principles surgeons no longer feared to venture into the peritoneal cavity, and operations for gallstones became common. A pioneer who scorned the benefits of antiseptic surgery was Lawson Tait, who in 1879 recorded his first case of cholecystotomy for gallstones. In the next four and a half years Tait did this operation fourteen times with but one fatality.

Marion Sims, remembered now chiefly as a distinguished gynecologist, did much to establish biliary surgery on a sound footing. His first recorded case (1878), one of operation for drainage of the gall bladder in a deeply jaundiced patient, was performed in Paris with antiseptic precautions and under the carbolic spray. Sims introduced the term "cholecystotomy," which has formed the basis for the nomenclature of the various operations on the biliary tract since introduced.

The operation of cholecystectomy was proved to be without notable ill effects on animals by Giuseppe Zambecarri in 1708 and even earlier by Teckof, a medical student in Leyden. In 1882 Carl Johann August Langenbuch recorded the first cholecystectomy on the human subject. The operation of opening the common bile duct to remove a stone was introduced by Adolf Kümmell and first successfully practiced by Courvoisier (1890).

Johann Nepomuk von Nussbaum in 1882 was the first to suggest that where an irremovable obstruction of the common duct existed an anastomosis might be made between the gall bladder and the intestine, and von Winwarter recorded the first example of such an anastomosis, the gall bladder being implanted into the hepatic flexure of the colon. Later, on the suggestion of Bernhard Bardenheuer, Cozi anastomosed the gall bladder to the duodenum.

During the past forty years progress in biliary surgery has been remarkable. Chiefly because of the work and writings of Sir Arthur Mayo-Robson and Moynihan in England, of the Mayo brothers in America, and Hans Kehr in Germany, what were formerly regarded as operations of hazard and uncertainty are now practiced the world over with safety and success.

Intensive studies of the physiology of the gall bladder by Francis

Peyton Rous and P. D. McMaster, Whitaker and Ivy, Mann and Bollman, and of its pathology by Karl Albert Ludwig Aschoff and his pupils have shown that the healthy gall bladder has an important function.

The history of gallstones as thus recorded by Wilkie is the background on which our present knowledge of diseases of the gall bladder is based. The vast literature of recorded clinical experience and experimental investigation in the past half century has established certain facts and principles of primary importance in the development of the medical and surgical management of the disease. These may be summarized as follows:

The incidence of gallstones in man has become more definitely established through better understanding of the symptoms associated with such concretions, through roentgenological examination, through abdominal operations, and through necropsy. From such sources of information it is now known that gallstones may occur at any age, but that they tend to occur most commonly after middle life. For example, necropsy performed on men and women past forty years of age showed that 20 per cent of them had had gallstones, men having had 16 per cent and women 32 per cent. On males and females of all ages, 16.3 per cent were found to have had gallstones. This figure does not, of course, represent the incidence of gallstones in the general population, since necropsy statistics are based chiefly on records of patients who had required admission to a hospital.

Primitive races, possibly because of simpler diet, supposedly had a high degree of immunity to calculous formations, but little statistical evidence is available to support this impression.

The incidence of gallstones in animals having gall bladders is low, but stones have been found in the ox, sheep, pig, and dog.

The morphological characteristics of gallstones were classified by Aschoff and A. Bacmeister[1] in 1909, and their classification has not been materially modified in the intervening years. Sir Humphry Rolleston and J. W. McNee[2] (1929) described the following types of gallstones:

Gallstones

§ TABLE OF CLASSIFICATION OF GALLSTONES

I. *Aseptic or Metabolic*
   (a) *Pure, solitary, radiate cholesterol stones.*
   (b) (probably) Pigment-calcium stones. Mulberry stones. "Pure pigment stones" of the older textbooks.
II. *Inflammatory or Septic*
   (a) *Cholesterol-pigment-calcium* stones. The common "multiple faceted gall-stones."
   (b) *Combination stones.* 1. The typical combination stone with a pure aseptic radiate cholesterol stone as center, surrounded by a dense laminated coat of mixed cholesterol-pigment-calcium of inflammatory origin. 2. The friable *earthy stone* of the bile ducts, with any sort of foreign body or gallstone as center, and loose crumbling cholesterol-pigment-calcium covering.
III. *Uncommon Forms of Calculi*
   (a) *Laminated cholesterol stones*—really *cholesterol-calcium* stones. Two varieties: (1) single stones, and (2) multiple small pearl-like calculi.
   (b) *Calcium-carbonate calculi*—never in the pure state. Rare.
   (c) *Calculi surrounding foreign bodies*—worms, ligatures.
   (d) *Casts of the bile ducts.* Rare in man.

The radiate cholesterol stone is composed almost entirely of cholesterol. It is usually single and is considered to be of metabolic origin, arising from gall bladders that are free from evidence of disease.

The cholesterol-bilirubin-calcium stones are usually found in gall bladders in which various stages of inflammation are present. When the cholesterol portion of such gallstone is dissolved with chloroform or ether, a protein framework remains, suggesting the formation of the stone in a milieu of inflammation. The average chemical composition of these stones, according to M. Pickens, G. O. Spanner, and L. Bauman,[3] is cholesterol, 94 per cent; calcium, 1.0 per cent; and pigment, 3.2 per cent.

The "combination" or "compound" stone usually has a center of cholesterol covered with a laminated shell. Of the rarer types, the calcium carbonate stones are particularly easy to depict on the roentgenographic film.

M. B. Dockerty[4] has classified the incidence of the various types of stone as follows: pure cholesterol, 10 per cent; pure pigment, 10.5 per cent; mixed, 78 per cent; and calcium carbonate, 1.5 per cent.

The incidence of gallstones in diseased gall bladders is between 80 (Bockus[5]) and 90 per cent and varies with the pathological changes in the gall bladder. Dockerty,[4] for example, found that stones were present in 50 per cent of the cases of cholesterosis (strawberry gall bladder), in 60 per cent of the cases of chronic catarrhal cholecystitis, in 90 per cent of the cases of chronic fibrous cholecystitis, in 96 per cent of the cases of acute or subacute cholecystitis, and in 96 per cent of the cases of empyema, hydrops, gangrene, and carcinoma.

The cause of gallstones concerns the actual and relative importance of the factors of metabolic changes, stasis, and infection, and is difficult to evaluate, as is true in any disease in which multiple factors are involved.

In a recent summary of the present concept of these etiological factors J. F. Weir[6] stated that the ratio of bile salts to cholesterol is 20:1, or even 30:1; that if the ratio decreases to 13:1, giving a supersaturation of cholesterol in the bile, cholesterol will crystallize out, and that this change in ratio occurs chiefly as a result of inflammatory changes in the wall of the gall bladder. Changes in the composition of the bile are seen in association with diseases of the liver, hemolytic diseases, and disturbances of general metabolism. In cases of congenital hemolytic jaundice, the excretion of bilirubin is increased, and in about 70 per cent of such cases gallstones are found, usually of the bilirubin-calcium type. This is also true in cases of sickle cell anemia. So there is strong presumptive evidence that bilirubin stones are of metabolic origin.

Changes in the cholesterol content of the blood have been noted in a number of conditions. Some investigators have noted a higher concentration of cholesterol in blood among patients who have gallstones than among normal persons, but this is by no means a constant finding.

In the condition known as "cholesterosis" in which the mucosa of the gall bladder is infiltrated with deposits of cholesterol, it is not understood whether the condition is a mild chronic inflammatory process or whether it is entirely metabolic in origin. Evidence at the time of this writing would certainly suggest that metabolic disturbances play an important role in the formation of certain types of stones, particularly of solitary cholesterol and pigment stones.

228

Gallstones

To what degree stasis is a factor in the production of gallstones is debatable, and many of the statements related to the role of stasis are conjectural. The effect of experimentally produced stasis in the gall bladder by partially obstructing the cystic duct was shown by W. H. Cole, M. V. Novak, and E. O. Hughes[7] to produce severe chronic cholecystitis. Such changes developed slowly, and infection, when it did occur, developed in only 30 per cent of the animals. They concluded that partial obstruction of the cystic duct is the likely mechanism in the production of chronic cholecystitis of man.

Much evidence supports the concept that the common mixed stone is the result of an inflammatory process, and the high incidence of cholecystitis in association with such stones emphasizes the direct relation between stone and infection. The probable sequence of events in the formation of new stones is initiated by a cholesterol stone plugging the cystic duct; this permits secondary infection followed by the pouring out of protein-rich exudate and calcium, absorption of bile salts, desquamation of epithelial cells, and precipitation and deposition of cholesterol, bilirubin, and calcium about the original cholesterol stone, all of which finally produces the laminated crust.

In bacteriological studies of surgically-removed gall bladders W. Magner and J. M. Hutcheson[8] have shown that positive cultures of fluid content could be obtained in such gall bladders in 63 per cent of the cases. It has, however, been shown by H. L. Bockus[5] and others that the incidence of sterile cultures in the presence of acute cholecystitis may be higher. Positive cultures yielded many types of bacteria, particularly *Escherichia coli,* streptococci and staphylococci. Experimentally, it is extremely difficult to produce infection of the gall bladder by the introduction of bacteria through the common or cystic ducts. Various other methods of producing cholecystitis have been used successfully, however, and prove that cholecystitis can be produced by factors other than infection, and that any infection is a secondary occurrence.

J. F. Weir[6] sums up the present concept of the etiology of stones as follows:

It thus seems reasonable to assume that because of the diversified composition of gallstones and the variability of their life history, there is more than one cause of them and that infection, stasis and metabolic disturbances, singly or in various combinations, as presently understood, do not explain adequately their formation. Furthermore, there is evidence that factors making for formation of stones appear to be periodic rather than continuous in their effects, even if not in their total mode of action. Incidentally, it is equally true that it seems impossible to prevent their formation.

Conspicuous advances in our knowledge of symptoms and complications of gallstones and their interpretation have been made in recent years. A typical gallstone attack is usually pathognomonic, but there are wide variations in the severity of the pain, its radiation, and in associated symptoms. For this reason it is difficult at times to distinguish between a gallstone attack, cholecystitis without stones, coronary disease, diaphragmatic hernia, peptic ulcer, and acute pancreatitis. The introduction of cholecystography with the use of a cholecystographic agent by E. A. Graham and W. H. Cole[9] was an advancement in radiology and an epoch-making contribution to the diagnosis of gallstones. Cholecystography has proved to be the most important diagnostic procedure for patients suspected of having gallstones, and it is estimated that the incidence of positive diagnosis of gallstones has been increased ten times by means of this procedure. With the development of other compounds and media similar to those used by Graham and Cole, phenomenal accuracy in diagnosis has been made possible; for example, in a series of 372 consecutive cases at the Mayo Clinic in which the diagnosis of gallstones was made by roentgenological examination, there was one error. Also, of more than eight thousand patients whose roentgenographic diagnosis was a normally functioning gall bladder, seventeen underwent explorations, and only four were found to have diseased gall bladders.

The incidence of stones in the common duct varies considerably, but averages from 12 to 15 per cent, while in only 5 per cent or less of all cases of gallstones are stones restricted to the common duct. The relationship of gallstones to inflammatory conditions of the pancreas probably exists in 25 per cent of the cases, and ocasionally acute pancreatitis is a complication. Changes in the liver occur commonly as slight atrophy of the hepatic cells in portal spaces, suppuration of the biliary tract, and formation of miliary abscesses, acute atrophy, or secondary biliary cirrhosis.

The complications directly caused by gallstones, such as jaundice, perforation of the gall bladder or ducts, stricture of ducts, internal or external fistulas, gangrene, and intestinal obstruction from impacted stone, are much less frequently seen today than they were in the early part of the century.

The manner in which the gall bladder functions has been summarized by J. L. Bollman[10] in the textbook of W. Walters and A. M. Snell on *Diseases of the gall bladder and bile ducts*. The gall bladder is caused to fill with bile during the interdigestive period of closure of the sphincter at the duodenal end of the common bile duct. The bile, owing to the secretory pressure of the liver, is thus forced to pass through the cystic duct into the gall bladder. The water content of the bile is absorbed by the mucosa of the gall bladder, which concentrates the bile and thus permits the storage of all bile secreted during the interdigestive period. The absorption of water is facilitated by small, rhythmic contractions of the musculature of the gall bladder, which gently stir the bile in the viscus. After the ingestion of food a reciprocal action takes place between the sphincter at the duodenal end of the common bile duct and the gall bladder that permits evacuation of the contents of the gall bladder into the duodenum at the initial stage of digestion. The tone of the sphincter is decreased or abolished by the passage of the gastric content into the duodenum. At the same time cholecystokinin is released from the duodenal mucosa and after absorption of this substance into the blood it stimulates the muscles of the gall bladder to contract and to force the contained bile into the duodenum.

The question of whether the function of the gall bladder is necessary must in the light of experience be answered in the negative, for there is no evidence to show that the gall bladder is essential to good health and a normal expectation of life.

In the evolution of the surgical management of gall bladder disease, certain basic principles have become well formulated. Probably the most important of these principles concerns the indications for the surgical removal of gallstones. The safety with which operations on the gall bladder can be done has established the general opinion that when gallstones are known to be present their removal is advisable, even if they apparently are not associated with any symptoms. The logic of this was pointed out by W. J. Mayo in 1911 in a classic paper entitled " 'Innocent' gallstones: a myth."[11] In the early history of operations for gallstones, cholecystotomy was soon looked on with disfavor because of the frequent recurrence of cholecystitis or stones, so that today the primary objective is removal of the gall bladder, which can be achieved with a mortality rate of less than 1.0 per cent.

Certain hazards in the conduct of the operation due to anomalies of the bile ducts, blood supply, and other circumstances occasionally may result in the unfortunate complication of injury to the common or hepatic bile ducts. Experience dictates an absolute rule in performing cholecystectomy: positive identification of cystic duct and artery before these structures are clamped or divided. The development of surgical procedures on the bile ducts, particularly reconstructive operations for stone, stricture, fistula, or malignant disease, has been one of the conspicuous achievements of modern surgery. At least 15 per cent of patients having stones in the gall bladder also have stones in the common bile duct, and in an additional 15 per cent the appearance of the common duct requires choledochotomy. The safety of operations on patients with jaundice has been greatly increased by pre-operative preparation and postoperative management. The administration of vitamin K, as shown by H. Dam,[12] reduces the coagulation time of the blood, and this together with combating dehydration, insuring adequate food intake, and transfusing blood, has largely eliminated uncontrollable bleeding as a cause of death in these cases. In the postoperative management of such patients cholangiography has become an important technical adjunct.

The chapter in the first edition of this book by Sir David Wilkie concludes as follows: "The work of the future must be to discover how we may prevent the metabolic disturbance which, together with infection and biliary stasis, leads to gallstone formation." In this era of preventive medicine this statement is as true today as it was when written.

§ REFERENCES

[1] Aschoff, L., and A. Bacmeister (1909): *Die Cholelithiasis*. Jena, Gustav Fischer.

[2] Rolleston, Sir. H., and J. W. McNee (1929): *Diseases of the liver, gallbladder and bile-ducts*. 3rd ed. London, Macmillan and Company.

[3] Pickens, M., G. O. Spanner, and L. Bauman (1932): "The composition of gall stones and their solubility in dog bile." *J. biol. Chem.*, 95, 505–507.

Gallstones

(4) Dockerty, M. B.: Personal communication to the author.

(5) Bockus, H. L. (1946): *Gastro-enterology*. Philadelphia and London, W. B. Saunders. Vol. 3.

(6) Weir, J. F.: "Gallstones." In *Vet. Admin. tech. Bull.*, Series *10*. Washington, D. C., Veterans Administration.

(7) Cole, W. H., M. V. Novak and E. O. Hughes (1941): "Experimental production of chronic cholecystitis by obstructive lesions of the cystic duct." *Ann. Surg., 114,* 682–96.

(8) Magner, W., and J. M. Hutcheson (1932): "Cholecystitis: a bacteriological and experimental study." *Canad. med. Ass. J., N. S. 27,* 469–77.

(9) Graham, E. A., and W. H. Cole (1924): "Roentgenologic examination of the gallbladder; preliminary report of a new method utilizing the intravenous injection of tetrabromphenolphthalein." *J. Amer. med. Ass., 82,* 613–14.

(10) Bollman, J. L. (1940): "Physiology of the gallbladder." In *Diseases of the gallbladder and bile ducts*. Edited by W. Walters and A. M. Snell. Philadelphia, W. B. Saunders. Pp. 41–54.

(11) Mayo, W. J. (1911): " 'Innocent' gall-stones: a myth." *J. Amer. med. Ass., 56,* 1021–24.

(12) Dam, H. (1935): "The antihaemorrhagic vitamin of the chick: occurrence and chemical nature." *Nature, Lond., 135,* 652–53.

§ REFERENCES ACCOMPANYING
SIR DAVID WILKIE'S TEXT

Charcot, J.-M. (1877): *Leçons sur les maladies du foie*. Paris, Bourneville et Sevestre.

Courvoisier, L. G. (1890): *Casuistisch-statistische Beiträge zur Pathologie und Chirurgie der Gallenwege*. Leipzig, F. C. W. Vogel.

Langenbuch, C. J. A. (1897): *Chirurgie der Leber und Gallenblase*. In *Deutsche Chirurgie*. Stuttgart, F. Enke. Forms 45, part 2.

Morgagni, J. B. (1767): *De sedibus et causis morborum*. Lugdunum Batavorum. Lib. iii, epistola 37, p. 127.

Naunyn, B. (1892): *Klinik der Cholelithiasis*. Leipzig, F. C. W. Vogel.

Pujol, A. (1823): *Mémoires sur la colique hépatique*. In *Oeuvres de médecine pratique*. Paris, Bechet jeune & J. B. Baillière. Vol. 4.

Thudichum, J. C. W. (1863): *A treatise on gall-stones*. London, Churchill and Sons.

BY WALTER R. BETT

M. R. C. S., L. R. C. P., F. R. S. L., F. S. A. Scot.*

chapter 14 / appendicitis

A DISEASE that so haunts the popular imagination and so perplexes the professional judgment may be expected to have an eventful and whimsical story. To a most peculiar degree appendicitis has tasted the fickleness of fashion and, by way of revenge, ever delights in changing its expression before an amazed and uneasy world. Its course may be so smooth that its operative prognosis is one of unrivalled safety. If it were otherwise the pride of surgeons would be grievously wounded. Yet it may leave in its train chronic ill health and suffering, or it may end abruptly in the tragedy of death.

It is fashionable to trace the history of disease back to the days of ancient Egypt and to try to discover in mummies, aloof, mysterious, and cynical, evidence of those ailments which afflict us today. There is nothing to suggest that the Egyptians knew of the existence of the appendix, though it has been claimed that viscera removed during the process of mummification have been found in jars with inscriptions mentioning the "worm of the bowel." References in the Ebers and other papyri to "worms in the belly" mean intestinal parasites. The sole unmistakable evidence of appendicitis in Egypt is furnished by a body belonging to the Christian (Byzantine) period; in accordance with contemporary practice it had not been eviscerated and shows the adhesions of an old appendicitis.[1]

The first serious description of the appendix as an anatomical organ was given in 1521 by Giacomo Berengario da Carpi, a good anatomist who wrote appalling Latin. The first picture of this organ

* Research librarian, National Association for the Prevention of Tuberculosis, London; bibliographer, British Association of Dermatology; and author of *Osler: the man and the legend* (1951) and *The infirmities of genius* (1952).

234

is contained in Johannes Dryander's illustrated edition of *Anatomia Mundini* (Marpurgi, 1531). The tongue of scandal insists this is an early unacknowledged sketch by Vesalius. Vesalius mentions and illustrates the appendix in the fifth book of *De humani corporis fabrica* (1543) under the name "the blind intestine" (*caecum intestinum*).[2]

While anatomists have been slow to appreciate the structural individuality of the appendix, physiologists have long debated its functions. In 1739 Johann Nathaniel Lieberkühn published in Leyden *De valvula coli et usu processus vermicularis*. Branded since as a vestigial structure, the appendix has by no means suffered such ignominy in silence. By no one is this fact more grimly appreciated than by the surgeon.

It is difficult to resist the temptation of introducing into the narrative, for completeness or polish, a learned, but dry catalogue of early clinical and pathological reports of what may or may not have been cases of appendicitis. The complicated terms and conceptions of "iliac passion" and "colic passion"[3] add further confusion to the picture. Critical examination of the documented material available suggests that, while the evacuation of encysted collections of pus from the right iliac fossa dates back to the dawn of the Christian era, what may be termed the deliberate surgery of the appendix is scarcely seventy-five years old. Aretaeus the Cappadocian in the second century A.D. gives the following equivocal case report: "I once made an opening into an abscess in the colon on the right side near the liver, and much pus rushed out, and much also by the kidneys and bladder for several days, and the man recovered."[4] Even in those cradle days of surgery, through the fog of vague surmises, we come face to face with the refreshing realization that the surgeon's hand has always been guided by the dogma: *Ubi pus, ibi evacua*.

One of the earliest accurate post-mortem reports of appendicitis occurs in Lorenz Heister's *Medical, chirurgical, and anatomical cases and observations* (translated from the German original by George Wirgman, London, 1755, observation CX). This description is all the more remarkable as he appears to have been first to advise his medical colleagues to bear a possible diagnosis of appendicitis always in mind:

In the month of November, 1711, as I was dissecting the body of a malefactor in the public theatre at Altdorff, I found the small guts very red and inflamed in several places, insomuch that the smallest vessels were as beautifully filled with blood as if they had been injected with red wax, in the most skillful manner, after Ruysch's method. But, when I was about to demonstrate the situation of the great guts, I found the vermiform process of the caecum preternaturally black, adhering closer to the peritonaeum than usual. As I now was about to separate it, by gently pulling it asunder, the membranes of this process broke, notwithstanding the body was quite fresh, and discharged two or three spoonfuls of matter. This instance may stand as a proof of the possibility of inflammation arising, and abscesses forming, in the appendicula, as well as in other parts of the body, which I have not observed to be much noticed by other writers; and when, in practice, we meet with a burning and pain where this part is situated, we ought to give attention to it. It is probable that this person might have had some pain in this part; but of this I could get no information. In such cases, I look upon clysters prepared with emollient and discutient herbs, such as mallows, marsh-mallows, and camomile-flowers, and the like remedies against inflammations, boiled in milk, and used frequently, to be of excellent use; as they reach the part, and may resolve the inflammation, or bring the abscess to a suppuration, partly by their warmth, partly by their resolving and discutient qualities, opening the abscess, that the matter may be discharged by stool, and the patient hereby may be saved; which, when the parts in the abdomen become corroded, can scarcely happen, but death must follow.

§ FIRST SUCCESSFUL APPENDECTOMY

Claudius Amyand, surgeon to St. George's Hospital, London, "Serjeant-Surgeon to His Majesty, and F. R. S.," in 1736 published the first recorded successful appendectomy (*Phil. Trans.*, 1736, *39*, 329–42) in a colorful account entitled "Of an inguinal rupture, with a pin in the appendix caeci, incrusted with stone ...."[5] This was twenty-two years before Mestivier (*J. Méd. Chir. Pharm. Paris*, 1759, *10*, 441), who merely drained an appendix abscess, but made no attempt to remove the offending appendix. His patient died.

In the following century James Parkinson, who has given his name to Parkinson's disease, presented a communication entitled "Case of diseased appendix vermiformis" (*Med.-chir. Trans.*, 1812, *3*, 57); and Thomas Hodgkin (*Lectures on the morbid anatomy of the serous and mucous membranes*. London, 1836) in lecture VI briefly but clearly described appendicitis. For many years Thomas Addison of

Guy's Hospital lectured on "caecitis" and in his published lectures (1836) used the term "perityphlitis," the most usual cause of which in his experience was a calculus in the appendix.[6]

In a paper published in 1827 François Mélier described the clinical features and the pathology of the perforated appendix (*J. gén. Méd. Chir. Pharm.*, 1827, *100, 317–45*). He recognized acute appendicitis as a clinical entity which, under certain circumstances, could prove rapidly fatal; he recommended early drainage and envisaged the possibility of early removal of the diseased appendix. Unfortunately, the great Baron Dupuytren ridiculed Mélier's views with the full weight of his authority and put back the clock of surgical progress.

In 1843 Adolph Volz introduced the opium treatment for perforated appendicitis, expressing the hope that one day the principle of rest for the intestines in inflammation of the appendix by means of this drug would be as clearly recognized as the same principle was recognized for a broken leg by means of splints.

Let us next peep for a moment into the fifth congress of the *Deutsche Gesellschaft für Chirurgie* in 1876. Georg Wegner of Berlin is speaking: "My contemporaries as well as myself have all been brought up in the fear of the Lord and of the peritoneum; the latter to many even today is a surgical *noli me tangere* of the worst kind."

§ AGGRESSIVE SURGERY OF THE APPENDIX

The operative story of appendicitis is intimately and impressively linked with the Listerian revolution in surgery. The aggressive surgery of the appendix is a posthumous child of this revolution.

In July, 1883, a twenty-three-year-old man with the diagnosis of "recurrent typhlitis" was warded at Guy's Hospital under Dr. Frederick Henry Horatio Akbar Mahomed. This physician, whose heart was in surgery, toyed with idea of operative interference, convinced that somewhere in the caecal region there was concealed an abscess cavity with a calculus or concretion in its depths. He carefully worked out the steps of the operation, which was performed by Sir Charters James Symonds, who removed a calculus from the much-twisted appendix. The case history ends somewhat lamely, though with grim humor: "When last heard of (April, 1885), though an inmate in the Barming Heath Lunatic Asylum, he was free from his old disease, and never had any trouble since Nov. 1883." The case is reported in *The Lancet*, 1885, *i*, 895.

Examples of deliberate interference with the appendix multiply rapidly. One of the first to remove a perforated appendix was Rudolph Ulrich Krönlein[7] of Zürich. His patient died two days after the operation. Heretical as it was, Lawson Tait's advice was beginning to become popular: "When the doctor is in doubt, and the patient in danger, make an exploratory incision, and deal with what you find as best you can."[8]

An editorial with the title "Timely operation for appendicitis" in the *Medical News, Philadelphia* (1892, 61, 153) next catches our eye. Here we make the acquaintance of Thomas George Morton, to whom "must be given the credit for having first deliberately sought out and removed an ulcerated appendix,"[9] and who introduced "what may justly be called one of the most important and radical advances of modern surgery." This editorial suggests that the operation be called "Morton's operation." Let us now turn to the correspondence column for November 5 (page 531) where we find a letter from the pen of Frederick Treves. He recalls that in 1886 he had under his care at the London Hospital a patient with "relapsing typhlitis," in whom he decided to "deliberately seek for and remove his appendix." The operation, performed on February 16, 1887, during an interval of apparently perfect health, consisted of correcting an appendicular distortion without actual excision. The patient recovered, and the case was reported to the Royal Medical and Chirurgical Society on February 14, 1888.[10] Those where the days when, to quote Treves: "Typhlitis, perityphlitis, and paratyphlitis are terms that, in the light of recent pathology, are losing no little of their original meaning. The distinctions that separated them have in great part vanished." It was Treves's policy to remove the offending appendix in selected cases of relapsing typhlitis during a quiescent period when peritonitis had become circumscribed. At first his suggestion met with a chilly welcome. "In due course, however, an exuberant reaction took place, and of late years appendices have been removed with a needless and illogical recklessness which has brought this branch of surgery into well-merited dispute." His loyalty to his surgical creed brought Treves many disappointments, many heartbreaking rebuffs, but none so cruel as the loss of his own daughter through perforation before the surgeon's knife could save her. Yet even that tragedy failed to shake his faith; he remained content to dwell in the paradise of his illusions, though he had seen the angel with the flaming sword.

§ "to be watched with knife in hand"

One of the most important names in the history of appendicitis is that of Reginald Heber Fitz of Boston, Massachusetts, for it was he who related the origin of the disease to the appendix, named it "appendicitis," stressed its diagnosis, and laid down its treatment. He impressed on his colleagues that it was their duty "to be mindful that, for all practical purposes, typhlitis, perityphlitis, perityphlitic tumor, and perityphlitic abscess mean inflammation of the vermiform appendix; that the chief danger of this affection is perforation; that perforation in the great majority of cases produces a circumscribed, suppurative peritonitis, tending to become generalized; that in the light of our present knowledge, the surgical treatment of this lesion offers the best chances for the life and future health of the patient, and that the progress of the disease needs to be watched with knife in hand."[11] How very modern all this sounds, yet it was written more than half-a-century ago![12]

§ "then, sir, you will go as a corpse"

One of the more dramatic factors in the rapid development of the operative treatment of appendicitis was an event in 1902 which greatly affected Britain. In June of that year elaborate preparations were being made for the crowning of Edward VII when it was suddenly announced that he suffered from perityphlitis and that the coronation was postponed. These, briefly, are the facts of this historic case: On June 13, while staying at Windsor, the royal patient had a sudden attack of abdominal pain, which was diagnosed as appendicitis by Sir Francis Laking and Sir Thomas Barlow. Treves was called in consultation five days later. The temperature gradually fell, and the local swelling and tenderness subsided. By June 21 the patient had sufficiently recovered to return to London. That same evening, however, there was a sudden rise in temperature, and a large painful swelling appeared in the right iliac fossa. The king was seen early on June 24 by Lord Lister, then seventy-five, and by Sir Thomas Smith, who advised immediate operation. Edward, however, was obstinate: "I must keep faith with my people and go to the Abbey." The distinguished physicians and surgeons were desperate. The fate of a nation hung in the balance, and the honor of their profession was in jeopardy. Finally Treves said bluntly: "Then, Sir, you will go as a corpse." Frederic Hewitt gave the anesthetic, and Treves operated upon his king—an elderly man, a stout man, and not a good surgical risk. Pus was found at a depth of four-and-a-half inches, and two large drainage tubes were inserted, surrounded by a pack of iodoform gauze. Nothing was reported concerning the appendix, which was probably not disturbed. The weight of responsibility on the surgeon's mind must have been enormous, for he did not go to bed for seven nights. The royal patient made an uneventful recovery. He had no further attacks of abdominal pain and died of bronchopneumonia in 1910.

Following that historic operation appendicitis became a fashionable disease, which filled the surgeon's pockets with happiness. Treves, who had been created a baronet, with honorable augmentation of a lion of England in his coat of arms, retired from practice in 1908, at the early age of fifty-five. He died—with tragic irony—of peritonitis in 1923.

§ MC BURNEY'S POINT

In 1889 Charles McBurney read before the New York Surgical Society his now classical paper on "Early operative interference in cases of diseases of the vermiform appendix,"[13] in which he stressed what is universally known as "McBurney's point": "The seat of greatest pain, determined by the pressure of one finger, has been very exactly between an inch and a half and two inches from the anterior spinous process of the ilium on a straight line drawn from that process to the umbilicus." McBurney's name is also frequently attached to the gridiron incision, but a facsimile letter published in 1937 (*Surg. Gynec. Obstet., 65,* 714) makes it clear that he himself acknowledged Lewis Linn McArthur's priority in describing this incision for approaching the appendix.

§ THE VOICE OF UNORTHODOXY

The diagnosis and treatment of acute appendicitis continues to be a favorite subject for discussion at medical meetings, and from time to time the voice of unorthodoxy is heard in the land. In his annual oration entitled "Fallen idols,"[14] delivered before the Medical Society of London, Sir James Berry advocated the policy of waiting and watching, and of exercising a wise discretion how and when to operate. In his opinion Edward VII owed his life to the fact that active treatment was avoided until the right time was judged to have come —nine days after he was first seen by the physician, and six days after he was seen by the operating surgeon. By way of contrast, the operation upon President Friedrich Ebert of Germany, performed three hours after he had first been seen by the surgeon, ended fatally.

The subject of delayed treatment of appendiceal abscess was reviewed in 1950 by P. Ladin,[15] who claimed that there is a markedly lower mortality with such treatment.

§ CHEMOTHERAPY

In 1950 G. E. Moloney, W. T. Russell, and D. C. Wilson[16] compared a series of Grey Turner's figures of the occurrence of acute appendicitis for a thirty-five year period ending in 1934 with the admissions for acute appendicitis to the Radcliffe Infirmary, Oxford, during the years 1945–48. The most striking difference was seen in the cases complicated by general peritonitis. The fatality in this group at the Radcliffe was 6.2 per cent, compared with Grey Turner's figure of 29.2 per cent. The authors concluded that the evidence strongly supported the employment of chemotherapy (sulphonamides and penicillin) in all cases in which inflammation had extended to the peritoneum.

§ REFERENCES

[1] *Bull. archaeol. Surv. Nubia*, 1908, *i*, 32. (plate xxv).
[2] Lambert, S. W. (1937): "Description of the vermiform appendix from the *De-fabrica* of Vesalius." *Ann. med. Hist., N. S. 9*, 422–27.
[3] Carson, H. W. (1931): "The iliac passion." *Ann. med. Hist., N. S. 3*, 638–49.

(4) *Aretaeus the Cappodocian* (1856): *The extant works of.* Edited and translated by Francis Adams. London, Sydenham Society. P. 312.

(5) See Creese, P. G. (1953): "The first appendectomy." *Surg. Gynec. Obstet., 97, 643–52.*

(6) See Brock, R. C. (1952): "One hundred volumes of the *Guy's Hospital Reports.*" *Guy's Hosp. Rep., 101, 235–50.*

(7) Krönlein, R. V. (1886): *"Ueber die operative Behandlung der acuten diffusen jauchig—eiterigen Peritonitis." Arch. klin. Chir., 33, 507–24.*

(8) Tait, L. (1883): "An account of two hundred and eight consecutive cases of abdominal section performed between Nov. 1st, 1881, and December 31st, 1882." *Brit. med. J., 1, 304.*

(9) Morton's case is reported in (1888) *Proc. Philad. Co. med. Soc., 8, 101.*

(10) Treves, F. (1888): "Relapsing typhlitis treated by operation." *Med.-chir. Trans., 71, 165–72.*

(11) Fitz, R. H. (1888): "The relation of perforating inflammation of the vermiform appendix to perityphlitic abscess." *N. Y. med. J., 47, 508.*

(12) See also Loveland, J. E. (1937): "Reginald Heber Fitz, the exponent of appendicitis." *Yale J. Biol. Med., 9, 509–20.*

(13) McBurney, C. (1889): "Experiences with early operative interference in cases of disease of the vermiform appendix." *N. Y. med. J., 50, 676, 693–95.*

(14) Berry, J. (1932): "Fallen idols." *Trans. med. Soc. Lond., 55, 261.*

(15) Ludin, P. (1950): "The delayed treatment of appendiceal abscess." *N. Y. St. J. Med., 50, 681.*

(16) Moloney, J. E., W. T. Russell, and D. C. Wilson (1950): "Appendicitis— a report on its social pathology and recent surgical experience." *Brit. J. Surg., 38, 52–64.*

§ FURTHER READING

Kelly, H. A., and E. Hurdon (1905): *The vermiform appendix and its diseases.* Philadelphia and London, W. B. Saunders & Company. (The historical introduction of this book occupies fifty-four pages.)

BY WILLIAM G. LENNOX
M. D.*

chapter 15 / epilepsy

WITH RESPECT to numbers, epilepsy is a common disease: one in two hundred among drafted adults in the United States of America is afflicted with it; the proportion is much higher in those below draft age. Yet in other respects it is uncommon. "Distinguished" is the word with respect to its scientific interest, its social treatment, and its place in the history of medicine.

The identity of many major diseases, viewed at a distance of time, is lost in the crowd of symptoms. Fever, pain, loss of weight—each of these is a chief symptom of various maladies. Consequently, many diseases now clearly distinguishable have only a brief history.

The chief symptom of epilepsy is both distinctive and dramatic— a sudden and devastating convulsion of body muscles, an abrupt loss of consciousness. Hence, for centuries before and after Christ, epilepsy carried the name of the "Falling Sickness." True, some physical phenomena such as syncope, hysterical fits, and insulin shock, are not epilepsy, and, conversely, modern study has enlarged the domain of epilepsy. These are modern refinements. For the ancients epilepsy meant a convulsion, a meaning almost always justified.

Throughout the centuries epilepsy has occupied a position of prominence in medical writings. Convulsions are dramatic and unmistakable, and opinions concerning them appear in the surviving fragments of the earliest medical literature. Indeed, relatively more space is devoted to epilepsy by ancient than by modern authors; for example, the Hippocratic writings give 2.6 per cent; Aretaeus, 3.4 per cent; Thomas Willis, 10 per cent; Osler, 0.8 per cent; Cecil (1951) only 0.5 per cent.

*Chief of seizure unit, Children's Medical Center, Boston, Massachusetts; president, International League against Epilepsy.

There is no mistaking the poetic description given by Lucretius (96–55 B.C.) in his *De rerum natura,* nor the moving account and demonstration of a child's convulsion in the presence of Christ (St. Luke 9:38–39).

§ DISEASE AND THE DISEASED

As a symptom, the disease of convulsions is static. Generalissimo Julius Caesar falls convulsing into the Tiber; Private Cesarè Antonio has a fit while driving his jeep. The convulsions are the same; the bystander's understanding of them is widely different. Symptoms remain, the individuals pass. The river is lasting, the particles of water go and never return. A history of epilepsy deals, therefore, with changing conceptions of the cause of convulsions, the cure of them, and the treatment, medical and social, of the persons afflicted. These three areas of change must be concurrently recorded. Change is not spontaneous. Knowledge advances in the wake of adventurers and explorers of physical events. These pioneers are countless in number, but, like steppingstones across a stream, certain individuals or schools of thought mark the principal points of advance.

There has been retreat as well as advance. Understanding has waited on the painfully slow progress of medical science, which stood virtually in its tracks for two thousand years. Negative treatment, which is worse than none, attended the expulsion of demons. Effective drug therapy lagged behind knowledge, and in recent decades social therapy has been static as compared with medical and surgical treatment.

Fragmentary references to seizures appear in the oldest of ancient medical writings. For a truly learned and fascinating account of conceptions and practices "from the Greeks to the beginning of modern neurology," the book by Owsei Temkin (1945) is strongly recommended. This book, like all epilepsy history with any substance, starts with the person (or the school) of Hippocrates nearly twenty-four hundred years ago.

The Hippocratic document is remarkable on two counts. First, the writer (*circa* 400 B.C.) attacked the conception that an epileptic is spirit-possessed. Spirits, both benignant and malignant, are important personages in primitive society. Usually those responsible for seizures are villainous, but among the ancient Greeks, perhaps because of the priest-physician influence, seizures were regarded as a manifestation of gods and goddesses. The Hippocratic writing is a vigorous and adroit rebuttal of this conception. "Those who first referred this disease to the gods, using the divinity as a pretext and screen of their own inability to afford any assistance, have given out that the disease is sacred, [and] have instituted a mode of treatment which is safe for themselves—purifications and incantations." From ignorance and wonder, men regarded the nature and cause of epilepsy as divine. But Hippocrates stated, "It appears to me to be nowise more divine nor more sacred than other diseases," for example the paroxysmal fevers. Furthermore, he argued, the origin of the disease is hereditary, like certain other diseases.

The second contribution by the Hippocratic writer is no less substantial: an explanation of the physiological pathology of seizures. The explanation forms an argument against the "sacredness" of epilepsy, since a physical cause makes a spiritual one less necessary. Hippocrates recognized that epilepsy had its seat in the brain, and as for mechanism:

The man becomes speechless when the phlegm, suddenly descending into the veins, shuts out the air, and does not admit it either to the brain or to the vena cava, or to the ventricles, but interrupts the inspiration. The air which enters the veins is of use [to the body] by entering the brain and its ventricles, and thus it imparts sensibility and motion to all members, so that when the veins are excluded from the air by the phlegm and do not receive it, the man loses his speech and intellect, and the hands become powerless and are contracted, the blood stopping and not being diffused as was its want.

Translated into modern speech, the fit, says Hippocrates, is due to cerebral anoxemia. Moreover, in goats seized with this disease, the brain is "humid, full of sweat and having a bad odor," *i.e.,* there is cerebral edema. The only case report by Hippocrates is a child treated by complete fasting—a preferred treatment in the nineteen twenties. He closes with these solemn and prophetic words: "But whoever is acquainted with such a change in man, and can render a man humid and dry, hot and cold by regimen, could also cure this disease—and without minding purifications, spells, and all other illiberal practices of a like kind." This emphasis on physiological processes that influence seizures is like one tower of a suspension bridge whose twin tower is more than two millenniums beyond; 400 B.C. and A.D. 1930 speak the same essential language, which says that epilepsy is influenced by alterations of brain physiology; by changes in the cerebral circulation, or in the oxygen supply, or in the fluid and acid-base balance of the body.

Galen, who lived some 500 years after Hippocrates (A.D. 130–200), though recognizing the essential fact that seizures arise in the brain, taught that the body outside the brain might play a role. He divides the epilepsies into three groups (Brock, 1929):

A. The cause of one group is a dyscrasia of the humors of the brain, brought on by cold. [This group he calls idiopathic.]

B. In a second group, the brain is stimulated by irritating substances brought to it from the body, and the convulsion is the brain's effort to repel the irritant. The analogy is the hiccough, which is a convulsive effort to the stomach to rid itself of offending matter. [This epilepsy he calls sympathetic.]

C. In a third group, a pathological humor is formed locally in an extremity and extends to the head. The analogy is the venom of the snake or insect, which spreads from the site of the bite to the brain. The proof lies in the preventive action of a tourniquet or amputation. "I once saw a rustic who, having had his whole finger bitter by a viper, took a pruning hook which he had by him—he was a vine dresser—and amputated the wounded portion at the last joint" and recovered. [Galen is speaking here of Jacksonian epilepsy.]

§ THE CAUSES OF EPILEPSY

For two thousand years and more, medical writers rang the changes on sayings of Hippocrates and Galen and minor authorities, annotating, interpreting, occasionally making a fresh observation. The background causes of epilepsy as viewed by the ancients were three: supernatural forces; phlegms or humors; and irritating or toxic substances, obstruction of air to the brain being the immediate cause of a convulsion.

Supernatural Forces. The concept of spirit possession, so neatly beheaded by Hippocrates, proved to be Hydra-headed. The satanic origin of seizures was accepted by the apostolic writers who described the miracles of Jesus. Medieval writers did not mention demons in their learned discussions about etiology, but they prescribed charms and holy ritual to ward off evil, nevertheless. As late as 1684 Thomas Willis excused Christ's biographers in these words:

> In truth, in this Distemper, no marks at all of the Morbisick matter appears, or are so very obscure, that we may have deservedly suspected it to be an inspiration of an evil spirit; at least it is probable that, as often as the Devil is permitted to afflict Miserable Mortals with his delusions, he is not able to draw more cruel Arrows from any other Quiver, or to shew Miracles by any better Witch, than by the assault of this monstrous Disease.

Fifty years later Gerard van Swieten (1744), commentator of Boerhaave, told of a convincing—to him—personal experience:

> The same diseases may be produced from supernatural, which we have known to arise from natural causes. I have seen an innocent boy of four years of age, who, as soon as be began to repeat the Lord's prayer was immediately convulsed and at the same time gave a loud frightful roar as seemed far to exceed his strength; after some minutes I desired his grandmother, who brought him to me, to order him again to repeat the same prayer, and thus four times running, always with the same success; and though I was forwarned of the event, and put on a strong resolution, yet I could not help being frightened at hearing him bawl out.

Demons are now dead, but the fear inspired by millenniums of demoniac possession still persists as a sort of embryonic thought in the unconscious minds of us moderns. How else is the unreasoning horror of convulsions to be explained?

Humors. The conception of "bad humor" requires explanation. There were four in number: blood, which is hot and moist; phlegm (inflammation or mucus), which is cold and moist; reddish bile, which is hot and dry; and black bile, which is cold and dry. As stated by Hippocrates, in epilepsy excessive phlegm obstructs the passage of air (oxygen) to the brain. Evidence of this is the saliva which flows from the patient's lips during a convulsion. This reasoning may explain the importance which many persons still attach to the question of whether the patient "frothed at the mouth." The arteries were believed to carry not blood but air, hence the ancient idea of an obstruction to an adequate supply of air to the brain approximates the modern idea of cerebral anemia.

Toxins. Although the influence of peripheral poisons or irritations is often mentioned by early writers, no better evidence is brought forward than the analogies advanced by Galen.

Epilepsy could hardly escape accusation of being contagious. The idea appeared in the Arabic writings of Rhazes (850–923). Bernard de Gordon (1304) in *Lilium medicinae* names epilepsy as one of the eight cardinal contagious diseases, the others being bubonic plague, phthisis, scabies, erysipelas, anthrax, trachoma, and leprosy. One miss out of eight was not bad.

§ GENERAL HYGIENE

Two thousand years ago, as now, co-operation with Nature, attention to hygiene, and the maintenance of morale constituted the backlog of enlightened treatment. Hippocrates was no advocate of a stagnant life: "Epilepsy in young persons is most frequently removed by changes of air, of country and of modes of life." The physician, moreover, said he, must use a rational therapy: "For in this disease as in all others, he must strive not to feed the disease, but endeavor to wear it out by administering whatever is most opposed—and not that which favors and is allied to it."

How attractive is the second-century advice of Aretaeus:

Promenades long, straight, without tortuosities, in a well ventilated place, under trees of myrtle and laurel, or among acrid and fragrant herbs, such as calamint, penny-royal, thyme, and mint; so much the better if wild and indigenous—it is a good thing to take journeys, but not by a riverside, so that he may not gaze upon the stream (for the current of a river occasions vertigo), nor where he may see anything turned round, such as a rolling-top, for he is too weak to preserve the animal spirits (pneuma) steady, which are, therefore, whirled about in a circle, and this circular motion is provocative of vertigo and of epilepsy . . . the exercise should be sharper, so as to induce sweat and heat, for all these attenuate. During the whole of his life [the patient] should cultivate a keen temper without irascibility.

In general, a life without excess or undue excitement was ordered. About the time of Christ, Celsus said the patient "should avoid sunlight, bathing, fire, and everything that may heat him; also cold, venery, looking from high places, terrifying sights, vomiting, lassitude, worries, business of all kinds." A thousand years later Bernard de Gordon repeated:

He should avoid all vegetables which are difficult to digest, he should avoid long sleep, lying on his back with his head inclined; when he is on top of mountains he should avoid looking downwards; he should avoid the sound of large bells; the roaring of lions, all terrifying things, the south; he should avoid anger and other disturbances of the soul, such as fear, worry, and in all those things which make for sudden intake and expulsion of breath.

The last warning, avoidance of hard breathing, has indeed a modern meaning, for this is a potent means of precipitating *petit mal*.

§ TREATMENT OF THE SUPERNATURAL

The aim of physicians in all ages has been to rid the body of the cause of seizures. But, alas! the causes have been numerous and diverse and hard to influence, especially when allied with malign and indestructible spirits. One form of treatment (very simple and most lucrative for the priest-physician) consisted of gifts or sacrifices made at the temple. Hippocrates had some caustic words for this practice. If, as seemed more reasonable, the seizures were more devilish than godlike, deliverance could be forced. Methods of exorcising the devil varied. Most simple was the direct command. What physician has not yearned for the power of Jesus as exhibited in the pathetic case so vividly described in the gospels (St. Mark, 9:17–27)! Though the disciples had tried to exorcise the boy's evil spirit and had failed, the glory of the deed carried vicarious power for many centuries. The earliest, and for a century the only, book on epilepsy from America (Pedro de Horta, 1763) is a vindication of demon possession.

§ RIDDING THE BODY OF POISONS

The aim of surgery was to release evil spirits or morbid secretions from the brain. The surest way was, of course, the trephine. Probably some of the hundreds of trephined prehistoric skulls which have been found belonged to persons with seizures. Ancient writers commonly advised the use of the cautery. (The cautery was "actual" when a hot iron, "potential" when a blistering ointment.) What suffering this treatment must have entailed! But as Aretaeus observed, "the habit of such persons renders them tolerant of pains, and their goodness of spirits and good hopes render them strong in endurance."

Ordinarily the actual cautery was applied to the occiput, where gravity would aid drainage of the "pernicious humor" (pus), which must have welled from the wound. Taxil (1602) said:

This sickness [epilepsy] occurs rather frequently in Florence, and the mothers keep certain iron buttons with which soon after the birth of the child they themselves actually make a rupture by pressing a hot button on the back of the head, and some take the infant to the priest to have it done with a glowing coal. (The French mothers on the contrary think it would kill their children if one only speaks of such a remedy.)

Independent and sensible minded French mothers! As late as 1861 Sieveking remarked: "The actual cautery deserves great commendation; whether acting by reflex or by the actual drain set up it sometimes appears to produce curative results which could scarcely be expected from milder remedies."

Medicine as well as surgery can be used for ridding the body of poisons. Therefore, bloodletting, purging, vomiting, diuretics, sweating—each or all together—have provided many a field day for the doctor and (more particularly) the patient.

§ DRUG TREATMENT

Distressing is the thought that seizured patients through the ages endured medicinal and other treatments prescribed by outstanding physicians, but all without value. It is intellectually, if not therapeutically, rewarding to follow the gropings of predecessor practitioners beset by needy patients. Between Hippocrates and the sixteenth century, advanced ideas were not only congregated in the latter part of the period, but in certain localities or in certain strata of society. The ancient Greeks scorned methods of treatment which today are popular among primitive people.

Thus, Aretaeus the Cappadocian in the second century said he had never given the brain of a vulture, the heart of a raw cormorant, or the liver of a man to an epileptic patient. "I leave these things to be described by those who would bear such means." But the first English court physician, John of Gaddesden, gave this advice (1314):

> The blood taken from a red-headed woman and dried is a sure cure. The brain of a camel or weasel, given with vinegar, cures epilepsy. Also the blood of a weasel saved and given in drink is a perfect cure. Also the dust of a burned weasel, and the dust of burned swallows are of the greatest benefit. The powdered bile of a kite is a very great remedy. The ashes of a stag's horn, when drunk, cures epilepsy.

Fifteen hundred years after Aretaeus the prescriptions of Thomas Willis, professor of physic at Oxford, contained such items as powdered human skull, dragon's blood, liver of wolf, the stones of swallows, and the gall of a boar fried with urine.

Again Aretaeus reported: "I have seen persons holding the cup below the wound of a man recently slaughtered, and drinking a draught of the blood! Oh, the present, the mighty necessity, which compels one to remedy the evil by such a wicked abomination! And whether even they recovered by this means no one can tell me for certain." Sixteen centuries later Hans Christian Andersen described witnessing as a child the execution of three persons, and seeing the parents of an epileptic boy make the boy drink a cupful of the blood. Physicians, modern as well as ancient, are under the compulsion of "doing something" for their patients. "More especially we must administer everything which will do the slightest good, or even that will do no harm." Also, when doctors (or their fees) are out of reach, non-doctors have advised. Thus, John Wesley, founder of Methodism, in his *Primitive physic: or an easy and natural method of curing most diseases* (1773 edition) gives thirteen cures for the "Falling Sickness," such as: "Be electrified: Tried; use the cold bath for a month daily; use an entire milk diet for three months, it seldom fails."

Reasons might be muddled and mixed, but the ancients had the advantage of authority. Galen said powdered human skull was good for epilepsy and for a thousand years and more the skull maintained its place in treatment. In the two thousand years between Hippocrates and the eighteenth century, many writers wrote of epilepsy. The book of Temkin quotes seven hundred authorities. Accounts are often picturesque, but rarely logical. "The cause of this disease," says Bernard de Gordon (1314), "is a humor or coarse windiness occluding the non-principal ventricles of the brain, impeding the passage of breath to the members." But immediately he affirms that if a person will repeat three times in the ear of a convulsing patient the words "Gasper bears the myrrh, Melchior, the frankincense, Balshasar the gold [names of the three Wise Men who fell down and worshiped the Christ child], undoubtedly the patient will arise immediately."

The Hippocratic scorn of meaningless prohibitions could not, however, withstand the practitioner's need of giving detailed advice. If the provisions were too difficult to fulfil, the patient and not the practitioner was to blame if fits continued. Every treatise on epilepsy from Galen to and including part of the present century specified articles of food that should or should not be eaten. "Of flesh meat the patient should eat small birds, except those which live in water or near lakes. Among quadrupeds, he should use kids, yearling lambs, veal, suckling pigs and young leopards. He should eat no fish; but if fish is necessary, he should use scaley fish from clean waters." A certain article might be praised by one and forbidden by another, but excessive use of alcoholic drinks was condemned by all, "since the many vapors which they generate fill the head."

Apparently there were critics of these minute and ceremonious prescriptions. Anthony Guainerius (about 1440) had an answer based on psychology:

Ceremonies are in order that greater confidence be placed in the medicine. The greater the affection with which the sick man takes his medicine, the more eagerly does nature receive it, and other things being equal, the better result is attained . . . we offer pills in unequal numbers, since the ignorant think that that number is much more perfect than an equal number.

Epilepsy

Animals provided treatment of epilepsy because of the belief in the transference of qualities, either to or from the patient. Said John of Gaddesden:

Some persons wear the head of the cuckoo about their neck . . . it alleviates and retards the paroxysms as I have often witnessed in children who cannot take medicine. The reason is because each month the cuckoo himself has epilepsy wherefore it cures epilepsy by drawing the matter to itself as rheubarb draws choler.

A poison must be fought with poison-killing substances. Anthony Guainerius defended his prescription of noxious substances:

Some men, thinking themselves to be wise, wonder that the disease can be removed by the things described. Know, however, that no poison is driven away by cold or dryness or moisture alone; you must find in the repellent some hidden counter-agent to the poison. Since, therefore, epilepsy is produced by reason of something poisonous, the thing which expels it must possess some quality opposed to the poison, and this can reside in the gall of a frog, the blood of a dog, or the urine of a man, or something else.

Every treatise on epilepsy ended with a list of double-barreled prescriptions, often containing both animal and vegetable materials. From five to twenty items, mostly herbs, would be named. Of the properties of these herbs we moderns are ignorant. Four enjoyed particular popularity: elder, garlic, mistletoe, and peony. Mistletoe was praised by such widely separated authorities as Paracelsus, Pliny, and Boerhaave. Sir James Frazer in *The golden bough* attributes its reputation to the fact that being rooted in the branches of the oak it cannot fall to the ground, therefore it must help falling sickness.

§ CARE OF THE PATIENT DURING CONVULSION

What is to be done for the patient in those agonizing minutes of a convulsion when he seems on the point of dying? Anthony Guainerius gave unusually specific directions:

. . . let it be your aim to prevent the ascent of vapors, and as far as possible, to draw the matter downwards. Therefore, perform vigorous rubbings or painful ligatures on the extremities, on the buttocks; under the knee make a slight incision with a cupping-glass; and call the patient in a loud voice by his own name. Place a wooden peg between his teeth; then with fumes of balsam rub his palate, his nostrils, and the veins pulsing at his temples. These things usually drive away the paroxysm at once, and retard it greatly, as I have learned by experience. Also, when an epileptic falls, at once kill a dog, and give the gall to the patient in any way that you can. If the one who first sees the attack urinates in his own shoe and then stirs it around, as if to wash it, then gives the urine to the patient to drink, afterwards the patient will be entirely delivered.

Thomas Willis describes the indignities heaped on the defenseless patient during seizure and then adds:

I say this kind of practice is often too roughly instituted or ordained; because after this manner is double trouble put upon nature, to wit, one from the disease, and the other not lighter from the standers by and helpers, when it were much better, for the fit to be suffered to pass over after its own manner, and the sick to endure but one trouble only.

§ THEORY AND PRACTICE AFTER THE RENAISSANCE

The fresh winds of the Renaissance cast ancient precepts adrift and filled the sails of original thought and investigation. Anchors aweigh for all of science and medicine! For epilepsy, transition from the old to the new may be marked by the writings of Thomas Willis (1621–75) of Oxford and London and Hermann Boerhaave (1668–1738) of Leyden. The thoughts of Willis were born from the union of busy consulting and autopsy room experiences. He argued that all seizures, hysterical as well as epileptic, arise in the brain, and muscular movements are not due to the mechanical traction of nerves, but to chemical reactions within the central nervous system. This chemical activity which ends in muscle movements is, he says, akin to the explosion of gunpowder.

Nor is this all. Born researchers, like born poets, may have illuminations of prophetic sight—arrival at the proof of which may require centuries of painful travel. In one such illumination Willis, a century before Galvani and nearly three before Hans Berger, compared the seizure to an electrical discharge:

For whosoever shall consider the sudden puffings up, the violent and strong Contractions in the members and the affected parts, yea, sometimes the most impetuous concussions, and violent throws of the whole body, can conceive no less, than that very many heaps of the animal spirits are exploded, or thrust out, even as lightning breaks forth from a Cloud.

In the nineteenth century interest followed the shifting developments of science. The pathologist, physiologist, chemist, psychologist —each had his turn, and with or without their inspiration the clinician has tried this and that and has reported results that in the main were very encouraging for his own treatment and unfavorable for some other. Cutting the spinal cord, exclaimed Radcliffe (1858), results in a spasm of the muscles supplied; epilepsy must then be due to a decrease (rather than an increase) of nervous activity; therefore, stimulate the patient. Spasm of the glottis, said Marshall Hall (1841), is the antecedent of which convulsions and stupor are consequences; therefore, dash cold water on the patient's face or, better still, give him a permanent tracheotomy opening. Obstruct the blood supply to the brain, reported Kussmaul and Tenner (1849), and animals have convulsions. Therefore, avoid bloodletting and cut the vasomotor nerves. But, argued the pathologists, the exposed brain of the epileptic is congested; patients are plethoric and too much blood overstimulates the brain; therefore, bleed or tie the carotid arteries. Patients have a retention of uric acid, observed Haig (1892). The leopard (like the convulsing patient) exhibits violent but short muscular activity and is meat-eating, said Hughlings Jackson. Therefore, advised both Haig and Jackson, forbid the patient to eat meat. Irritating the skin of an animal when half the spinal cord is cut results in a spasm, says Brown-Séquard; so clinicians hurried to remove sources of peripheral irritation (intestinal worms, teeth, uteri) and to amputate extremities in which seizures start.

§ THE MODERN ERA

However, change of ideas is a blessed relief from the prolonged period of stagnant concepts. The modern era for epilepsy and the precipitous betterment of knowledge and treatment began a century ago. The place was a hospital "for the paralyzed and epileptic," at Queen Square, London. The impetus for this hospital came from two poorly circumstanced maiden ladies. The shining lights of the hospital, epilepsy-wise, were John Hughlings Jackson (1835–1911) and Sir William Richard Gowers (1845–1915). Their contribution was from the bedside and not the laboratory. Jackson defined and interpreted what doctors from Hippocrates onward had watched in wonder. Epilepsy, he said, "is the name for occasional, sudden, excessive, rapid and local discharges of the grey matter." He never dreamed that these electrical discharges could or would be recorded on moving paper. He postulated three evolutionary levels for the mechanism of fits. He thought an instability of nerve cells might be due to their malnutrition, which caused a nervous discharge from certain focal areas of the brain. Jackson's was a great contribution to the understanding of epilepsy, yet the reader of his works does not see the patient, only the disease. The defect was remedied by Gowers. His textbook (1885 and 1901) winnowed the experiences of nearly twenty-five hundred patients.

Effective treatment may not follow improved understanding of disease. But in this same period and city an effective remedy was at long last found. In the year 1857 Charles Locock, obstetrician to Queen Victoria, was knighted, and he stated at a medical meeting that use of bromides had stopped the seizures of a group of his patients. For fifty-five years bromides were the only drugs at all effective against convulsions. Yet they often failed, and dismally so if attacks were *petit mal* or psychomotor. Also, they tended to dull the mind and disfigure the skin of the patient.

Then in 1912 a German, Alfred Hauptmann, announced that luminal (phenobarbital) would stop convulsions. This proved more effective than bromides and less unpleasant in its reactions, and for twenty-six years phenobarbital occupied the throne of therapy. But these sedatives controlled no more than a minority of attacks. More important, they did not throw light on the mechanism of seizures.

Help came from an unexpected direction. A food faddist claimed that epileptic seizures, among other diseases, were controlled by a period of starvation. In desperation, responsible doctors tried the scheme and were surprised to find that it worked. However, the period of starvation was limited to three or four weeks. Could acidosis, the prominent feature of starvation, be induced in other ways? Geyelin in

Epilepsy

New York and Wilder at the Mayo Clinic suggested that a high fat, low carbohydrate diet which could be maintained for long periods be substituted for the consumption of body fat. Other studies demonstrated that acidosis, however induced, was indeed an inhibitor of seizures, especially of the transient blackouts of consciousness called *petit mal*. Here at last was evidence that pointed to epilepsy as a metabolic disorder. With great joy Lennox and Cobb (1928) summarized these newer developments. Years later Putnam and Merritt (1938) announced a remarkably effective and non-sedative anticonvulsant, sodium diphenylhydantoin (Dilantin, Epamin or Epanutin). This and yet newer drugs have displaced the ketogenic or dehydration treatments. However, demonstration of the value of acidosis induced by muscular and mental work encourages patients to participate in life's activities instead of merely looking on.

The most decisive break-through in the ages-long fight against epilepsy came in 1929 when Hans Berger announced his observations with the electroencephalograph. This instrument gave the brain a means of written communication. From within its bony castle the brain proclaims its epileptic misbehaviors on a moving strip of paper. The most distinctive brain wave pattern is an alternate dart and dome formation recurring at the rate of three per second, which coincides with the period of unconsciousness of the type of seizure called *petit mal*.

The work of the pioneering Dr. and Mrs. F. A. Gibbs (1952) depicts the great variety of electrical expressions of this once "Sacred Disease," now called a "symptomatic paroxysmal cerebral dysrhythmia." The domain of epilepsy has been enlarged beyond mere convulsions to include transient impairment of consciousness, periods of automatic activity, and even subjective phenomena (hallucinations of sight, smell, taste, or hearing) and paroxysmal disturbances of the autonomic centers of the brain with resulting attacks such as migraine.

The electroencephalograph, or, as it is often called, the E. E. G., helps in the diagnosis, prognosis, and medical treatment of patients and may even assist in advice about marriage and children, since the brain wave pattern is a hereditary trait. Brain surgery, crudely attempted in ancient times, is now a fine art. Recording of electrical messages from the surface or even from the depths of the brain helps the surgeon to identify the epileptogenic focus.

Effective medicines have increased in number and specificity—
the diones (Tridione and Paradione) for *petit mal,* and Phenurone
for psychomotor seizures. Various experimental drugs are in the testing stage.

Thus, instead of being the stepchild of medicine, epilepsy has become a fairy princess. Epilepsy is the chief beneficiary of the electroencephalograph. Study of epilepsy increases our understanding of
that most intricate and important of all contrivances, the human brain.
If abnormal brain function can be remedied, all mankind will benefit.

In the past thirty years more has been learned about the essential
nature of epilepsy and about means of control than in the preceding
three thousand. Unfortunately, social esteem of the epileptic has not
kept pace with improved knowledge and medical treatment of
seizures. Many medieval ideas persist in the public mind; therefore,
the complete conquest and history of epilepsy will be the happy task
of some future historian.

§ REFERENCES

Aretaeus (1856): *The extant works of Aretaeus the Cappadocian*. Edited and translated by Francis Adams. London, Sydenham Society.

Brock, A. J. (1929): *Greek medicine*. London and Toronto, J. M. Dent & Sons; New York, E. P. Dutton & Co.

Celsus (1756): *Of medicine in eight books*. Translated by James Greive. London, D. Wilson and T. Durham.

Gibbs, F. A., and E. L. (1952): *Atlas of electroencephalography*. Cambridge, Massachusetts, Addison-Wesley Press. Vol. II.

Gowers, Sir W. R. (1901): *Epilepsy and other chronic convulsive diseases*. London, J. and A. Churchill.

Hippocrates (1849): *The genuine works of Hippocrates*. Translated from the Greek by Francis Adams. London, Sydenham Society. Vol. II.

Jackson, J. H. (1931): *Selected writings of John Hughlings Jackson*. Edited by James Taylor. London, Hodder and Stoughton. Vol. I.

Lennox, W. G. (1939): "John of Gaddesden on epilepsy." *Ann. med. Hist.*, *1*, 283–307.

Lennox, W. G. (1940): "Antonius Guainerius on epilepsy." *Ann. med. Hist.*, 2, 482–99.

Lennox, W. G. (1941): "Bernard of Gordon on epilepsy." *Ann. med. Hist.*, *3*, 372–83.

Lennox, W. G., and S. Cobb (1928): *Epilepsy*. London, Baillière, Tindall & Cox.

Swieten, G. van (1765): *Aphorisms of Hermann Boerhaave*. London, J. Knapton. Vol. X, p. 335.

Taxil, M. J. (1602): *Traité de l'epilepsie*. Tournon, Claude Michel.

Temkin, O. (1945): *The falling sickness*. Baltimore, Johns Hopkins Press.

Willis, T. (1684): *Practice of physick*. London, T. Dring, C. Harper and J. Leigh.

BY HAROLD BURROWS

C. B. E., Ph. D., F. R. C. S. Eng.*

chapter 16 / CANCER

CANCER is not a modern evil: its treatment was a problem in remote ages. Herodotus tells of a Greek physician, Democedes, who was captured by the Persians and quickly rose to wealth and influence at the Persian court through attending Darius for an injury to the ankle. His good luck, however, did not long endure, for Atossa, the queen, had a growth in her breast which was ulcerated and spreading. While the tumor had been small, she had been too modest to show it to any one. Now, as it had become worse, she consulted Democedes, who undertook to cure her if she would grant him a request. She agreed, and Democedes proceeded with the treatment. His request was that she should persuade Darius to invade Greece. This was already much in the King's mind, and Atossa's advocacy brought him to a decision. Sent by Darius with a preliminary surveying expedition to Greece, where his knowledge of the language would be useful, Democedes deserted and eventually reached his home in Calabria. He had exchanged his prosperity in Asia Minor for a perilous adventure, no doubt because he understood Atossa's condition and the fate which would await him when his inevitable failure to rid her of the cancer should become known. His predecessors at court had been sentenced to impalement because their handling of the King's injured ankle had been deemed unsatisfactory.

The vague hearsay of history yields other tales suggesting that cancer occurred among the ancients. Here is one from the Bible (II Chronicles 21:18–19): "And after all this the Lord smote him [Jehoram] in his bowels with an incurable disease. And it came to pass, that ... after the end of two years ... he died."

*Former experimental pathologist, Research Institute, The Cancer Hospital (Free), London.

Cancer

§ GENERAL PATHOLOGY

Before writing of cancer it may be well to explain what is meant by the term. Cancer is a tumor formed by the uncontrolled growth of certain cells that not only destroy their neighbors, but may enter adjoining lymphatics and blood vessels and be dispersed through them to form secondary tumors in other parts of the body.

Anatomical and Pathological Knowledge. Throughout the Dark Ages every medical thought was governed by "authority," and it was not until the Renaissance that men once again sought the springs of reality. After this awakening, dissection and experimentation revealed many anatomical facts, and the grosser features of cancer were exposed by post-mortem examination. Discoveries of the circulation of the blood (1628), the lymphatic system (1652), and the blood-capillaries (1661) showed how the disease could be carried to distant parts of the body.

Henry François Le Dran (1757) seems to have been the first to appreciate the spread of cancer by the lymphatics to the nearby lymphatic glands: "It is well, before deciding to operate on a cancer of the breast with enlarged glands in the axilla to consider whether the disease may not have already passed into the blood stream."

Many of John Hunter's (1728–93) notes were destroyed without any transcript, yet in those that remain he added to our knowledge of cancer. He drew attention to the hardness of malignant growths as a diagnostic character, and to the central necrosis which is common in these tumors. He also recounted the odd phenomenon of dormant cancer, referring to cases of his own in which, years after an apparently successful removal of a cancerous breast, enlarged glands in the armpit displayed a recrudescence of the disease.

A further advance was made by Marie François Xavier Bichat (1801), who distinguished between the cancerous parenchyma and the noncancerous stroma by which it is supported and nourished.

Invasion of the veins by cancer and its consequent dissemination by the blood stream was first described by Joseph Claude Anthelm Récamier (1829), and it was he who introduced the term "metastasis" for a secondary growth at a distance from the primary one.

Until this time the pathology of tumors had received no histolog-

261

ical study: the cellular nature of animal tissues had not yet been recognized, although in 1665 Robert Hooke had already discovered the cell as the unit of vegetable structure. Examining thin slices of cork, he found that they contained numerous separate compartments, and by making sections in different planes he learned that these compartments were not tubes cut across, but were what he named "cells." He then examined the pith of elder and the stalks of various plants and found that they, too, were largely made up of cells; and the pith of a feather also was seen to be cellular. His observations were greatly extended by Nehemiah Grew between 1672–74, whose illustrations published in 1682 exquisitely show the foundations of vegetable structure.

Though at this period Anton van Leeuwenhoek (1632–1723) had recognized spermatozoa, and both he and Jan Swammerdam (1637–80) had perceived the red blood corpuscles, the cellular composition of animal tissues was not revealed until the nineteenth century because attention had always been focused on the cell wall—a structure not readily visible in animal tissues. Great advances in animal histology were impossible until the introduction of achromatic microscopy—including the use of water immersion and compound objectives—by Giovanni Battista Amici (1812), Arthur Chevalier (1820), and others. The first step forward in histology was made by René Joachim Henri Dutrochet (1824), who announced that organs of animals, like those of plants, are composed of *vésicules agglomérées,* though unlike vegetable cells they cannot always be distinguished by the eye. The cellular structure, he said, is especially easy to see in the liver, testes, or salivary glands of certain molluscs, for the *vésicules* in them are larger than those of vertebrates. At about the same time M. Raspail (1827), when examining adipose tissue, found it to consist of globules composed of a cell wall insoluble in alcohol and the contained fat, which is soluble: *"Donnez-moi une vésicule dans le sein de laquelle puissent s'élaborer et s'infiltrer à mon gré d'autres vésicules; et je vous rendrai le monde organisé."* Raspail asserted also that muscle tissue consisted of bundles of elongated cells.

Not long after these discoveries Johannes Müller was rearranging the collection of tumors in the Royal Museum of Berlin. Dissatisfied with the classification previously adopted, he began to arrange tumors according to their histological appearances. The first results of his work were published in 1836 and 1837. At this time he had both seen and depicted animal cells, though perhaps he had not yet fully appreciated their significance.

Meanwhile, the nature of the cell, whether animal or vegetable, was being better understood. Robert Brown, whose name is associated with "Brownian movement," while studying the fertilization of plants and the developments which follow the application of pollen to the stigma, had already recognized (1831) that each vegetable cell has an areola or "nucleus" as he termed it. Six years later, as the story goes, while Theodor Schwann and Matthias Jakob Schleiden—both pupils of Müller—were dining together, conversation turned on the nuclei of vegetable cells. Schwann remembered having seen similar structures in the cells of certain animal tissues and at once guessed the connection between the two phenomena. The resemblance was quickly confirmed by both observers. Schleiden affirmed that a nucleated cell is the only constituent of the plant embryo and that the development of all vegetable structures must be referred to such cells—a principle afterwards embodied in Virchow's phrase *"omnis cellula e cellula"* (1858), which reminds one of William Harvey's dictum *"ex ovo omnia"* (1651). Schleiden thus established the cell as the unit of physiological activity in plants, and he was the first to describe the "nucleolus." Until this time the growth of animals, whose tissues were furnished with obvious vessels, had been commonly regarded as essentially different from that of plants. Schwann pointed out that there are some animal cells which grow without vessels, mentioning the ovum and epidermis as examples, and he concluded that there was only one original element, namely the cell, of all organized bodies, whether animal or vegetable.

The observations of Schwann and Schleiden were published in 1838, and in the same year appeared Müller's great work on the nature and structural characteristics of cancer (*Über den feinern Bau und die Formen der krankhaften Geschwülste*). Müller's understanding of this disease was far in advance of the general knowledge of his day; for example, he pointed out that a cancer contains within itself the principle of its further development and that cancer cells do not differ in appearance from those of benign tumors or of embryonic tissues. He also called attention to anaplasia as a frequent characteristic of malignant cells. Müller's influence bore remarkable fruit, culminating in Rudolf Virchow's work on cellular pathology and in Julius Friedrich Cohnheim's hypothesis of "resting" cells; for not only Schleiden and Schwann, but Virchow and Cohnheim also had studied under Müller.

Grades of Malignancy. David Paul von Hansemann in 1902 called renewed attention to anaplasia as a feature of many tumors and tried to correlate the degree of anaplasia—the failure of its cells to reach an adult, highly differentiated form—with the degree of clinical malignancy. J. Schottlaender and F. Kermauner (1912), regarding uterine cancer, concluded that the most anaplastic tumors were the most malignant. On this foundation endeavors were made to grade the malignancy of a cancer before operation by the degree of differentiation present in its cells (A. C. Broders, 1920; W. C. MacCarty, 1925, and others). This attempt at grading a tumor before its removal is independent, of course, of the presence or absence of detectable metastases.

Propagation of Tumors by Transplantation. In the early days of cancer research much was learned by grafting portions of a tumor from one animal into another of the same species. The first successful operation of this kind was done by Arthur Nathan Hanau (1889), who grafted pieces of a subcutaneous cancer from one rat into two other rats. Leo Loeb (1901) went further: he transplanted portions of a spontaneous thyroid cancer into other rats, and by repeating the performance he maintained the tumor for fifteen months, using 360 transplants in 150 animals; throughout this period the morphological and physiological characters of the original cancer were preserved. Carl Oluf Jensen (1903) amplified this method of study: he carried a mouse tumor unchanged through nineteen generations of graft and showed that the daughter growths consisted of cells derived from the graft and not from those of the host, though the latter supplied the stroma by which the tumor cells were maintained. As A. M. Cloudman (1932) states, all the detectable physiological characteristics of tumors carried on by a succession of grafts are under an orderly genetic control which is specific for each tumor and is unaltered by the host.

The irreversibility of the cancerous change has been proved not only by the long successions of tumor grafting just mentioned, but also by cytological practice. Albert Fischer (1948) maintained by artificial culture the cells of an Ehrlich mouse carcinoma for fifteen years, and in all this time the numerous subcultures retained their malignant character, as shown by their producing cancer when inoculated into mice (A. Fischer and F. Davidsohn, 1939).

Growth of Malignant Tumors. The transition from innocence to malignancy appears to be a graduated change and not a sudden one. As Sir Henry T. Butlin (1892) pointed out, soot does not immediately induce cancer; it brings about a precancerous condition which seems to go no further at the time and perhaps never becomes malignant. Experiments in the laboratory show that, if a carcinogen is repeatedly applied to the dorsal skin of a mouse until warts appear, and then no more applications are made, one of three things may happen: the warts may disappear; they may persist as simple warts; one or more of them may become malignant. The successive stages, as Alexander Haddow has remarked, are hyperplasia, innocent neoplasia, cancer—an ordered development particularly well seen in the neoplasias produced by estrogens (H. Burrows and E. S. Horning, 1952).

Criteria of Malignancy. The facts just mentioned raise a doubt as to the reliability of our customary tests for cancer, which depend on the presence or absence of invasion by the tumor of the adjacent tissues; for the innocent tumor of today may be cancerous in the future.

Multifocal Cancer. Surgeons used to be taught that every cancer has a single point of origin, and though this notion has been helpful in practice, it is no longer acceptable as a generalization. Sir George Lenthal Cheatle, by his large sections of breast tissue, showed that the early changes of mammary cancer in women may be more diffuse than had previously been believed (Cheatle and Max Cutler, 1931); and several human tumors, e.g. hereditary polyposis of the large intestine and epitheliomata due to arsenic or sunlight, are often multiple. In the laboratory the simultaneous appearance of cancer in two or more of the mammae is a familiar occurrence among mice.

Respiration of Malignant Tissues. In 1926 Otto Warburg reported that cancer cells obtain part of their energy, like those of the embryo, not only by oxidizing glucose, but also by splitting it without oxidation into lactic acid. In fact, cancer cells can live anaerobically in the presence, though not in the absence, of glucose.

§ CAUSATION OF CANCER

The notion that cancer was a constitutional or "humoral" disorder caused by an excessive accumulation of "black bile" was accepted and tenaciously held through many centuries. Once the inadequacy of this idea was recognized, a search began for some alternative view of its causation.

§ *Exogenous Carcinogens*

Soot, Tar, and Mineral Oils. Our recognition of chemical carcinogens as such begins with Percivall Pott's account of scrotal cancer in chimney sweeps (1775), in which he attributed the disease to a lodgement of soot in the rugae of the scrotum. Pott's observation was added to in the following year by Manouvriez (1776), who reported the occurrence of scrotal cancer in fuel briquette makers. Sir James Earle (1808) in a second edition of Pott's works mentioned two patients with soot cancer who were not chimney sweeps. One of the men, with a scrotal cancer, had never swept a chimney, but had lodged with a chimney sweep in whose house soot bags were deposited. The other patient was a gardener who had often sprinkled soot among young plants; he used to carry the soot in a garden pot slung to his left hand by a loop, and the cancer appeared where the loop had rested on the back of his hand.

The long interval which may occur between the last exposure to soot and the appearance of cancer was pointed out by Thomas Blizard Curling (1853), who had noticed that men who had been chimney sweeps when young, but had since been long removed from contact with soot, might nevertheless come to have a scrotal cancer.

Our knowledge of the causation of cancer by particular materials was enlarged by Richard von Volkmann (1875), who described three instances of scrotal cancer in laborers at a brown-coal tar works, and in 1876 by Joseph Bell—the prototype of Sherlock Holmes—who reported two examples of scrotal cancer affecting shale-oil workers in Scotland.

The greatest advance in our knowledge of cancer in the nineteenth century was made by Sir Henry Butlin (1892), whose observations may be summarized as follows:

(1) Scrotal cancer is not brought about by mechanical irritation as had been thought. More irritation of the scrotum is caused in several occupations than those of a chimney sweep without producing cancer.

(2) The peculiar frequency of sweeps' cancer in England as compared with that in the United States of America or the continent of Europe is due to personal uncleanliness and other local circumstances and not to a difference in the quality of the soot.

(3) Sweeps' cancer is heralded by precancerous warts which may long exist in a benign state before becoming malignant.

(4) Soot prepares the tissues for cancer because of some chemical influence. For one hundred years, he says, we have seen the human experiment of "the repeated applications of a chemical substance, or a mixture of chemical substances, to a particular part of the integument which is not at all predisposed to cancer, with the effect of rendering it pre-eminently disposed to the occurrence of cancer."

(5) On one occasion Butlin noticed that the men in a gas works who were particularly subject to warts were those employed with the last products of coal-tar distillation, that is to say, with those compounds which had been distilled at the highest temperature.

Attempts to learn the cellular reactions to tar were made by H. P. G. Bayon (1912), who injected it with lanolin into the ears of rabbits; and when the animals were killed two months later, the tar was found to have caused pronounced epithelial proliferation with the formation of cell nests, whereas lanolin alone had no such result. In private correspondence Bayon informed me that before his own experiments, though he had been unaware of it at the time, Hanau had induced some cutaneous proliferation by repeated applications of tar to rats' scrota. Bayon said that he had afterwards examined Hanau's specimens and could confirm his results. Here, as an incidental matter of general interest, it may be mentioned that Hanau's suicide was not, as some have stated, attributable to any lack of appreciation of his work by others, but to cancer.

The experimental production of cancer was first achieved by Katsusaburo Yamagiwa and Koichi Ichikawa in 1916 by repeated application of tar to rabbits' ears, and in 1918 Tsutsui caused epitheliomata in mice by painting coal tar on their backs. Because of its speed, cheapness, and ease, this is a common method of testing the capacity of any substance to induce cancer of the skin. By means of it Passey (1922) produced tumors in mice with domestic chimney soot, and in a comparable way with tar he brought about epitheliomata in dogs (1938).

Attempts were soon begun to discover which of the very numerous constituents of tar were able to induce cancer. A pointer was given by Ross (1918), who noticed that occupational cancer was more readily caused by gas-works tar than by blast-furnace tar, which is distilled at a lower temperature. Bloch and Dreifuss (1921) also found that the carcinogenic agent of coal tar lay among the highest boiling constituents: it was a neutral, nonnitrogenous substance which could be distilled without decomposition. A notable advance was made by Sir Ernest L. Kennaway (1924), who showed that carcinogenic tars could be produced by submitting acetylene or isoprene to high temperatures in an atmosphere of hydrogen, thus proving that some carcinogens are pure hydrocarbons. Furthermore, Kennaway (1925) heated acetylene, isoprene, yeast, and human skin to various temperatures and found that the carcinogenic potency of the resultant tar depended largely on the degree of heat which had been used.

Synthetic Carcinogens. Fruitful pioneer work was initiated by Mayneord in 1927 when he examined the fluorescence and fluorescence spectra of tars and observed three distinct shadows in the spectra of every carcinogenic tar examined. The short wave-length edges of these bands were at 4,000, 4,180, and 4,400 A. In this work he was joined by Hieger, and they found that the intensity of these bands predominated over the combined bands of all the other fluorescent substances in tar. Having received from de Barry Barnett various specimens of hydrocarbons, they discovered that 1:2 benzpyrene had the spectrum of cancer-producing tars; when tested on mice this compound was proved to be carcinogenic. Subsequently, by a fractional analysis of a carcinogenic pitch guided by the characteristic spectrum, Hieger (1937) found that 3:4 benzpyrene was a predominant, though not the only, carcinogen in tar (Cook, Hewett, and Hieger, 1933). A further observation was that 1:2:5:6 dibenz-anthracene also had the characteristic fluorescent spectra and was carcinogenic.

The molecular structure of these and chemically allied carcinogens led to a search for some connection between them and the naturally occurring sterols and bile acids; though no connection was found, the search brought about the synthesis from deoxycholic acid of the very potent carcinogen methylcholanthrene (Cooke and Hasle-wood, 1934).

These discoveries by Kennaway, Mayneord, and their colleagues have been followed by the synthesis of numerous carcinogens, and they are not all pure hydrocarbons.

Azo-compounds and Tumors of the Liver. The first chemical compound to be recognized experimentally as a cause of cell proliferation was not a hydrocarbon, but an azo-compound. B. Fischer (1906) injected the dye scarlet red into rabbits' ears and in this way caused tumor-like proliferations of epithelium, which resembled early cancer but always receded after a time, and no cancer was produced by scarlet red until Yamagiwa and Ohno (1918), by injecting it into the wall of the hen's oviduct, induced cancer in three of the forty-one hens so treated. A little later, Schmidt (1924), when trying to follow the progress of fats stained with scarlet red and given orally to mice, observed a hepatoma in one of the animals at the end of thirteen months. Pursuing the subject further, Yoshida (1932) gave o-amido-azotoluol —which had been found by Hayward (1909) to be the active component of scarlet red—by the mouth to rats with the consequence that adenomas of the liver appeared in some of them within five to eight months, and eventually hepatic cancers were found in four of the nine survivors. Later reports (Yoshida, 1934; Nishyama, 1935; Sasaki and Yoshida, 1935; Hashimoto, 1935) showed that hepatic cancer was the usual result of giving o-amido-azotoluol to rats, mice, and rabbits; and the same effect was produced by introducing the compound subcutaneously in mice (Shear, 1937). Surprisingly, it has been found that the ability of o-amido-azotoluol and some related compounds to cause liver tumors depends largely on the nature of the animal's diet (Maisin, Pourbaix, and Cuvelier, 1939).

Bladder Tumors in Dye Workers. In 1895 Rehn reported the occurrence of vesical tumors in three of forty-five workmen employed making fuchsin, and he says that Granhomme had already noticed hematuria in dye workers, though he does not give the reference. Experimentally, Hueper and Wolfe (1937), and Hueper, Wiley, and Wolfe (1938) induced tumors of the bladder in dogs by giving them beta-naphthylamine by the mouth. The same result may be caused in rats by repeated subcutaneous injections of the compound. Another compound now known to cause tumors of the bladder is benzidine (Hueper, 1950).

Apropos of bladder tumors regarded generally, Henry, Kennaway, and Kennaway (1931) learned from the death certificates for England and Wales during 1921–28 that tumors of the bladder in tar distillery workers were five times as frequent as in farmers.

Metallic Carcinogens. The capacity of arsenites to cause epithelioma in man was first noticed by Jonathan Hutchinson in 1887, and it has been confirmed since by clinical experience. The disease has appeared in patients who have had prolonged treatment with arsenic for psoriasis, for the bromide rashes in epileptics, or for other skin troubles. Today it is a recognized item of public health that arsenic acquired accidentally through the water supply or in handling arsenical preparations, including sheep dip, may bring about skin cancer in man (Neubauer, 1947).

From certain limited factory experiences it seems that some compounds of nickel may cause malignant disease, especially of the nasal mucous membrane, and recently Hueper has reported the induction of sarcoma in the mouse by injections of powdered nickel. Hitherto, arsenic has failed to induce cancer in laboratory animals.

Parasites. The possibility that cancer of the bladder might be caused by Bilharzia was suggested by R. H. Harrison in 1889. He described the pathological findings in five patients who had died in Alexandria with Bilharzia-infected bladders, and in four of the cases carcinoma was present. Since then the association of bilharzial infection with cancer of the bladder has been accepted by some as an instance of cause and effect. Thus, Afifi (1947) reported that eighty patients with vesical cancer seen at the Kasr-El-Ainy Hospital in Cairo between the years 1905 and 1930 all had bilharzial lesions in the bladder. Yet, as a specific cause of cancer, the role of bilharziasis may be doubted, for the incidence of this infection in the native population of the Egyptian delta has been found to be very high, and its association with cancer may, therefore, be merely a matter of chance. However, if not the cause, Bilharzia may perhaps have some influence on the incidence of bladder cancer through the chronic irritation which it provides.

A great sensation was caused when Johannes Fibiger (1913) reported the occurrence of papillomata in the stomach of rats which had been fed on cockroaches infected with a nematode (*Gongylonema neoplasticum*). The diet of these rats had been unsupplemented white bread, and some years later Fibiger's conclusions were controverted, for it was found that the lesions, which had sometimes been regarded as cancer, were in fact the nonmalignant metaplastic changes brought about in the gastric epithelium by a deficiency of vitamin A in the diet. The same results could be obtained in rats maintained on white bread alone, whether or not cockroaches were supplied in addition (Passey, Leese, and Knox, 1935).

Cysticercus fasciolaris is the only animal parasite proved by experiment to cause cancer. This parasite is the larval stage of *Taenia crassicolis,* a tape worm of cats. Bullock, Curtis, and Rohdenburg (1920) infected five hundred rats with the *cysticercus* by adding to their food the eggs of *Taenia crassicolis* obtained from cats' feces. An outcome of this experiment was the occurrence of sarcomata in many of the rats, the tumors arising in every instance in the wall of a parasitic cyst. The observation has been abundantly confirmed by others, and an interesting sequel has been recorded by Dunning and Curtis (1946), who gave intraperitoneal injections of a saline suspension made from cysts of *Cysticercus fasciolaris* to 103 rats, among which peritoneal sarcomata developed in 51.

Viruses and Cancer. Many years ago it was learned that human warts were caused by a filterable agent, and later experiments have shown that in laboratory animals tumors may sometimes be caused by a virus. In 1911 F. Peyton Rous announced that he had propagated a sarcoma growing in a chicken to other fowls by a cell-free tumor filtrate; and later Rous and Murphy (1914) reported the propagation of three different fowl sarcomas by cell-free filtrates. In each instance the inoculation had caused the quick appearance of a sarcoma precisely like that from which the filtrate had been obtained. Since then, viruses have been shown to cause malignant disease in other animals, e.g. the mouse (Bittner, 1936, 1940), the rabbit (R. E. Shope, 1932, 1933), the frog (Lucké, 1934). In causing the Shope tumor by the cell-free agent there is no great delay, but in other instances there is a peculiar time lag between the introduction of the virus and the appearance of the tumor. This curious phenomenon is seen in mammary cancer of mice (Bittner, 1936), renal tumors of the leopard frog (Lucké, 1934), and in mouse leukemia (Gross, 1952).

§ *Carcinogenic Irradiations*

Ultraviolet Light. Paul Gerson Unna (1894) was the first to attribute skin cancers to sunlight, and mentioned a particular liability to the disease among sailors. His observations have been confirmed by others (Shield, 1899; Hyde, 1906; Dubreuilh, 1907; Paul, 1918), who have shown that fair people are more subject to the disease than dark ones and that the condition is commonest in agriculturists and others who are most exposed to direct sunlight, especially in those parts of the world where the actinic rays are most plentiful. Areas of skin directly exposed to the rays, e.g. the backs of the hands, tips of the ears, nose, and lower lip, are most often affected; and not only are the thickness and pigmentation of the epithelium protective factors, but the angle of incidence of the rays on the skin is a regulating condition (Magnuson, 1935); for example, the lower lip is affected nearly ten times as often as the upper one.

Epitheliomata have been produced in the laboratory by subjecting albino mice, rats, and rabbits to repeated exposures to the ultraviolet rays of a mercury-vapor lamp (Findlay, 1928, 1930; Holtz and Putschar, 1930). *Xeroderma pigmentosum* in man appears to be a special instance of sunlight cancer in patients who have inherited a Mendelian recessive character, which renders them unusually susceptible to the malady (Macklin, 1936).

X Rays. Soon after Roentgen's discovery in 1895 it became apparent

that X rays, like excessive sunlight on a fair skin, caused dermatitis
(Gilchrist, 1897), and a few years later the first case of X-ray cancer
was shown by A. Frieben at a meeting of the Hamburg Medical
Society in 1902. The patient, thirty-three years old, had been employed
for four years in making X-ray tubes, which he habitually tested with
his own hand, on the back of which, after a severe dermatitis, an ulcer
appeared and was diagnosed by Unna as a cancer. The patient's arm
was amputated that year, but death occurred in 1906 from metastasis.
Thereafter, nearly every one who had made frequent use of X rays
for medical purposes early in this century became, after a period of
intractable dermatitis, afflicted with cancer of the hand. Experiments
have shown that the rat, rabbit, guinea pig, and mouse are all susceptible to cancer under the influence of X rays (Marie, Clunet, and
Raulot-Lapointe, 1910; Block, 1923; Goebel and Gérard, 1925; Lüdin,
1934; Furth and Butterworth, 1936). Experiments on animals have
shown that a single dose of X rays is more likely to induce cancer
in a tissue which is already inflamed at the time of exposure than in
one that is not inflamed.

Radium and Other Radioactive Substances. As long ago as 1879 the
frequency of pulmonary cancer among workers in the Schneeberg
and Schwartzenberg mines was demonstrated by F. H. Härting and
W. Hesse, though obviously at that time the cause could not be veri-
fied. The dust of the mines includes cobalt, nickel, bismuth, arsenic,
and radioactive substances, and the air contains radon; and there is
little doubt that the lung cancer is attributable to the radiations.

The carcinogenic action of radium was first shown by epithelioma
of the thumb in men who frequently handled it (MacNeal and Willis,
1923; Wakeley, 1927), and the subject received acute attention through
a disaster in the United States of America, where girls had been employed in applying luminous paint to the dials of watches. The paint
consisted of zinc sulphide containing minute amounts of radium,
mesothorium, and radiothorium. The girls gave a fine point to their
brushes with their lips and so continually swallowed tiny doses of
radioactive materials which became permanently deposited in their
bones, in which sarcomata thereafter arose (H. S. Martland and
Humphries, 1929; Martland, 1931). Since then sarcomata have been
induced experimentally by radium and other radioactive minerals in

the rat, rabbit, mouse, and fowl (Daels, 1925; Daels and Biltris, 1931; Mottram, 1931, 1935; Sabin, Doan, and Forkner, 1932).

§ ENDOGENOUS CARCINOGENS

Estrogens, unlike the exogenous carcinogens, are normal products of life and are secreted by the ovaries, adrenals, testes, and placenta. Their pathological effects are vastly important, for they are frequent causes of neoplasia in women. The first experimental indication of their carcinogenicity was the fact that by spaying newborn mice of a strain very subject to mammary cancer, their liability to this disease was almost abolished (Lathrop and Loeb, 1916). Goormaghtigh and Amerlinck (1930) refined the problem: they injected daily into female mice an extract of follicular fluid from sows' ovaries, and in time the mice displayed cystic mastopathy, adenomata, and in one instance cancer of the breast. From similar follicular fluid, Mac-Corquodale, Thayer, and Doisy (1936) isolated alpha-estradiol. Already estrone in pure form had been extracted by Doisy, Veler, and Thayer (1929), and by Butenandt (1929), from the urine of pregnant women. The numerous estrogens, natural and synthetic, which are now known, all have biological effects which are qualitatively alike, even as carcinogens.

In women and several mammals the main secretion of estrogen occurs in brief recurrent periods, a larger output being followed by a smaller one; and the histological changes normally caused by estrogen are reversible and last only as long as there is enough of the hormone to maintain them (H. Burrows, 1935). To induce any tumor, estrogen must be supplied in effective quantity without intermissions long enough to permit reversion of its effects (Lipschutz, Rodrigues, and Vargas, 1939, 1941). With this proviso and the choice of a suitable animal, the persistent administration of estrogen will induce tumors in the pituitary (Cramer and Horning, 1936; Zondek, 1936; H. Burrows, 1936); the breast (Lacassagne, 1932; H. Burrows, 1935); the uterus [including fibromyomata (Nelson, 1937; Moricard and Cauchoix, 1938; Lipschutz and Iglesias, 1938), endometrial cancer (Greene and Saxton, 1938, H. Burrows, 1940), cervical cancer (Gardner and Allen, 1939)]; the ovary (Champy, 1937; Mosinger, 1947); the testicle (H. Burrows, 1935, 1936, 1937; Gardner, 1937); the adrenal

(Gardner, 1947); the kidney (Matthews, Kirkman, and Bacon, 1947); the bones (Pybus and Miller, 1938, 1940); and subcutaneous tissues (Cori, 1927; Suntzeff, Burns, Moskop, and Loeb, 1936; Gardner, Smith, Strong, and Allen, 1936; Lacassagne, 1937).

Estrogens have also been thought to take part in the causation of tumors of the prostate (H. Burrows, 1949; Teilum, 1950); the bladder (Dunning, Curtis, and Segaloff, 1947); epididymis (Vasquez-Lopez, 1944); and some forms of leucosis. (For a fuller account of the neoplastic effects of estrogen see Burrows and Horning, 1952.)

One of the factors in the causation of tumors by estrogen is the quantitative balance between this hormone and those secreted by the other endocrine organs, for one hormone may inhibit the production of another, or may increase or lessen its action according to the relative concentrations in which the two are present.

Murray (1937) established parabiosis between male and female mice so that there was a continual exchange of hormones between them, and in 189 such pairs, although the mice belonged to a strain peculiarly liable to mammary cancer, not one instance of this tumor occurred. Others have shown that cancer of the breast in mice can be prevented by repeated injections of androgen (Lacassagne, 1939; Nathanson and Andervont, 1939); and either androgen or progestin can prevent the development of abdominal and uterine fibromata in guinea pigs (Lipschutz and Schwartz, 1944; Lipschutz, Bruzzone and Fuenzalida, 1944; Courrier, 1950).

§ Ancillary Agents of Neoplasia

Certain conditions that do not themselves induce cancer may nevertheless encourage its development.

Heredity. In man a familial tendency to some special kind of cancer has long been recognized, e.g. polyposis of the large intestine, some tumors of the eye, and the occurrence of tumors in identical organs in uniovular twins. In mice two kinds of cancer inheritance are known: the first is genic, and the second is a virus infection carried to the infant in the mother's milk.

Nutrition. A predilection to affect otherwise healthy people has been traditionally attributed to cancer, probably with some truth. Human statistics show that the liability to this malady rises with the proportion of weight to height (Dublin, 1929; Tannenbaum, 1940); and in the laboratory most tumors are seen to grow more readily in well-fed than in ill-nourished animals (Loeb, Blumenthal, and Kirtz, 1944; Tannenbaum and Silverstone, 1946, 1949). On the other hand, as already remarked, certain kinds of malnutrition are apt to cause tumors of the liver.

Chronic Irritation. For centuries cancer was attributed to chronic irritation without which, Theodor Billroth affirmed, it does not occur. Johannes Müller (1838) questioned this idea; he pointed out that a scirrhous cancer of the breast develops without any preceding inflammation and that its structure differs *ab initio* from that of inflammatory induration. As to the tendency of certain innocent lesions to become cancerous, he remarked that some of them, including nevi, are less prone than normal tissues to inflammation.

The favoring effect of inflammation in precipitating cancer was shown by Berenblum (1949), using chemical carcinogens, and by Lacassagne and Vinzent (1929), and Burrows, Mayneord, and Roberts (1937), with X rays. There are two possible explanations: (*a*) Any carcinogen present in the circulation will pass most readily into an inflamed tissue and be retained there by inflammatory fixation. Such an event has been demonstrated by Brunelli (1935), using estrone, and can be regarded as a principle of pathology (H. Burrows, 1932). (*b*) Inflammation causes an increased rate of cell division.

Accelerated mitogenesis, whatever its cause, may be an important factor in cancer, for chemical agents have been shown to act with special facility on cells which are dividing. Various influences affecting mitogenetic activity have been detailed in a fine series of papers by Bullough (1949, 1950, 1952; Bullough and Eisa, 1950).

Cell Rests. Cohnheim (1877), like his teacher Müller, found it hard to attribute cancer purely to chronic irritation, and he suggested that during embryonic growth more cells may be produced here and there than are immediately required, and that, although quiescent, they may yet retain a special capacity for proliferation in response to some stimulus in later life. Whether some forms of cancer, especially teratomata, have such an origin remains to be proved. Nevertheless it has been demonstrated (H. Burrows, 1944) that such embryonic cells do exist and may remain in a dormant state throughout life, retaining all the while an ability to multiply and differentiate if a suitable stimulus is provided.

§ TREATMENT OF CANCER

Surgical removal. Attempts were sometimes made even in remote ages to get rid of a cancer by excision or cautery; yet the failure of these methods was already perceived by Hippocrates, who says (Aphorism 38) that they are more apt to shorten than to prolong the patient's life.

Today a surgeon's ideal would be, of course, to operate during the precancerous stage. F. J. V. Broussais advocated this as long ago as 1816. He complained that the practitioners of his day were too fatalistic about cancer: when an organ or tissue remains indurated, he declared, they await the issue before making a diagnosis, and when the tumor has become obvious they claim that it could not have been foretold, and having reached this stage it is pronounced incurable.

Modern operations for cancer have been governed by the details of its pathological anatomy, the purpose being to eradicate the tumor before it has extended too widely either by direct spread or by metastasis through the vessels; and the main epochs of this work are those concerning all surgical interference. The use of anesthesia (Morton, 1846) allowed a more elaborate dissection than could be performed on a sentient patient, and the introduction by Lister of antiseptic surgery in 1860 made operations comparatively safe which till then had been hazardous or impossible.

Irradiation. The discovery of X rays (Roentgen, 1895) and the radio-activity of uranium (Becquerel, 1896), and the isolation of radium (M. and P. Curie, 1898), led almost at once to experimental applications of the newly discovered irradiations to diseased tissues. The first successful treatment of cancer by X rays was reported by T. Sjögren in 1899: the patient had an epithelioma of the cheek. Four years later S. W. Goldberg and E. S. London (1903) showed two patients in whom basal-cell carcinoma had healed after treatment with radium; and in 1904 R. Abbe was already able to state from personal experience that superficial epitheliomata, rodent ulcers, and small recurrent cancer nodules would disappear under the influence of radium. Since then the application of X rays or radium has become the accepted treatment for superficial cancer.

The use of irradiation for other than surface growths has not been so straightforward. If, as was done at first, X rays were given to a deeply situated growth through a single portal, the skin through which they entered was liable to severe damage because it received larger doses of irradiation than the underlying tumor—the softer rays, then in common use, having relatively small powers of penetration. Several ways of avoiding this complication were devised. One of these was invented by Henri Dominici (1908) who interposed a sheet of lead between the X-ray tube and the patient so as to arrest the softer rays. Subsequently the screen of lead was replaced by one of copper because this provides a more homogeneous wave length in the beam of rays.

Another way to avoid superficial damage when irradiating a deeply seated tumor was to direct the beam of rays successively on to it through different areas of skin so that the tumor and its immediate surroundings received a larger total dose than that to which the various superficial tissues were subjected. Yet an additional method of achieving this end was by using the hardest, most penetrating rays, obtained either from radium or from X-ray machinery with extremely high voltages and other devices.

For a long while a persistent obstacle to accurate radiotherapy was the absence of any precise measurement of the radiation used. This difficulty disappeared when in 1937 the "roentgen" was universally accepted as the unit for estimating the doses of X rays or radium.

Hormonal therapy. John Hunter (1728–93) long ago saw that castration led to a progressive atrophy of the prostate, and subsequent attempts to cure prostatic enlargements by removal of the testicles were founded on this observation (Wood, 1900; White, 1893, 1895, 1904). Though some good results were reported, the operation was soon abandoned for reasons which now seem inadequate. The operation has been revived for the treatment of prostatic cancer with success (Huggins and Stevens, 1940; Huggins, Stevens, and Hodges, 1941).

278

Cancer

Though it does not provide a permanent cure of prostatic cancer, it gives great temporary relief and some prolongation of life. The recurrence of the trouble which happens after a while may be due to a compensatory secretion of gonadal hormones by the adrenals, for this is known to occur; and to overcome the drawback the operation of double adrenalectomy has been introduced.

Beneficial treatment for cancer of the prostate may be induced in another way, namely, by administering estrogen: this reduces the output of androgen from the testicles and to some extent may neutralize its action (Kahle and Maltby, 1940; Herrold, 1941; and many others).

A comparable train of thought arose about cancer of the breast in women, and it was hoped to retard the disease by removing the ovaries (Sir G. T. Beatson, 1896, 1902, 1910; Boyd, 1900; Thompson, 1902; Lett, 1905; and others). After a brief experience of oöphorectomy, often combined with dosages of thyroid extract—a method of treatment which was said to benefit about 30 per cent of the cases—the procedure became obsolete.

Instead of reducing the supply of estrogen by removing the ovaries, its secretion may be diminished by prolonged treatment with androgen, and this will prevent the development of mammary cancer. The effect was shown by Murray (1937) who joined together male and female mice like Siamese twins. A strain of mice was used among whose females spontaneous mammary cancer was very common; and yet among 189 pairs living parabiotically not a single tumor of the breast appeared. The prevention of mammary cancer in mice by repeated injections of androgen was demonstrated by Lacassagne (1939); Nathanson and Andervont (1939); Heiman (1944); and Gardner (1947). Still another way of preventing mammary cancer in mice was shown by Huseby, Smith, and Bittner (1946): they grafted ovaries into male mice, some of which were castrated. The ultimate percentages of cancer in the breasts of these mice was 84.0 in the castrated ones and 2.5 in those with testes.

Chemotherapy. The possibility of preventing or curing certain kinds of tumor by the use of appropriate hormones, vitamins, aminoacids, and other biological and nonbiological materials is being investigated with vigor in many parts of the world. Perhaps the most promising

279

inquiry is based on Alexander Haddow's observation that many carcinogenic agents will retard for a time the growth of existing tumors, and this is true to some extent of hydrocarbons whose carcinogenic potency is feeble (Haddow, 1935; Haddow and Robinson, 1937; Haddow, Scott, and Scott, 1937). Haddow had already noticed in bacteria that an increased rate of proliferation is apt to follow a long continued period of growth inhibition. The important significance of these two facts in their application to cancer can be readily apprehended.

§ REFERENCES

Abbe, R. (1904): *Yale med. News, 10,* 433.

Afifi, M. A. (1947): *Cancer Res., 7,* 537.

Amici, G. B. (1890): *Ann. Chim. Phys., 13,* 384.

Bagg, H. J. (1936): *Amer. J. Cancer, 26,* 69.

Bayon, H. (1912): Lancet, *ii,* 1579.

Bell, J. (1876): *Edinb. med. J., 22,* 135.

Berenblum, I. (1949): *The Biological Mechanism of Carcinogenesis.*

Bichat, M. F. X. (1801): *Anat. gén., 1,* 99. Part 1.

Biskind, M. S., and G. R. (1945): *Proc. Soc. exp. Biol. Med., N. Y., 39,* 4.

Bittner, J. J. (1931): *Amer. J. Cancer, 15,* 2202.

Bittner, J. J., and C. C. Little (1937): *J. Hered., 28,* 117.

Bloch, B. (1923): *Congrès Cancer, Strasbourg, 2,* 31.

Bloch, B., and W. Dreifuss (1921): *Schweiz. med. Wschr., 2,* 1033.

Boyd, S. (1900): *Brit. med. J., ii,* 1161.

Brambell, F. W. R., A. S. Parkes, and U. Fielding (1927): *Proc. roy. Soc., B, 101,* 29.

Broders, A. C. (1920): *J. Amer. med. Ass., 74,* 656.

Broussais, F. J. V. (1816): *Examen de la doctrine médicale généralement adoptée et des systèmes moderne de nosologie.* Paris.

Brown, R. (1833): *On the organs and mode of fecundation in Orchideae and Asclepiadiae.* London.

Brunelli, B. (1935): *Arch. int. Pharmacodyn., 49,* 214, 243, 262.

Bulloch, F. D., M. R. Curtis, and G. L. Rohdenburg (1920): *Proc. Soc. exp. Biol. Med., N. Y., 18,* 29.

Bullough, W. S. (1949): *J. exp. Biol., 26,* 261, 287.

Bullough, W. S. (1949): *Brit. J. Cancer, 3,* 275.

Bullough, W. S. (1950): *Nature, Lond., 165,* 493.

Bullough, W. S. (1950): *J. Endocrinol., 6,* 340, 350.

Bullough, W. S. (1952): *J. Endocrinol., 8,* 265.

Bullough, W. S. (1952): *Biol. Rev., 27,* 133.

Bullough, W. S., and E. A. Eisa (1950): *J. exp. Biol., 27,* 257.

Cancer

Bullough, W. S., and E. A. Eisa (1950): *Brit. J. Cancer, 4,* 321.

Burrows, H. (1932): *Some factors in the localisation of disease.* London.

Burrows, H. (1935): *Amer. J. Cancer, 23,* 490.

Burrows, H. (1935): *J. Path. Bact., 41,* 218.

Burrows, H. (1936): *Amer. J. Cancer, 28,* 741.

Burrows, H. (1936): *J. Path. Bact., 42,* 161.

Burrows, H. (1937): *J. Path. Bact., 44,* 699.

Burrows, H. (1940): *J. Path. Bact., 51,* 385.

Burrows, H. (1944): *Yale J. Biol. Med., 17,* 397.

Burrows, H. (1949): *Biological actions of sex hormones.* Cambridge.

Burrows, H., and E. S. Horning (1952): *Oestrogens and neoplasia.* Oxford.

Butenandt, A. (1929): *Dtsch. med. Wschr., 55,* 2171.

Butlin, Sir H. T. (1892): *Brit. med. J., i,* 1341–46; *ii,* 1–6, 66–71.

Champy, C. (1937): *C. R. Soc. Biol., Paris, 125,* 634.

Cheatle, Sir G. L., and M. Cutler (1931): *Tumours of the breast.* London.

Cloudman, A. M. (1932): *Amer. J. Cancer, 16,* 568.

Cohnheim, J. F. (1877): *Vorlesungen über allgemeine Pathologie.* Berlin.

Cook, J. W., and G. A. D. Haslewood (1934): *J. chem. Soc.,* 428.

Cook, J. W., C. L. Hewett, and I. Hieger (1933): *J. chem. Soc.,* 395.

Cori, C. F. (1927): *J. exp. Med., 45,* 983.

Courrier, R. (1950): *Vitam. & Horm., 8,* 191.

Cramer, W., and E. S. Horning (1936): *Lancet, i,* 247.

Curling, T. B. (1853): *A practical treatise on the diseases of the testis.* London, Vol. II, p. 459.

Daels, F. (1925): *Brit. J. Radiol., 30,* 474.

Daels, F., and R. Biltris (1931): *Bull. Ass. franç. Cancer, 20,* 32.

Doisy, E. A., C. D. Veler, and S. Thayer (1929): *Amer. J. Physiol., 90,* 329.

Dominici, H. (1908): *Congr. franç. Méd.,* 9th session, 429.

Dublin, L. I. (1929): *Trans. Life Insce med. Dir. America, 15,* 402.

Dubreuilh, W. (1907): *Ann. Derm. Syph., Paris, 8,* 387.

Dunning, W. F., and M. R. Curtis (1946): *Cancer Res., 6,* 668.

Dunning, W. F., M. R. Curtis, and A. Segaloff (1947): *Cancer Res. 7,* 511.

Dutrochet, H. (1824): *Recherches anatomiques et physiologiques sur la structure intime des animaux et des végéteaux, et sur leur mobilité.* Paris.

Earle, Sir J. (1808): *The chirurgical works of Percivall Pott.* 2nd ed. London. Vol. III, p. 180.

Falin, L. I. (1940): *Amer. J. Cancer, 38,* 199.

Fibiger, J. (1913): *Z. Krebsforsch., 13,* 217.

Findlay, G. M. (1928): *Lancet, ii,* 1070.

Findlay, G. M. (1930): *Lancet, i,* 218.

Fischer, A. (1948): Personal correspondence.

Fischer, A., and F. Davidsohn (1939): *Nature, Lond., 143,* 436.

Fischer, B. (1906): *Münch. med. Wschr., 53,* 2041.

Frieben, A. (1902): *Dtsch. med. Wschr., 28,* 335.

Furth, J., and J. S. Butterworth (1936): *Amer. J. Cancer, 28,* 54, 66.

Gardner, W. U. (1937): *Anat. Rec., 68,* 339.

Gardner, W. U. (1947): *Recent Progr. Hormone Res., 1,* 217.

Gardner, W. U., and E. Allen (1939): *Yale J. Biol. Med., 12,* 213.

Gardner, W. U., G. M. Smith, L. C. Strong and E. Allen (1936): *Arch. Path., 21,* 504.

Gilchrist, T. C. (1897): *Bull. Johns Hopk. Hosp., 8,* 17.

Goebel, O., and P. Gérard (1925): *C. R. Soc. Biol., Paris, 93,* 1537.

Goldberg, S. W., and E. S. London (1903): *Derm. Z., 10,* 457.

Goormaghtigh, N., and A. Amerlinck (1930): *Bull. Ass. franç. Cancer, 19,* 527.

Goss, C. M. (1937): *Yale J. Biol. Med., 10,* 65.

Graham, J. B., and J. V. Meigs (1952): *Amer. J. Obstet. Gynec., 64,* 1159.

Greene, H. S. N., and J. A. Saxton (1938): *J. exp. Med., 67,* 691.

Grew, N. (1682): *Anatomy of plants.* London.

Gross, L. (1952): *Ann. N. Y. Acad. Sci., 54,* 1184.

Gross, L. (1953): *Cancer, 6,* 153

Haddow, A. (1935): *Nature, Lond., 136,* 868.

Haddow, A., and A. M. Robinson (1937): *Proc. roy. Soc., B, 122,* 442.

Haddow, A., and C. M. and J. D. Scott (1937): *Proc. roy. Soc., B, 122,* 477.

Hanau, A. (1889): *Arch. klin. Chir., 39,* 678.

Hanau, A. (1889): *Fortschr. Med., 7,* 321.

Hansemann, D. von (1902): *Die Mikroskopische Diagnose der bösartigen Geschwülste.* Berlin.

Harrison, R. H. (1889): *Lancet, ii,* 163.

Hashimoto, T. (1935): *Gann, 29,* 306.

Hayward, E. (1909): *Münch. med. Wschr., 56,* 1836.

Heiman, J. (1944): *Cancer Res., 4,* 31.

Henry, S. A., and N. M. and Sir E. L. Kennaway (1931): *J. Hyg., Camb., 31,* 125.

Hertig, A. T., and S. C. Sommers (1949): *Cancer, 2,* 946.

Hertig, A. T., S. C. Sommers, and H. Bengloff (1949): *Cancer, 2,* 964.

Hieger, I. (1937): *Amer. J. Cancer, 29,* 705.

Holtz, F., and W. Putschar (1930): *Münch. med. Wschr., 77,* 1039.

Hooke, R. (1665): *Micrographia, or some physiological descriptions of minute bodies made by magnifying glasses, with observations and inquiries thereupon.* London.

Hueper, J. E. W. (1950): *Sth. med. J., Nashville, 43,* 116.

Hueper, W. C. (1952): *Texas Rep. Biol. Med., 10,* 167.

Hueper, W. C., F. H. Wiley, and H. D. Wolfe (1938): *J. industr. Hyg., 20,* 46.

Hueper, W. C., and H. D. Wolfe (1937): *Amer. J. Path., 13,* 656.

Hunter, J. (1837): *The works of John Hunter.* Edited by J. F. Palmer. London.

Huseby, R. A., F. W. Smith, and J. J. Bittner (1946): *Cancer Res., 6,* 494.

Hutchinson, J. (1887): *Brit. med. J., ii,* 1280.

Hyde, J. N. (1906): *Amer. J. med. Sci., 131,* 1.

Jensen, C. O. (1903): *Z. Bakt., 34,* 28, 122.

282

Cancer

Jungch, E. C., C. G. Heller, and W. O. Nelson (1947): *Proc. Soc. exp. Biol. Med., N. Y., 65,* 148.
Kennaway, Sir E. L. (1924): *J. Path. Bact., 27,* 233.
Kennaway, Sir E. L. (1924): *Brit. med. J., i,* 564; (1925): *Ibid., ii,* 1.
Lacassagne, A. (1932): *C. R. Acad. Sci., Paris, 195,* 630.
Lacassagne, A. (1933): *C. R. Soc. Biol., Paris, 112,* 562; (1937): *Ibid., 126,* 190, 385; (1939): *Ibid., 132,* 365, 395, 431.
Lacassagne, A., and R. Vinzent (1929): *C. R. Soc. Biol., Paris, 100,* 249.
Lathrop, A. E. C., and L, Loeb (1916): *J. Cancer Res., 1,* 1.
Lathrop, A. E. C., and L. Loeb. (1918): *J. exp. Med., 28,* 475.
LeDran, H. F. (1757): *Mém. Acad. roy. Chir., 3,* 1.
Lett, H. (1905): *Lancet, i,* 227.
Lipschutz, A., and R. Iglesias (1938): *C. R. Soc. Biol., Paris, 129,* 519.
Lipschutz, A., F. Rodriguez, and L. Vargas (1939): *C. R. Soc. Biol., Paris, 121,* 939.
Lipschutz, A., F. Rodriguez, and L. Vargas (1941): *Endocrinology, 28,* 664.
Lipschutz, A., and J. Schwarz (1944): *Cancer Res., 4,* 24.
Little, C. C. (1933): *Science, 78,* 465.
Loeb, L. (1901): *J. med. Res., 6,* 28.
Loeb, L., H. T. Blumenthal, and M. M. Kirtz (1944): *Science, 99,* 230.
Lucké, B. (1934): *Amer. J. Cancer, 20,* 352.
Lüdin, M. (1934): *Acta radiol., Stockh., 15,* 553.
MacCarty, W. C. (1925): *Surg. Gynec. Obstet., 41,* 783.
MacCorquodale, D. W., S. A. Thayer, and E. A. Doisy, (1936): *J. biol. Chem., 115,* 435.
MacNeal, W. J., and G. S. Willis (1923): *J. Amer. med. Ass., 80,* 466.
Maguson, A. H. W. (1935): *Acta radiol., Stockh.* Suppl. XXII.
Maisin, J., Y. Pourbaix, and E. Cuvelier (1939): *C. R. Soc. Biol., Paris, 132,* 315.
Manouvriez, A. (1876): *Ann. Hyg. publ., Paris, 45,* 459.
Marie, P., J. Clunet, and G. Raulot-Lapointe (1910): *Bull. Ass. franç. Cancer, 3,* 404.
Martland, H. S. (1931): *Amer. J. Cancer, 15,* 2435.
Martland, H. S., and R. E. Humphries (1929): *Arch. Path., 7,* 406.
Matthews, V. X., H. Kirkman, and R. L. Bacon (1947): *Proc. Soc. exp. Biol. Med., 66,* 195.
Michalowsky, I. (1928): *Virchow's Arch., 267,* 27.
Moricard, R., and J. Cauchoix (1938): *C. R. Soc. Biol., Paris, 129,* 556.
Mosinger, M. (1946): *Le problème du cancer.* Paris.
Mottram, J. C. (1931): *Brit. J. exp. Path, 12,* 378.
Mottram, J. C. (1935): *Proc. R. Soc. Med., 29,* 15.
Müller, J. (1838): *Über den feinern Bau und die Formen der krankhaften Geschwülste.* Berlin.
Nathanson, I. T., and H. B. Andervont (1939): *Proc. Soc. exp. Biol. Med., 40,* 421.
Nelson, W. O. (1937): *Anat. Rec., 68,* 99.

Nelson, W. O. (1939): *Endocrinology, 24, 50.*

Neubauer, O. (1947): *Brit. J. Cancer, 1, 192.*

Nishiyama, Y. (1935): *Gann, 29, 285.*

Parkes, A. S. (1927): *Proc. roy. Soc., B, 101, 71.*

Passey, R. D. (1922): *Brit. med. J., ii, 1112.*

Passey, R. D. (1938): *J. Path. Bact., 47, 349.*

Passey, R. D., A. Leese, and J. C. Knox (1935): *J. Path. Bact., 40, 198.*

Paul, C. N. (1918): *The influence of sunlight in the production of cancer of the skin.* London.

Pott, P. (1775): *Chirurgical observations.* London.

Pybus, F. C., and E. W. Miller (1938): *Amer. J. Cancer, 34, 248, 252.*

Pybus, F. C., and E. W. Miller (1940): *Amer. J. Cancer, 40, 47.*

Raspail, M. (1827): In *Répertoire général d'anatomie et de physiologie pathologiques et de clinique chirurgicale.* Paris. Vol. III, p. 165.

Récamier, J. C. A. (1829): *Recherche sur le traitement du cancer.* Paris.

Rehn, L. (1895): *Arch. klin. Chir., 50, 588.*

Rehn, L. (1906): *Verh. dtsch. Ges. Chir., 35, 313.*

Ross, H. C. (1918): *J. Cancer Res., 3, 321.*

Rous, P. (1911): *J. Amer. med. Ass., 56, 198.*

Rous, P., and J. Murphy (1914): *J. exp. Med., 19, 52.*

Sabin, F. R., C. A. Doan, and C. E. Forkner (1932): *J. exp. Med., 56, 267.*

Sasaki, T., and T. Yoshida (1935): *Virchow's Arch., 295, 175.*

Schleiden, M. J. (1838): *Arch. Anat. Physiol. wiss. Med., 137–76.*

Schmidt, M. B. (1924): *Virchow's Arch., 253, 432.*

Schottlaender, J., and F. Kermauner (1912): *Zur Kenntnis des Uterus Karzinoms.* Berlin.

Schwann, T. (1839): *Mikroskopische Untersuchungen über die Uebereinstimmung in der Struktur und dem Wachstum der Thiere und Pflanzen.* Berlin.

Shear, M. J. (1937): *Amer. J. Cancer, 29, 269.*

Shield, A. M. (1899): *Lancet, i, 22.*

Shope, R. E. (1932): *J. exp. Med., 56, 793, 803;* (1933): *Ibid., 58, 607.*

Sjögren, T. (1899): *Förhandlingar vid Svenska Läkaresällskapets sammankomster.* Stockholm. P. 208.

Smith, W. E., D. A. Sunderland, and K. Sugiura (1951): *Arch. industr. Hyg., 4, 299.*

Suntzeff, M. D., and C. Carruthers (1946): *Cancer Res., 6, 574.*

Tannenbaum, A. (1940): *Arch. Path., 30, 509.*

Tannenbaum, A., and H. Silverstone (1946): *Cancer Res., 6, 499;* (1949): *Ibid., 9, 162, 403.*

Teilum, G. (1950): *Acta endocrinol., 4, 43.*

Thomson, A. (1902): *Brit. med. J., ii, 1538.*

Tsutsui, H. (1918): *Gann, 12, 17.*

Twort, C. C., and J. D. Fulton (1930): *J. Path. Bact., 33, 119.*

Unna, P. G. (1894): In *Orth's Lehrbuch der speziellen pathologischen Anatomie.* Berlin. P. 719.

Cancer

Vasquez-Lopez, E. (1944): *J. Path. Bact., 56,* 1.
Virchow, R. (1858): *Cellular-pathologie.* Berlin.
Volkmann, R. von (1875): *Beiträge zur Chirurgie.* Leipzig.
Wakeley, C. P. G. (1927): *Brit. J. Surg., 14,* 677.
Warburg, O. (1925): *Klin. Wschr. 4,* 534.
White, J. W. (1893): *Trans. Amer. surg. Ass., 11,* 167; (1895): *Ibid., 13,* 103.
White, J. W. (1904): *Ann. Surg., 40,* 782.
Wood, A. (1900): *Ann. Surg., 32,* 309.
Yamagiwa, K., and K. Ichikawa (1916): *Mitt. med. Fak., Tokio, 15,* 295.
Yamagiwa, K., and K. Ichikawa (1918): *J. Cancer Res., 3,* 1.
Yamagiwa, K., and S. Ohno (1918): *Gann., 12,* 3.
Yoshida, T. (1932): *Proc. imp. Acad. Japan, 8,* 464.
Yoshida, T. (1933): *Trans. Jap. path. Soc., 23,* 636.
Zondek, B. (1936): *Lancet, i,* 776.

BY EDWARD L. MURPHY

M. D., M. R. C. P.*

chapter 17 / malingering

It is certain that there were brave men before Agamemnon. It is equally certain that, before and after, there existed men who could not accumulate enough resolution to reach the level of behavior commonly accepted as that expected from one who is not a coward, but one without any aspirations to heroism either. So it will ever be. If we agree with Thackeray that "bravery never goes out of fashion," so also we must subscribe to Voltaire's *"un des plus grands malheurs des honnêtes gens c'est qu'ils sont de lâches."* Dislike of death or the more dreaded mutilation must always exist, but a public avowal of this is necessarily an antisocial act in a society whose members are voluntarily or compulsorily engaged in activities fraught with these very hazards. Thus, to avoid punishment at the hands of one's fellows, or to evade their contempt, some cloaking of the real desire must be in evidence; illness is often the only excuse valid enough to prevent ostracism. However, escape from martial duties and dangers is only a small part of the total problem. The varieties of malingering are far more complex than any single problem such as cowardice, although the accusation in peacetime may comprise all that is understood by the term to those upholding military discipline, and in war the substitution of the one aspect for the whole may seem obvious to all. To an insurance assessor the word may imply nothing but the assumption of nonexistent symptoms in order to gain financial compensation. No effort need be made to force the possible reasons for the simulation of disease into any rigid classification. This will be obvious to readers, who will find later in this section many strange and

* Physician, neurological department, St. Vincent's Hospital, Dublin.

286

inexplicable reasons for malingering. Effort is better spent on defining our terms of reference.

The exact meaning of malingering is often confused in lay opinion and even in medical circles; a similar difficulty has always been associated with the differentiation of hysteria. Reference to the usual sources of information may not be very helpful. One dictionary gives a totally erroneous definition of malingering: "Simulation of illness to avoid duty." Lexicographical bias in another work produces another incorrect interpretation when it is stressed that the assumption of ill health was always for financial gain. Perhaps the most helpful elucidation is that of R. N. De Jong (1950) in his monumental treatise, *The neurologic examination*. He defines malingering as "a willful, deliberate, and fraudulent imitation or exaggeration of illness, usually intended to deceive others, and, under most circumstances, conceived for the purpose of gaining a consciously desired end." We need not occupy ourselves with his consideration of "negative malingering" (i.e., dissimulation), which is described as the concealment of existing symptoms by various methods of deception. Although an entity, its appearance is rarely noted, except in such uncommon events as the suppression of truth about one's age, in an attempt to enter the armed services in defiance of the regulation age limits. De Jong lists three varieties of pure malingering, i.e., the deliberate and designed feigning of disease or disability. This may be done by (1) false allegations (untrue attestations that symptoms exist, or spurious denial of previously existing diseases); (2) imitation, i.e., simulation of signs and symptoms of genuine ailments may be employed; or (3) provocation, generally held to be of greater culpability, which is the deliberate production of organic signs or symptoms by artificial means.

It is a common claim that almost every form of human activity can be found in the Old Testament, and proof that a subject has a real historical validity is often afforded by search of Holy Writ. Even for such an unlikely aspect of medical history as malingering the generalization holds good. Thus we find that the simulation of disease can be identified as far back as Jacob whose eventful life was lived around 2000 B.C. We read of his wife Rachel pretending illness to escape detection as responsible for the unfilial larceny of her father's lares and penates. Sitting on her spoils, she pleaded: "Let it not displease my lord that I cannot rise up before thee; for the custom of women is upon me." David eluded the wrath of Achish, King of Gath, by "swooning" and resisted removal by "scrabbling on the doors of the gate," even going so far as to imitate the drooling mouth of a senile dement. These histrionic efforts were successful in making the unsuspicious King exclaim: "Lo, ye see the man is mad: Wherefore then have ye brought him to me? Have I need of mad men, that ye have brought this fellow to play the mad man in my presence?" At this stage of our examination of the historical evidence of malingering it is necessary to seek some explanation for the neglect of the fraudulent syndrome in its importance in the literature, with the expansive treatment awarded to other symptom-complexes of the general corpus of medical knowledge—syndromes whose importance and interest are much less obvious to the impartial observer than that of pretended illness. The reader need have no doubt about this comparative neglect.

The late Sir John Collie (1934), an undisputed expert on the historical aspect, admits in the first edition of the present work: "There are very few recorded instances of feigned sickness or injury in medical literature." Even in modern times this wilful or unconscious neglect reaches heights unlikely to be suspected by those who have not devoted intensive study to the question. The *Encyclopaedia Britannica* (1952 edition) does not include any article under the heading of malingering—a strange lack of information in a work popularly supposed to take all knowledge for its province. An even stranger omission is to be noted in Garrison's *An introduction to the history of medicine* (1929), where malingering is absent from a subject index occupying thirty pages. This lapse comes strangely from the "incomparable" Garrison, whose value to medical historians is easily demonstrated on every other possible aspect of their speciality. A more modern master of general medical history, Douglas Guthrie (1945), also omits malingering from his very detailed subject rota. That the fault lies in omission and not in incompetence is shown by Arturo Castiglioni (1941), who lists the word twice. The first makes reference to a condensed résumé of Galen's aphorisms on feigned illness, while a hopeful perusal of the second is ill rewarded with the mention of Giambattista Silvatico (1550–1621) as having written the parent monograph on malingering (*De iis qui morborum simulant deprehensis,* 1595). In a detailed volume of one thousand pages, such scanty mention seems cavalier treatment of an important subject, especially

288

when we note that there is total neglect of the matter after 1595—a time when the spread of knowledge was beginning to produce the sources from which our history must derive.

The neglect of malingering seems peculiar when we have evidence of contemporary social recognition of fraudulent disease. As far back as the late Middle Ages it was common knowledge that deliberate performance of surgical operations was going on. The unfortunate children selected for these mutilations were being prepared for a life of begging from the public charity, whose largesse was artfully excited by the pitiable and horrible deformations of the face or limbs. Victor Hugo showed one aspect of the subject in *L'homme qui rit,* and in *Notre-Dame de Paris* listed a large number of fraudulent illnesses which were prevalent among the medieval beggars of Paris. Despite this, it is not until the end of the eighteenth century that any real scientifically trended writing appeared, while a thorough study of the speciality had to wait until 1843. In 1913 Collie lamented that no definitive work on malingering had appeared since H. Gavin's essay of 1843.

It may be worth mentioning some causes which have been operative in this neglect of feigned disease. Primarily it is to be remembered that medical writing as we know it is a growth of comparatively modern origin. Up to 150 years ago the absence of technical periodicals ensured that appearance in print was rare and justified only by the importance of the material. The initial description of common diseases usually appeared in book form. Even more important were the general standards and morale of the "doctors" placed in charge of those people liable to malinger because of their occupational hazards. In the Royal Navy, doctors of commissioned rank did not appear until well into the nineteenth century. Their predecessors wore no special uniform and held warrant rank only, and while their official status was graded as equal to carpenters or master gunners, an equal generosity was not granted in matters of pay. They also acted as barbers (as did the Prussian military surgeons up to the time of Frederick the Great), and with rare exceptions were little known except possibly for their notorious tendency to drunkenness and debauchery. Doctors like these were not the most likely of their profession to engage in literary descriptions of their charges' psychical ailments. Again, since malingering in that era was almost inevitably associated with the shirking of military employment or the dangers of war service, it would seem inevitable that those with the care of these poltroons would have hesitated before publishing to the world the true state of national morale. This spirit of foolish nationalism, which is only seen sporadically in modern times, shrank from fouling its own nest, just as the first descriptions of syphilis were written by physicians who hastened to christen the disease with the name of a country other than their own. In Italy the "French evil" was rampant, while in France the sufferers were gratified by the knowledge that they were afflicted with the "Italian pox."

Needless to say, our knowledge of medicine in prehistoric times must always be limited, but if we are to judge it by the customary anthropological method in which the behavior of modern natives is taken as an extension of the ancient way of life, it would seem obvious that malingering (save in those really insane) must have been very rare. In savage societies, where the modern creed of civilization giving as its sacred duty the succor of the afflicted has not permeated, the assumption of false illness must have been a perilous endeavor. In these societies the sick man is felt to be weak and helpless, like a child or an old man. He may not be able to move around, hunt, or attend to his customary occupations—serious defects in a close-knit group whose communal activities are all necessary, if the malice of Nature is to be combated. The sick and the senile are both unable to contribute their share of labor to the common welfare. In some cultures the acceptance of this helplessness is part of the credo, and the ill are treated with an unexpected charity. However, these are exceptions, and in the great majority of aboriginal societies a logical but cruel treatment awaits the afflicted. The handicapped are jettisoned or murdered; sometimes they are eaten—as the Bobos of the western Sudan, who pursue the matter in a pitiless environment to its logical conclusion. When a tribesman or woman is noticed to be ill of a disease, thought to be incurable or prolonged, he is killed and eaten before he has had time to lose much flesh. Apart from these economic reasons there are other causes for the sick native's lot being indeed undesirable. The magico-religious concept of illness, almost obligatory in primitive cultures, usually ordains the belief that lapse from health is due to direct action by some malevolent deity; the resultant belief is that the sick one has become possessed by a devil. A fear of possible

contagion is the reason why various savage tribes kill the seriously
ill and often do so by burial when alive, thus making sure that the
evil spirit is not allowed to escape and infect others. In general, however, the treatment of the sick is that of desertion or neglect, which
we have come to believe as the customary fate of the "old man of
the tribe."

Little is known of simulated illness in ancient Egypt. Herodotus,
writing in the fifth century B.C., states that its inhabitants were, next
to the Libyans, "the most healthy people in the world"—a verdict
which could not possibly be given twenty-five hundred years later.
The dictatorships of the Pharaohs necessarily included the acceptance
of military service, but no record is known of the fellahin adopting
simulation to escape it. Perhaps the endeavor was too subtle a matter
for hieroglyphic recording. The civilization showed a ruthless aspect
when engaged in the construction of the many gargantuan attempts to
immortalize the Pharaohs; a pitiless form of slave labor must have
been necessary to allow the limited resources of the country the erec-
tion of a tomb made up of 230,000 blocks of solid limestone, weighing
on an average two and one-half tons each. There would have been
little opportunity or hope of success for the workers malingering,
and such a conclusion is borne out by the observation of Diodorus
Siculus. He visited some of the penal settlements, such as those where
gold was mined, and in a heartbreaking account of the workers' terrible conditions mentions that "there is no forgiveness or relaxation
at all for the sick or the maimed, or the old, or for women's weakness,
but all with blows, are compelled to stick to their labor until worn out
they die in servitude." Despite the enormous mass of knowledge accumulated by the acumen of the Egyptologists in medical as in all
aspects of life, our knowledge must be limited, and, apart from this,
the system of medicine in the civilization of the Nile valley was too
much dominated by magic and religion for us to accept any evidence
relating to complicated psychical matters such as malingering. The
same objection applies to the Babylonian and Hittite cultures. On the
face of it these civilizations would seem to have offered little encour-
agement to the malingerer. In their religious creeds the view, Judaic
in origin, was held that a sick man was a sinner, meriting an isolated
position in society because of his disgrace. Deliberate eschewing of
labor must have been rare in countries which rigidly enforced the

Ius Talionis to a degree of legal cruelty seldom surpassed since then. That punishment would have been severe we can judge by that meted out to women procuring abortion: they were impaled alive and left to rot on their stakes.

We are on much firmer ground when we come to study Greek medicine, and a breath of common sense is welcome after the sinister mumbo-jumbo of the Semitic cultures. Galen is strangely modern in his views on malingering and its detection. To the reader who notes that Galen was born in A.D. 130 at Pergamum in Asia Minor and that his medical practice was almost entirely conducted in Rome, his selection as the spokesman of Greek medicine may appear as a misnomer. It is to be remembered that Roman medicine did not exist as an endogenous mode of culture; all fashionable Roman medicine was Grecian, and its practitioners were Greeks. Galen wrote: "People pretend to be ill for many reasons, and it would seem a physician's business to discover the truth in all such cases." He recognized simulated hemoptysis, the frauds being clever enough to produce the blood only at the end of a severe bout of coughing. One of his patients had been summoned to an assembly (his attitude was comparable to the modern citizen's reluctance for jury service), and the complaint of painful intestinal colic which ensued was easily recognized by Galen. He notes dryly that when the assembly dissolved the cries of pain ceased also.

If patients are really in great distress, they are prepared to put up with any remedy; in fact, they are the first to beg the doctor to do anything he chooses, so long as their trouble is cured. On the other hand, they flee from such remedies if they are only in slight pain or not at all. They will not endure prolonged fasts or bitter medicines. We ought to tell them, when they say that they have great pain, that these are the only things that will cure such conditions, or else advise cutting or burning operations and abstinence from all articles of food and drink to which we see them addicted. Medical experience was, of course, essential, but plain common sense, "by few possessed so perfectly," would usually detect the malingerers. Galen's neologism "pathomimes" never came into general use and is today unknown— a pity, since the nomenclature of malingering suffers from having few synonymous usages. Lampooning his less erudite colleagues, he sneered: "The laity also reckon him the one to distinguish those who

Malingering

are lying from those who are speaking the truth." The deliberate production of fraudulent signs had reached a high degree of skill if we are to judge by the Pergamite's statement: "An inflammation, an erysipelas, or a swelling produced purposely by external application of drugs can be detected and distinguished by the physician from affections arising from within the body." Some of Galen's patients feigned mania or depression, but one feels that his intellectual snobbery forced him to overstatement when he announced: "All these conditions the laity think ought to be discovered and distinguished from one another by the doctors."

We have traveled a long way since Galen, and today even the most astute psychiatrist still finds difficulty in unveiling some clever malingerers. It would be interesting to know if Galen gained his knowledge from his experiences as surgeon to the gladiatorial training schools. One presumes that some of these warriors may have shown evidence of simulated ailments, especially the pitiable captives who, having graced a proconsul's triumph, were spared the disgrace of slavery for the much more terrible fate of allotment to the training schools. That these unhappy men did not accept their compulsory participation in the arena's blood-lust is evident from the finding in the fighter's academy at Pompeii of the trainees being incarcerated with heavy manacles, although it is not possible at this date to deny that this fettering may have been punitive. However, reluctance to act as the arena expected is well shown by the contemporary descriptions of the poor wretches' reluctance to face the terrors awaiting them and having to be conquered by their keepers beating them with whips or red-hot irons—treatment not very different from that which we shall see recommended for unwilling warriors in the eighteenth century. Perhaps the most telling proof of the likelihood of malingering in gladiators was the extreme precaution which was needed against a more dignified method of escape from an intolerable existence—suicide.

Among the freemen of early republican Rome cowardice or malingering must have been rare indeed. *"Dulce et decorum est pro patria mori"* was the genuine sentiment, and without the disciplined, unthinking courage of the legions their small army groups would never have been able to compass the annihilation of the huge tribal hordes of Gaul and the desert. Of course there must have been malingerers as well as poltroons in the Roman levies, but the former crime must have been as rare as the latter if its discovery earned the same punishment—that of decimation in the true meaning—the execution of every tenth man in the unit displaying unjustified tendencies to disengage from battle. It is a commonplace of military history that soldiers fight best when they are sure of their leaders providing adequate medical care for the wounded. In this respect it is to be remembered that the greatest development of the early system of hospitals was a product of the Roman Army. In the first years of empire-building, sick and wounded soldiers had to be sent home to Rome for treatment, but as the legions extended their rule to the farthest corners of the known world the lines of communication became too long, and hospitals were erected at sites near the divisional headquarters. Civil illness was also catered to in Rome, where a hospital was erected as early as 293 B.C. This foundation's history forms a useful reminder that the simulation of disease was not likely to be a profitable procedure in those times. The first hospital was located on an island which also fulfilled another purpose: to it were deported slaves who had become too old or ill to earn their keep. Suetonius says of this island, named (sacrilegiously, one feels) after Aesculapius, that it was the favorite site for the abandonment of ill or worn-out slaves, "so as to avoid the trouble of caring for them at home." The Emperor Claudius gave these poor wretches the dubious gift of their freedom if they survived their marooning. There are few, if any, indications that the pagan Romans felt it their duty to provide any care for the sick poor.

That the great period of Arabian medicine saw some malingering seems established when we read of the conduct of medical practice in Bagdad. Besides the many learned physicians who resided there, an equal army of quacks or unscrupulous "licensed" doctors found employment also. Some of the graduate practitioners resorted to pernicious methods of "puffing" their professional success by hiring "patients" who were well coached in their complex ailments and equally voluble in their public praise of the doctor who had so brilliantly cured them.

Returning to the West, we note a modern historian's dictum: "From the fall of the Roman Empire beyond the thirteenth century —nearly a thousand years—there is no advance in medical science to record in western Europe." (H. W. Haggard, 1934). The advent of Christianity as a wide-spread religion produced one result which influences our present summary. The nobility of the novel doctrines led to their practical implementation. Instead of the harsh treatment of the poor and the sick under pagan influences there arose systems for relief of the poor and the treatment of illness-systems whose origins stemmed from the teachings of one who in His life never rejected the poverty-stricken and who did not shun the company of those affected with loathsome diseases. The very excess of charity itself was later to cause abuses tending to encourage the cultivation of false illness. New traditions of healing became associated with saints and their relics. This development grew to extravagant heights, and the monasteries and cities vied with each other in the number and importance of their relics. Halfway through the Middle Ages the craze had extended so freely that a small German town, Halle, boasted 21,000 genuine relics! A great increase in the number of beggars was seen, who earned their living by begging at the shrines of relics to whose aid in their "cure" they publicly gave testimony. As for the saints themselves, tradition began to give them a reputation for healing, and hagiological Harley Street in London had saints specializing in all the common ailments. St. Blaise dominated disorders of the throat, and his reputation has persisted to the present day, while his fellow thaumaturge, St. Erasmus, an abdominal man, has long been forgotten. All these reliquaries, "holy" wells, and shrines were supplied with malingerers who excited the hopes of the pilgrims by exaggerated accounts of the symptoms which had been cured by prayerful intercession. G. G. Coulton (1935) quotes a churchman of the eleventh century who bluntly accuses the abbot of one French monastery of encouraging a fabrication of miracles. The vulgar herd were impressed by "feigned deafness, affected madness, fingers purposely cramped into the palm, and soles twisted up under men's thighs," so that the very depths of men's purses were emptied by lies.

In England the very comforts of the hospitals were eventually to be accused of creating illness instead of curing it. All medical institutions were necessarily owned and administered by religious orders whose successful pursuit of devotions, allied to the many legacies bequeathed to them by pious friends, produced an income sufficient to keep the patients in what was comparative luxury for those spartan times. We read of some hospitals in which a gallon of beer, a loaf of bread, herrings, cheese, butter, and vegetables were given daily to each inmate. In days of starvation and cruelty at the hands of feudal barons such largess must have tempted large numbers of the struggling peasants to engage in a career of fraud undetectable by the primitive diagnostic methods then prevailing. The leper houses must have long outlived their original purpose at a time when two hundred of them were noted as being in activity when the reformation under Henry VIII purged them. Hatred of the sufferers arose not only from the Biblical tradition, but from the *"terribilis aspectus"* of the leper. To become a beggar was his natural fate, and it is undoubted that the privilege of begging was abused and claimed by numbers who pretended to be lepers.

Sir Thomas More (no enemy of the old religion) wrote on the question of fraud: "Some priest, to bring up a pilgrimage in his parish may devise some false fellow feigning himself to come seek a saint in his church and there suddenly say, that he has gotten his sight." (G. G. Coulton, 1935.) Then the bells are rung for a miracle, and foolish people are taken in by frauds who keep a plentiful supply of crutches, so that they satisfy the pious credulity of the numerous visitors with these tangible proofs of the cure. It is gratifying that one observer was able to unmask an impostor. A pilgrim claimed that he had his vision, congenitally absent, suddenly restored by the intercession of St. Alban. The Duke of Gloucester, overjoyed at this proof of the shrine's sanctity, interviewed the fellow and, becoming suspicious, casually asked him to name the colors of the clothes which he (the Duke) was wearing. Proud to show his miracle, the fraud named them all correctly; his chagrin was great when the nobleman asked him how he could know them all since he had never seen them before. It is good to read that the blasphemer was sent to the stocks for prolonged punishment.

Malingering seems to have reached a high degree of perfection in the Paris of the late Middle Ages. Victor Hugo's *Notre-Dame de Paris,* set in the times of Louis XI, gives almost a clinical description of the mendicants who lived in the fortress-like "Court of Miracles." He lists the daylight nightmares, such as one man without arms or legs who jumped along on his two hands like a "mutilated daddy-long-legs." Another's mass of crutches and wooden legs made him look like a perambulating scaffolding"; he walked with a blind man whose huge hound was more for protection than guidance, since the loss of vision was just as feigned as his companion's mechanical appeals to compassion. Other spectacular malingerers were to be seen also. One sort of "fake soldier," a *"narquois"* as he was termed in the argot, was undoing the bandages of his false wound and limbering up his healthy limb, which had been bound in a thousand ligatures. Another *"malingreux"* was preparing with celandine and ox-blood his *jambe de Dieu* or sore leg for the morrow's begging. A *coquillart* was dressing in his pilgrim's outfit, designed to add the appeal of religious fervor to the charity excited by his illness. In another corner a young apprentice was taking a lesson in epilepsy from an old *sabouleux* (false epileptic), who was teaching him the art of foaming at the mouth by chewing a piece of soap.

About the same time a rather different type of mendicant malingerer was to be seen in all the English traveling fairs, or tramping alone to the most remote villages. These "Tom O'Bedlams" had their origin in the financial chaos of Bethlehem Hospital, which had received more patients than money and, being originally unendowed, was forced to discharge harmless lunatics as collectors of charity. These poor maniacs soon became a part of the English rural scene, and no wake or fair was complete without its Tom, who, wearing a turban, a fantastic attire decked with ribbons, weeds, and flowers, went through his pitiful role as a zany. His passport was his collector's badge and collection box, and thus it was soon established that the imposters, delighted with such an easy way of gathering their livelihood, may have outnumbered the real seekers after charity. Even as late as 1674 a work with the engaging title *The Canting Academy* (Whitwell, 1946) mentions the "Abram-men otherwise Tom-of-Bedlams" who "very strangely and antickly garbed," travel the land and "for all their seeming madness, they have wit enough to steal as they go." Another contemporary author dismisses their pranks and ridiculous clothing as being mere devices to make them seem mad or distracted when they were only "dissembling knaves."

In the Renaissance an epileptic was considered to be a poor wretch deserving pity and special consideration. This being so, some people found it profitable to simulate the convulsive disease. How cunning beggars used to give a good imitation of an attack is described by Ambroise Paré (1951) who speaks of: ". . . such as falling down counterfeit the falling sickness, binde straitly both their wrests with plates of iron, tumble and rowl themselves in the mire, sprinkle and defile their heads and faces with beasts' bloud, and shake their limbs and whole bodie. Lastly, by putting sope into their mouths, they foam at the mouth like those that have the falling sickness." English malingerers developed a jargon in which epilepsy was the "cranke." There is a record dated 1556 which describes a pretended epileptic who was in rags, had his face covered with blood, and gave a fraudulent account of himself: " 'Syr,' saythe he, '. . . my name is Nycolas Genings, and I have had this falling syckness viii. yeares, and I can get no remedy for the same; for I have it by kinde, my father had it and my friendes before me; and I haue byne these two yeares here about London, and a yeare and a halfe in bethelem.' 'Why, wast thou out of thy wyttes?' quoth I. 'Ye, syr, that I was.' " Cheats of this type were not confined to England and France. In Germany about the same time they were known as *"Grantners"* and in Italy as *"Accadenti,"* one of the thirty-four classes of malingering vagabonds in that country. Often they co-operated with other criminals by simulating an attack while their colleagues would pick the pockets of the curious or compassionate onlookers.

Evasion of punishment or torture was a powerful stimulus towards feigning epilepsy. As late as the eighteenth century a case was referred to the medical faculty of Halle University for definitive diagnosis. A woman threatened with torture had exhibited realistic attacks while claiming she had them since childhood. The professors considered her fraudulent and turned her over to the torturers, as the torments would not endanger the general health. As Owsei Temkin (1945) points out, feigned convulsions did not really come into their own until the European nations introduced compulsory military service. Deception of medical men continued to be seen throughout the years, and no doubt occurs at the present time. In 1880 a large number of experts were fooled by one "dummy-chucker" who was real enough to cut his tongue with a concealed knife and risked serious injury in falls to add verisimilitude to his impersonation. Objective tests were necessary, and for many centuries the physicians put their faith in actual infliction of pain or at least, sinister hints of its immediate necessity. When the patient was apparently unconscious, the medical attendant would explain to his retinue that castration or a general use of the hot cautery was absolutely imperative.

Very often this maneuvre had the desired result: the "patient" would jump to his feet and beg to be spared the new therapy.

As the knowledge of nosology grew, the disentangling of simulated, hysterical, and real epilepsy became an important problem. Hermann Boerhaave cured most of his cases with threats of flogging. On one occasion an entire orphanage in Haarlem was preserved from an epidemic of seizures by his heating irons and making a show of applying them to each sufferer. Indeed, it mattered little what etiology the attacks had, since widespread use of the cautery was the indicated therapy.

It is well known that eighteenth-century London was notorious for its quacks. "Spot" Ward and James Graham of "Celestial Bed" notoriety won public fame to a much greater degree than the reputable physicians. Quacks and malingering seem to be necessary bedmates, and London was no exception. The public appearances of the fraudulent leeches were always graced by large numbers of patients who were only too willing to testify to the marvelous cures worked on them. These wretches were termed "decoy ducks" and were hired for a half crown a week. For this stipend they had to attend two gatherings per week and give public proof of their having been relieved of whatever common disease they had been coached to imitate. Less commonly employed were better-dressed people who arrived in carriages. They were demonstrated as "private patients" and for this upgrading in social status earned a crown per week, exclusive of the coach fare.

Anyone who has read H. Mayhew's (1950) gigantic survey of *London Labour and the London Poor* will have no difficulty in believing that the tradition of simulation was passed from generation to generation of rogues, whose frauds Mayhew classified in his racy, fascinating chapters on the London of 1851. The first variety of cheat identified by Mayhew were those with real or simulated sores. The great majority had skin lesions which were unreal, and the device responsible was known in the thieves' argot as the "scaldrum dodge." This was brought about by covering a portion of a limb with soap to the thickness of a "plaister" and then saturating the whole with vinegar. The latter caused the soap to blister and assume a festering appearance, which on examination was undetectable from a true ulcer. Mayhew grimly describes the deception as a new method: "It came in with penny postage, daguerreotypes, and other modern inventions." In less scientific epochs he had known the skin lesions to have been produced by burns, scalds, and lacerations which the mendicants inflicted on themselves with a ruthless hand. Our author tells of a long conversation he had with a beggar who used a nail or pin to prick his flesh all over to procure blood and give the appearance of a generalized ulceration. He told of the "scaldrum dodge" with scorn and sighed for the days when the beggars slowly scraped the skin off their feet with glass—a procedure that had to be repeated every few days to attain the desired effect. Beggars with swollen legs, which they took care to exhibit on the pavement, were, according to Mayhew, the most evident of frauds. His pathology was not on a par with his social detection since he states that a "mere swelling cannot be a normal or chronic condition of the human body." A swelling of several years' standing could only be due to the continued application of a poisonous ointment or to the compression of the limb with ligatures.

Cripples were of all sorts, such as the man with crutches and his foot in a sling, another wretch without hands who attempted to paint with his stumps, the crab-like man without legs who sat on a board and walked on his hands, etc. London also contained legless men who propelled themselves in little primitive carriages and idiotic-looking youths who "stand pad with a fakement,"† shaking in every limb as if under the influence of galvanism. Some of these were tolerated by the police as being genuine, but Mayhew doubted the reality of some of the mutilations. At any rate he knew them to be a public danger because he had personal knowledge that the sight of one of the "crab-like" creatures had so frightened a pregnant lady that her child was born in all respects similar to him. In some cases the "missing" arms were strapped to the side, and the "stumps" were cloth stuffed with bran. One feels that the beggar who pretended to have a missing leg by doubling back his foot to his thigh earned his pittance. Men who feigned paralysis were constantly appearing, and the police had orders to bring them to the district surgeon, who speedily produced alleviation.

That begging in Victorian London was lucrative seems established by the publication in the papers of how a respectable young lady ran away from home and lived in sin and luxury with a "blind" mendi-

† Criminal argot for a beggar who stands with a written appeal hanging on him.

300

cant. Long before the police found him out, he had been detected by the local boys, who were accustomed to stealing the alms from the bowl of any blind man they met. They were very surprised when their game was stopped by the "blind" victim of poverty, who punished them with his stout cane.

Epileptic beggars were fraudulent to a man. Some of them were co-workers with bands of pickpockets, who set about their work when a crowd had collected around the victim of a seizure. Others were alone and depended on the charity of bystanders to help them in their "fit." Of all the arts of deception, pretence of convulsive disease reached the highest levels of cheating. The pallor of the face was prepared with chalk, and the stages of the episode were copied to a nicety. One incorrigible old woman persisted in falling down with the one object of obtaining brandy. She always staged her attacks near a public house, into whose open doors she would inevitably be carried. Besides planning the scene of her illness, she also timed her fits, waiting until a well-dressed pair approached. This was repeated so often during the day that towards night she could be found lying in the gutter, unable even to mutter "brandy," as she did when that remedy did not immediately suggest itself to her benefactors. It is doubtful if the malingerers should be stretched to include the man who kept falling into the Serpentine in Hyde Park so that he could be revived with the brandy supplied for that purpose by the Humane Society. Eventually his rescuers took no notice of his danger of drowning, and he was forced to revive himself.

No form of misfortune was better calculated to appeal to charity than that demonstrated by young men giving the appearance of "being in a decline." Mayhew had noticed that all these pitiable-looking fellows wore a white cloth around their head, surmounted by a black cap. It was this contrast in combination with a little rouge around the eyes that produced the woeful faces. Of course, dramatic action was also necessary; there was a noisy panting for breath and a hacking cough, and the head was bowed in intolerable misery. Mayhew lists four other types of malingering beggar, but they can all be classed as those portraying starvation. "Shallow coves" was the cant name given to the beggars who exhibited themselves half-clad, especially in winter. Even the hardened journalist admitted that they presented a spectacle of wretchedness the imagination could never conceive. The almost naked state (the missing shirt made as obvious as possible), a hollow, glaring eye ("like that of a famished dog") were nearly always to be seen outside a pastry cook's, into whose windows he directed his hungry look. Other frauds, as if ashamed of their poverty, depended on placards around their necks with statements that they were starving along with a large dependent family. The script of all these appeals was universally copper plate, adding a subtle suggestion that their education was good. However, this was as fraudulent as their other claims. Either their placards were written for them or certain rogues instructed them to trace the letters mechanically. Indeed, one of the scriveners who drew the pavement appeals could only write backwards. There were the "choking dodgers" who ostentatiously produced the dryest of crusts, one of obvious stone-like consistency which was dirty with street mud. An allied class were the "offal-eaters," who searched the garbage cans and with pretended shame tried to devour some food remnant planted, no doubt, by his accomplices. All in all, London seems to have become a much more moral city than it was in the days when Mayhew saw a beggar with a grossly swollen leg covered with bloodstained bandages use this limb in a gay dance when his "work" was done.

Of recent years malingering has been common in convicts, usually those sentenced to long imprisonments. Apart from the infirmary being the goal, there is the inevitable desire to best the authorities. Writing in 1893, A. Griffiths states that the most frequent methods of simulation were imbecility, hemorrhage from the nose and lungs, and paralysis, but a prison physician in 1863 described one old "lag" who had sewn up his mouth and eyelids with a large needle and coarse thread. Another man with realistic paraplegia was given light duty until his discharge, when, roaring with laughter, he smashed his crutches across his "paralyzed" legs. In later years interstitial emphysema was found to result from the patients puncturing their lungs with pins. It is interesting to note that in many cases the suffering endured was out of all proportion to the anticipated gain. One patient who ate a pound of candles as an appetizer and who preferred blankets cut into squares to prison diet might in these more charitable days be treated as psychotic. The obstinacy of the malingerers was well nigh incredible: one prisoner was persistent enough to have needed forcible feeding on eight thousand successive occasions! One feels after reading Griffiths' authoritative work that the scepticism of the doctors was greatly increased by their experiences with malingering convicts.

Modern penological memoirs are not reassuring on the problem of psychiatric patients in prison. One episode described by W. Macartney, in which castor oil was given in a dosage more suitable for torture than purgation, makes a bad impression; and it should be remembered that Michael Davitt's account of his imprisonment in Dartmoor and other English prisons is little more than fifty years old. His inquiring mind led him to investigate the process by which a convict was tested before he was grudgingly accepted as a genuine psychotic. The final and "acid" test consisted of substituting for the patient's dinner a plate of human excrement; if this was eaten and enjoyed, the poor victim was allowed to exchange his prison cell for an almost equally grim apartment in an asylum. Fedor Dostoyevsky has given a graphic picture of a Russian prison hospital in 1850. Contrary to one's expectations, the doctors were most humane and adored by their patients. Knowing the rigors of the prison, they tolerated the hospitalization of men whom they knew to be healthy, no matter what the simulated symptoms were. Febrile Catharalis [sic] was the classical diagnosis, and for this a week's stay was allowed. Obstinate cases, ungrateful enough to persist in their faking, were "treated" with a seton. The procedure consisted of seizing the nape of the neck, piercing it, and threading a skein of cotton wool about as thick as the finger through the tunnel. Every day at fixed hours this skein was pulled backwards and forwards so the wound would not heal. Men endured this horrible suffering for several days before giving in. The Russian soldiers' malingering was not undertaken because of any service difficulties, but to avoid or postpone the execution of a court martial sentence condemning them to flogging with the knout or, even more feared, the running of the gauntlet.

Human inconsistency seems well established when we read of the divine tokens of sanctity being simulated for reasons of spiritual pride. In 1546 a Spanish nun, Magdalena de la Cruz, was brought before the Inquisition and found guilty of the deliberate production of stigmata. Fr. Herbert Thurston, S. J. (1952) mentions this case as well as a similar *cause célèbre* of the same blasphemous fraud—*Sor María de la Visitación,* the nun of Lisbon. Thurston points out that the wounds in the hands, feet, and chest were painted on by the stigmatic herself, but was unable to identify the mechanism producing the bleeding wounds of the young girl whom he personally examined in London in 1920. Thurston is not blind to the possibilities of malingering and/or hysteria in these people claiming to be afflicted with supernatural wounds. He points out that all the known stigmatics have been female, except for the first example, St. Francis of Assisi, and the present-day case of Padre Pio, which is still *sub judice* and without the slightest official recognition by the Vatican.

In other centuries, too, religion and its excesses have tempted malingerers to imitate the devotees solely for ulterior purposes of gain or sexual excess. The strange mass movement of the Flagellants, which spread so quickly through Europe after the Black Death, is stated by J. F. C. Hecker (1884) to have included many fraudulent mendicants who satisfied their wanderlust at the expense of public charity without having anything of the epidemic masochism which their fellow travellers displayed. Towards the end of this short-lived sectarian movement the sessions of penitential scourging often terminated in the grossest of sexual orgies; this motive attracted fraudulent penitents just as similar ruffians adapted the Anabaptist ideas to their own immoral ends. St. Vitus's dance in its mass-affliction form was also brought into disrepute in the same way. Even the tarantela had malingerers among those exhibiting the classical forced movement of the limbs.

War and its potential dangers have always been a fruitful source of malingering. For those admirers of the "young eagle who tore the very heart out of glory" it is advisable to read the fuller story as described in Erckmann-Chatrian's *Conscript: a tale of the French war of 1813* (1870). Though fictional, the treatment is documentary in this picture of Napoleon's army between the Russian debacle and the battle of Leipzig. Every effort was made to fill the ever-thinning ranks. Many young men refused to enter the army, giving trivial reasons such as the minor degree of limping from which they suffered. Some broke their teeth so they could not bite the cartridges, others shot away their thumbs so they could not handle a musket. Some swallowed unwholesome things to make their faces pale or tied up one of their limbs to make their veins swell, and some pretended to be deaf or blind or insane. Remembering some story they had heard, some drank quantities of vinegar to produce pallor.

From such cowardice it is pleasant to pass for a moment to examples of malingering for more noble ends. In both world wars some of the most interesting personal odysseys have been those of the gallant officers and men who escaped from prisoner-of-war camps. In many cases these men feigned symptoms of disease in order to gain a transfer to a less heavily guarded hospital or some respite in the watch constantly kept on them. E. H. Jones (1920) in *The road to En-dor* has written one of the classical examples of escape literature. He and C. W. Hill, after valiantly bearing many hardships, were released from their captivity in Turkey by various masterpieces of deceipt played on their captors. Coached by a doctor who was a fellow prisoner, they simulated general paresis and depression; so good was the coaching and so realistic were the pretended symptoms that their investigation by competent but puzzled Turkish neurologists makes fascinating reading.

Unfortunately, the pleasing tales of malingering form only a short portion of its history; there are far too many examples of malingering for an ulterior motive, no matter where the country or when the period. Purposive mutilation of the thumbs was mentioned above as a feature of Napoleonic days. Nothing is new under the sun, and in a short note by Montaigne (very appropriately the previous essay is entitled "Of not malingering. How a man should not counterfeit to be sicke!") we learn that a similar vicious custom was well known to Romans who lacked virtue. These skulkers were astute enough to suffer the mutilations, even if the lottery of fate directed their war service to the naval forces. Inability to hold a sword or spear was not the only reason for the action of these degraded cowards; they recognized that the use of an oar necessitated the same digits. In later centuries the thumb's action in pulling back the bowstring was responsible for its deliberate amputation. The modern war of machines did not thwart the planners of organized criminal surgical amputations, for they soon learned to promote "accidents" requiring removal of the great toe with the subsequent loss of the plantar arch, making walking impossible. The relatively low incidence of such degraded self-injuries and malingering in its other manifestations in the wars

305

of the present century has many explanations offered by exponents of such widely different theories as that which ascribes the phenomenon to the success of mass propaganda inculcating the justice of the combatants' cause, or, in complete contrast, the unpleasantly cynical suggestion that malingering is as widespread as ever but is now disguised under the cloak of such psychiatric diagnoses as "battle-neurosis."

It has been mentioned above that service morale has always depended on the opinion held by fighting men of their care if wounded. Efficient succor of the stricken in battle is a feature of warfare found only in modern times. Field ambulances first appeared in the Napoleonic wars as a product of Baron Larrey's consecrated zeal for his soldiers' welfare. Fifty years later the battle of Solferino resulted in such a stricken field that Henri Dunant had the inspiration for adequate military medical practices that was to conquer the civilized world. The prodigious success of modern military medicine and surgery, combined with the increasing interest in the provision of decent living conditions for soldiers and sailors, are very important factors in the maintenance of modern morale. There is no doubt that the frequency of such obvious crimes as the mutilations of the foot noted above was ridiculously exaggerated during World War I by the sensationalism inherent in the organization of modern news reporting. The present-day newspaper has increasingly manifested a tendency to linger on the unpleasant matters of all it illuminates, as if it wished to confirm the adage of bad news travelling fast.

It would be invidious to discuss the differences between the malingering activities of World War I and II or to contrast the frequencies in the hostile nations. The historian of the subject can note with interest the introduction of novel methods of "making a separate peace," as the amusing slang phrase has it. It was not long after the introduction of cordite as a rifle bullet propellant that some brave researcher was able to spread the knowledge of its action in producing signs and symptoms of cardiovascular ailments, and the issue of picric acid as an antiseptic soon led by an obvious association of ideas to its use in the artificial appearance of jaundice. Modern belief of the nature of contagious diseases and the means of infection was the cause, no matter how indirect, of the popularity of one ancient *fille de joie* who flourished in Kiel during the last few years of World War I. Sailors of the submarine flotillas learned to find temporary release from their doomed voyages in the neisserian infection certain to be the result of commerce with this disease-ridden drab whom, in derision, they honored as Madam Gonococca of Kiel. As a contrast to these "advances" in the science, or rather art, of malingering, it gives the impartial observer great pleasure to record a discovery of equal merit in the detection of such devices. Soon after the advent of electroencephalography as a useful means of investigation in various cerebral dysfunctions, it was pointed out that the wave patterns could be applied to the detection of shammers claiming total loss of vision in one or both eyes. If with the eyes open the alpha waves persist, it is certain that true blindness exists, but if these waves vanish, it is equally certain that the subject of the test is seeing something. It is gratifying to learn that re-examination with the electroencephalogram has shown some pensioners to be simulating blindness when every other means of estimating vision had tended to confirm their fraud.

Many papers and medical monographs having the pretence of disease as their subject dwell with great emphasis on the opportunity for fraud inherent in the introduction of such socially beneficial legislation as the National Health Insurance schemes and the Workmen's Compensation Act. Similar Cassandra-like predictions have been made about compulsory automobile insurance regulations and the present-day Health Services in Britain The author cannot subscribe to these jeremiads. He believes that these merciful laws have shown from their published results as well as from the experience of the medical men who implement them that their exploitation has not been any greater than one would expect from consideration of the precarious balance of virtue and evil in human nature. Certainly any experienced examiner of automobile casualties would declare that deliberate malingering is excessively rare. Optimism in thinking that a new morality has come into being is foolish and to be deprecated. The attractions of evil are still very much with us, and care will always be necessary against such mercenary ruffians as the author's personal patient who charged two guineas for his sputum, guaranteed positive for tubercle bacilli, so that pretenders to "chest troubles" resulting from World War I could start prolonged epochs of robbery at the expense of H. M. Ministry of Pensions.

§ REFERENCES

Castiglioni, A. (1941): *A history of medicine.* Translated from the Italian and edited by E. B. Krumbhaar. New York, Alfred A. Knopf.

Collie, Sir J. (1913): *Malingering and feigned sickness.* London, Edward Arnold.

Collie, Sir J. (1934): "Malingering." In *A short history of some common diseases.* Edited by W. R. Bett. London, Oxford University Press. Pp. 191–201.

Coulton, G. G. (1935): *Life in the middle ages.* Cambridge, Cambridge University Press. P. 361.

Coulton, G. G. (1938): *Medieval panorama.* Cambridge, Cambridge University Press.

Creighton, C. (1891): *History of epidemics in Britain.* Cambridge, Cambridge University Press.

Davitt, M. (1885): *Leaves from a prison diary.* 2 vols. London, Chapman and Hall.

DeJong, R. N. (1950): *The neurologic examination.* London, Cassell & Co. P. 932.

Dostoyevsky, F. (1911): *The house of the dead.* London, J. M. Dent and Sons.

Erckmann-Chatrian, M. M. (1870): *Conscript: a tale of the French war of 1813.* London, Smith, Elder & Co.

Galen (1929): In *Greek medicine.* Translated and annotated by A. J. Brock. London and Toronto, J. M. Dent.

Garrison, F. H. (1929): *An introduction to the history of medicine.* 4th ed. Philadelphia and London, W. B. Saunders.

Gavin, H. (1843): *On feigned and factitious diseases.* London, John Churchill.

Griffiths, A. (1893): *Secrets of the prisonhouse, or gaol studies.* London, Chapman and Hall.

Guthrie, D. (1945): *A history of medicine.* London, Thomas Nelson and Sons.

Haggard, H. W. (1934): *The doctor in history.* New Haven, Yale University Press. P. 164.

Hecker, J. F. C. (1844): *The epidemics of the middle ages.* London, Sydenham Society.

Jones, E. H. (1920): *The road to En-dor.* 5th ed. London, John Lane.

Mayhew, H. (1950): *London's underworld: selections from London labour and the London poor.* London, William Kimber.

Macartney, W. (1936): *Walls have mouths: a record of ten years' penal servitude.* London, Victor Gollancz.

Paré, A. (1951): *The apologie and treatise of Ambroise Paré.* Edited and with an introduction by G. Keynes. London, Falcon Educational Books.

Temkin, O. (1945): *The falling sickness: a history of epilepsy from the Greeks to the beginnings of modern neurology.* Baltimore, Johns Hopkins Press.

Thurston, H. (1952): *The physical phenomena of mysticism.* Edited by J. H. Crehan. London, Burns Oates.

Whitwell, J. R. (1946): *Analecta psychiatrica.* London, H. K. Lewis. P. 8.

Malingering

For a general survey of the medicine of prehistoric times and the early civilizations, use has been extensively made of Sigerist, H. E. (1951): *A history of medicine*. New York, Oxford University Press. Vol. I. This work is of incomparable value to all writers on medicine of the epochs surveyed, and its merit causes the other six volumes which are contemplated to be eagerly awaited. To those interested in the infinite varieties of service malingering, Gavin's book will be found to be of absorbing interest. The work is not generally available, so see résumé Murphy, E. L. (1953): *J. Irish med. Ass., 32* 9–17.

GLOSSARY OF MEDICAL TERMS

achondroplasia: Congenital dwarfism caused by disordered bone formation.

acromegaly: Progressive enlargement of head, hands, feet, and chest, as a result of hyperactivity of the pituitary gland in the brain.

adenitis: Inflammation of a lymph gland.

adenoma: Tumor composed of glandular tissue, usually innocent.

aegophony (egophony): Bleating character, like a goat, of the patient's voice heard when listening to the chest over a compressed lung, at the upper border of fluid.

agranulocytosis: Febrile disease characterized by marked reduction of granulocytes (white blood cells).

albuminuria: Excretion of albumin (a protein substance) in the urine.

albumosuria: Presence of albumose (an albuminous substance) in the urine.

anaerobic: Growing in the absence of oxygen or air.

anaplasia: Reversion of cells to the embryonic type.

anastasis: Recovery, convalescence.

anastomosis: 1. Communication between two blood vessels. 2. Establishment of a communication between two hollow organs.

aneurysm: Circumscribed dilatation of the wall of an artery, forming a pulsating tumor.

angina pectoris: Attacks of severe constricting pain in the chest.

ankylosing spondylitis: Arthritis of spine with ossification of ligaments and complete stiffness of back.

anorexia nervosa: Hysterical aversion to food.

anoxemia: Lack of oxygen in the blood.

antigen: Substance stimulating production of antibodies.

anuria: Suppression of urine.

aortic stenosis: Abnormal narrowing of the orifice of the aorta at the base of the heart.

arrhythmia: Variation from normal rhythm of the heartbeat.

atheroma: Fatty degeneration of the walls of the arteries.

auscultation: Examination of an organ (heart, lungs) by listening to the sounds arising from it.

basal cell: One of the cells of the deepest layer of stratified epithelium.

Bilharzia: Blood fluke responsible for hematuria.

bubo: Inflamed lymph gland in groin or armpit.

bulbus cordis: Part of the embryonic heart.

bursitis: Inflammation of sac over bony prominences.

cachexia: Weakness and wasting caused by some chronic constitutional affection such as cancer.

carcinogen: Cancer-producing agent.

carcinoma: Malignant epithelial tumor.

cardiolipin antigens: Substances extracted from beef hearts and used in serological tests for syphilis.

carpopedal: Affecting wrist and foot, or fingers and toes.

cataplasm: Poultice.

cholangiography: X-ray visualization of gall bladder and bile ducts.

cholecystitis: Inflammation of gall bladder.

choledochotomy: Incision into common bile duct.

cicatrix: Scar

cirrhosis: Degenerative disease of the liver.

clyster: Enema.

collagen: Albuminoid constituent of fibrous tissue, converted into gelatin on boiling.

coronary thrombosis: Clotting of blood in a coronary artery of the heart muscle.

cribriform: Perforated like a sieve.

cyanosis: Bluish discoloration of skin and mucous membranes.

cynanche: Old name for severe sore throat with threat of suffocation.

cystic mastopathy: Cystic disease of breast.

desquamation: Shedding of superficial epithelium.

dysostosis: Defective formation of bone.

dyspnea: Difficulty in breathing.

edema: Excessive accumulation of fluid in the tissue spaces.

emphysema: Abnormal distension of tissue by air or gas.

empyema: Presence of pus in pleural or other cavity.

endemic: Said of a disease constantly prevalent in a particular locality.

Glossary of Medical Terms

eosinophile cells: Cells readily stained with eosin or other acid dyes.

epithelioma: Tumor derived from epithelium.

erysipelas: Acute infectious disease of skin and subcutaneous tissues caused by a streptococcus.

erythema: Redness of skin.

etiology: Study of causation of disease.

exanthema: Eruption of skin.

extravasation: Passing of body fluid out of its proper place.

fibrillation: 1. Formation of fibrils. 2. Local twitching of muscle fibers.

fibromyoma: Innocent tumor consisting of fibrous tissue and muscle.

fibrositis: Inflammatory proliferation of fibrous tissue.

galbanum: Gum resin used as expectorant and stimulant.

hematuria: Passing of blood in urine.

hemoglobinuria: Presence of hemoglobin (red blood-cell pigment) in urine.

hemolytic: Relating to liberation of hemoglobin.

hemoptysis: Spitting of blood.

hepatization: Conversion of tissue into a liverlike substance, e.g. lungs in pneumonia.

hepatoma: Tumor of liver.

hermodactyl: Root formerly used in medicine.

hydrarthrosis: Accumulation of fluid in a joint.

hyperplasia: Increase in size of a tissue or organ, because of increase in number of cells.

hypochondrium: Upper lateral region of abdomen below lower ribs.

hypoglycemia: Low sugar level in the blood.

infarct: Area of necrosis (local tissue death) due to complete interference with blood flow.

ischemia: Local diminution in blood supply.

laryngismus: Spasm of larynx.

leucosis (leukemia): Disease of blood-forming organs with excessive proliferation of white blood cells.

linctus: Sirupy medicine.

macrogenitosomia: Precocious development with large genitals.

mesenchyme: Part of mesoderm (embryonic tissue) producing connective tissue, blood, etc.

metastasis: Spread of disease from a primary focus to distant parts of the body through blood or lymph vessels.

microcephaly: Abnormal congenital smallness of head and brain.

mitral stenosis: Narrowing of mitral valve of left side of heart.

morbilli: Measles.

moxa: Combustible material applied to the skin to produce a scar.

myeloma: Malignant tumor of bone marrow.

myocardium: Muscular tissue of heart.

myomalacia cordis: Softening of heart muscle.

myositis: Inflammation of muscle.

necropsy: Post-mortem examination (autopsy).

neisserian: Genus of bacilli (cocci) named after Max Neisser.

neoplasia: Formation of new tissue or of tumors.

neurogenic arthropathy: Osteoarthritis with nutritional (trophic) disturbance.

nevi: Circumscribed pigmented or vascular areas of skin; a birthmark, mole, or vascular tumor.

nosography: Systematic description of disease.

nosology: Science of classification of diseases.

oöphorectomy: Removal of ovary.

osteitis fibrosa cystica: Inflammation of bone with fibrous degeneration and cyst formation (von Recklinghausen's disease).

osteochondrodystrophy: Degeneration of bone and cartilage.

osteogenesis imperfecta: Hereditary abnormal brittleness of long bones (*fragilitas ossium*).

otitis: Inflammation of ear.

oxymel: Mixture of honey, water, and vinegar.

pandemic: Epidemic over a wide geographical area.

papilloma: Tumor derived from superficial epithelium—benign, but tending to recur.

parabiosis: Union of two individuals in several or all of the vital processes, as in the case of joined twins.

parenchyma: Essential tissue of an organ as opposed to the supporting connective tissue.

paresis: Slight paralysis.

paries: Enveloping structure or wall.

pathogens: Agents capable of causing disease.

314

pathognomic (pathognomonic): Characteristic of a disease, distinguishing it from other diseases.

pectoriloquy: Distinct transmission of the voice on listening to the chest (heard over solid lung).

pericardium: Membranous sac enveloping the heart.

peripneumonia: Old term for lobar pneumonia involving the membrane of the lung.

perityphlitis: Old term for appendicitis.

phaeochromocytoma: Tumor of sympathetic nervous system, found in adrenal glands.

pineal *pubertas praecox:* Puberty at an early age, caused by tumor of the pineal gland.

polyposis: Presence of polypi (projecting masses of swollen and hypertrophied mucous membrane).

polyuria: Excessive excretion of urine.

precordia: Area of chest overlying the heart.

prodromal: Relating to early manifestations or symptoms of a disease.

prolan: Hormone derived from the pituitary gland.

puerperal: Relating to childbirth.

pyrexia: Fever.

râle: Abnormal sound in the chest heard on auscultation.

rubefacient: Agent causing the skin to redden.

sarcoma: Malignant tumor composed of connective tissue.

scleroderma: Disease marked by hardening of the skin.

scorbutic: Pertaining to scurvy.

scrofula: Formerly applied to a variety of conditions, most of which are now considered to be tuberculous glands of the neck.

septum: Dividing wall between two cavities or spaces.

sequela: Abnormal state following as a consequence of a disease.

seton: Thread drawn through the skin as a means of counter irritation.

spirillum: Genus of spiral bacilli.

spirochete: Spiral organism of the family Spirochaetaceae.

status thymicolymphaticus: Condition marked by increase in size of the lymphatic structures, and especially by persistence of the thymus gland.

stroma: Supporting framework of an organ.

struma: Goiter.

suppuration: Formation of pus.

syndrome: Group of symptoms and signs characterizing a disease.

teratoma: Congenital tumor containing substances not normally found in the part where it grows, and resulting from embryonic misplacement of tissue.

tophaceous: Gritty (as in gouty deposits).

traumatism: Condition produced by injury.

trephine: 1. Instrument for excising a circular piece of bone, usually from the skull. 2. Operate with the trephine.

treponemal: Relating to a genus of spiral microorganisms of the family Treponemaceae.

trypanosomes: Genus of protozoal parasites causing sleeping sickness, etc.

valgus: Bowlegged or knock-kneed (talipes valgus; *genu valgum*).

varus: Turned inward (talipes varus).

venesection: Opening of a vein in order to let blood.

wet cupping: Application of a cup to the incised skin in order to abstract blood.

xerophthalmia: Dry, thickened state of the conjunctiva.

xiphoid articulation: Sword-shaped process at lower end of sternum (breastbone).

index of subjects

Acromegaly, tumor removal in: 211–12
ACTH, discovery of: 122
Addison's disease: 209
Adenoids: first description of, 176; association with mental retardation, 177
Adenoma, toxic, differentiated from Graves' disease: 206
Adiposogenital dystrophy, Babinski's description: 212
Adirondack Cottage Sanatorium: 109
Adrenalectomy, development in England: 210
Adrenalin, rickets treated by: 195
Albuminuria, classification of: 166–67
Angina: Bard's monograph on *angina suffocativa,* 13; relieved by vasodilators, 148; ischemia of heart muscle as cause, 148; Osler's Lumleian lectures on, 150
Ankylosing spondylitis, first account of: 121
Appendectomy: first recorded success, 237; first deliberate, 238
Appendicitis: etiology of, 239; term first used, 239; operation on Edward VII, 239–40; waiting policy in, 241
Arsenites, causing epithelioma: 270
Arthritis: rheumatoid, differentiated from osteoarthritis, 120–21, 133; juvenile rheumatoid, 122; psoriasis in, 133–34; "infectious arthritis," 136; gonorrheal, 136
Arthritis deformans, term suggested: 133
Arthropathia psoriatica: 134
Auricular flutter, first described: 145

"Back pressure" theory of heart failure: 154
Bismuth, in treatment of syphilis: 186
Blood pressure, high, in kidney disease: 151, 165
Bright's disease: 163–69

Index of Subjects

Goiter: iodine for, 208; surgery of, 208; burnt sponge and seaweed for, 208
Gonococcus, identification of: 182
Gout: term first used, 115, 128; Sydenham on, 117; colchicum in, 119; urates in blood of gouty, 130
Graves' disease: 205; differentiated from toxic adenoma, 206; iodine in, 206

Heart: disease following acute rheumatism, 117; heart block, 144–45; relationship between renal and cardiac disease, 151; congenital diseases of, 152–53
Heberden's nodes: 121, 132, 135
Hematuria, distinguished from hemoglobinuria: 167
Hemoglobinuria, distinguished from hematuria: 167
Hemophilus influenzae, description of: 78
Hemophilus pertussis, observation and cultivation of: 63
Hemorrhage, cerebral, connected with renal disease: 166
Hyperpiesia: 151–52

Influenza: epidemics, 71–72; discovery of influenza virus A, 78; of virus B, 78; *Hemophilus influenzae* described, 78; observations on swine influenza, 79
Inoculation: for smallpox, 51; of Catherine II, 53; in America, 54
Insulin, discovery of: 214
Internal secretion, doctrine of: 204
Iodine: in Graves' disease, 206; for goiter, 208

Kidneys: arterial thickening in kidney disease, 151; high blood pressure, 151, 165; relationship between renal and cardiac disease, 151; Hippocrates on, 157; hardening of, 159–60; in dropsy, 162; cerebral hemorrhage and renal disease, 166; phenolsulphonephthalein test of renal function, 167
Koplik's spots: 45

Lancefield group of streptococci: 37
Luminal, in treatment of epileptic convulsions: 256

Measles: confused with scarlet fever, 29, named, 39; epidemic in Faroes, 42–43; first successful transmission of, 44; Koplik's spots, 45; first clear account of German measles, 45–46
Miners' phthisis, described by Paracelsus: 102
Mitral stenosis, bruissement in: 141
Mumps, discovery of causative agent: 60

index of names

Abbott, Maude, *Atlas of congenital cardiac disease:* 153
Abraham, J. Johnston, on sale of sarsaparilla in London streets: 185
Adams, Robert, advocates term "chronic rheumatic arthritis": 132
Addison, Thomas: on origin of pneumonia in air cells of lungs, 92; Addison's disease, 209
Aëtius of Amida: description of disease resembling diphtheria, 7; of kidney sclerosis, 159
Alibert, Jean Louis Marc, first notes psoriasis in arthritis: 133–34
Allbutt, Sir Clifford, recognizes "hyperpiesia": 151–52
Amyand, Claudius, first recorded successful appendectomy: 236
Andrewes, Christopher Howard, discovery of influenza virus A: 78
Aretaeus: description of Egyptian or Syriac ulcer, 6–7; of peripneumonia, 85; on arthritis, 127; on gout, 129; on diabetes, 213; on epilepsy, 248–51
Arnold, Thomas, death from myocardial infarction: 149
Astruc, Jean, writes treatise on syphilis: 182
Auenbrugger, Leopold: discovery of percussion as diagnostic aid, 89, 105, 141; detects fluid in pericardial sac, 153
Avicenna, on hardening of kidneys: 160

Babinski, Joseph, describes adiposogenital dystrophy: 212
Baillie, Matthew, on hepatization of lungs in pneumonia: 88
Baillou, Guillaume de: description of diphtheria, 9–10; detailed description of whooping cough, 61–62; differentiates gout from rheumatism, 116; uses "rheumatism" in sense of acute polyarthritis, 116, 129
Balzer, Félix, advocates bismuth for treating syphilis: 186
Bannatyne, G. A., differentiates rheumatoid arthritis from osteoarthritis: 120
Banting, Sir Frederick Grant, discovery of insulin: 214
Bard, Samuel, monograph on *angina suffocativa:* 13
Barlow, Sir Thomas, separates scurvy from rickets: 194

Index of Names

Broussais, François Joseph Victor, advocates operation in precancerous stage: 277

Browne, Sir Thomas, on rooks' livers for rickets: 199

Brunton, Sir Thomas Lauder, relieves angina pectoris by a vasodilator: 148

Bumstead, Freeman, uses term "chancroid": 178

Burns, Allan, recognizes ischaemia of heart muscle as cause of angina: 148

Butlin, Sir Henry Trentham: on malignant changes, 265; on scrotal cancer, 267

Caelius Aurelianus, on arthritis and rheumatism: 127

Carpi, Giacomo Berengario da, describes appendix as anatomical organ: 234

Carson, James, recommends artificial therapeutic pneumothorax: 104

Cedrenus, on cynanche in Byzantine Empire: 8

Celsus: first description of tonsillotomy, 171; on phimosis, 179–80; on epilepsy, 249

Charcot, Jean-Martin, regards rheumatoid arthritis and osteoarthritis as variants of one disease: 121

Chauffard, Anatole, describes juvenile rheumatoid arthritis: 122

Chick, Harriette, studies on rickets: 198

Churchill, Edward Delos, operative release of constrictive pericardial adhesions: 154

Churchill, Sir Winston, probably saved by sulphapyridine: 96

Cohnheim, Julius, notes "forward failure" theory of heart failure: 154

Coindet, Jean François, iodine treatment of goiter: 208

Cole, William Harder, introduction of cholecystography: 230

Colles, Abraham, "Colles's law": 183

Collip, James Bertram, discovers parathormone: 216

Connor, Bernard, first account of ankylosing spondylitis: 121

Cooke, William, recognizes female *pubertas praecox* connected with adrenocortical hyperplasia: 210

Cortesius of Messina, on contagiousness of diphtheria: 11

Corvisart, Jean Nicolas: describes thrill (bruissement) of mitral stenosis, 141; studies size and shape of heart, 142

Coulton, George Gordon, on faked cures and malingering: 295–96

Courvoisier, Ludwig George, on gallstones: 223–24

Crafoord, Clarence, excision of coarctation in aorta: 153

Cullen, William: on pneumonia, 87; treatment by bleeding, 87–88

Cummins, S. Lyle, on Trudeau's contribution to tuberculosis management: 110

Cushing, Harvey: Cushing's disease, 211; applies X-rays to pituitary, 211; on hypersecretion of growth hormone in acromegaly, 211

Index of Names

John of Gaddesden: introduction of term "measles," 39; on treatment of epilepsy, 251

Johnson, C. D., discovers causative agent of mumps: 60

Kendall, Edward Calvin, discovery of cortisone and ACTH: 122

Kilpatrick, James, revives practice of smallpox inoculation: 52–53

Kirkes, William Senhouse, connects cerebral hemorrhage with renal disease: 166

Kitasato, Shibasaburo, discovery of tetanus antitoxin: 21

Klebs, Edwin: discovers causal organism in diphtheria, 19–20; proves existence of bovine tuberculosis, 107

Koch, Robert: discovery of tubercle bacillus, 108; *The etiology of tuberculosis,* 109

Kölliker, Albert von, microscopic study of faucial tonsils: 175

Koplik, Henry, notes importance of buccal spots in diagnosis of measles: 45

Laënnec, René Théophile Hyacinthe: discovery of the stethoscope, 89–92; studies on tuberculosis, 106–107; describes heart sounds, 142; studies size and shape of heart, 142; describes signs of active pericarditis, 154

Laidlaw, Sir Patrick Playfair, discovery of influenza virus A: 78

Lancefield, Rebecca C., grouping of streptococci: 37

Landré-Beauvais, Augustin Jacob, describes rheumatoid arthritis: 119, 132

Lanz, O., thyroid treatment of rickets: 195

Le Dran, Henry François, on spread of cancer by lymphatics: 261

Leichtenstern, Otto, on influenza epidemics: 71–72

Levaditi, Constantin, revives bismuth treatment for syphilis: 186

Levison, George, clinical observations on scarlet fever: 32–33

Lewis, Sir Thomas: on auricular fibrillation, 144; on electrocardiography, 150

Locock, Sir Charles, on bromides for epilepsy, 256

Loeffler, Friedrich, cultivates *C. diphtheriae:* 20

Louis, Pierre Charles Alexander, supports unitarian theory of tuberculosis: 107

McArthur, Lewis Linn, describes gridiron incision: 240

Macaulay, Thomas Babington, on smallpox: 49

McBurney, Charles, "McBurney's point": 240

Mackenzie, Sir James: *The study of the pulse,* 144; on angina, 149–50; supports "forward" theory of heart failure, 155

Maclagan, Thomas John, discovers salicin as remedy for rheumatic fever: 122

Index of Names

Traube, Ludwig, on relationship between renal and cardiac disease: 151

Treves, Sir Frederick: on "relapsing typhlitis," 238; operates on Edward VII, 239–40

Trudeau, Edward Livingston: founds Adirondack Cottage Sanatorium, 109; cultures tubercle bacillus, 110; contribution to tuberculosis management, 110

Unna, Paul Gerson, attributes skin cancers to sunlight: 272

Vierordt, Karl, invents instrument for estimating blood pressure: 165

Villemin, Jean-Antoine, proves that tuberculosis is a specific infection: 105

Virchow, Rudolph: opposes unitarian theory of phthisis, 107; suggests term *arthritis deformans,* 133; cellular pathology, 264

Volhard, Franz, classification of albuminuria: 166–67

Voltolini, Frederick Edward Rudolph, introduces posterior rhinoscopy: 176

Wagner von Jauregg, Julius, introduces fever therapy in syphilis: 186

Waksman, Selman Abraham, discovers streptomycin: 113

Wallace, William, introduces potassium iodide in treatment of syphilis: 185

Wassermann, August von, evolves complement fixation test for syphilis: 183

Waterhouse, Benjamin: introduces Jennerian vaccination into North America, 56; on *tussis convulsiva,* 62

Watson, Sir Patrick Heron, performs partial thyroidectomy: 206

Waugh, George Ernest, method of tonsil dissection: 174

Wells, William Charles, on urine and kidneys in dropsy: 162

Whistler, Daniel: thesis on rickets, 191; on origin of name "rickets," 191

White, Paul Dudley, operative release of constrictive pericardial adhesions: 154

Wilbraham, Anne, on rickets in England during periods of dearth: 193

Willcox, Sir William, theory of "focal sepsis": 120

Williams, Francis Henry, introduces X-ray treatment of thyroid diseases: 207

Willis, Thomas: on age and seasonal incidence of whooping cough, 62; on cause of consumption, 103; on epilepsy, 254–55

Wiseman, Richard: on tuberculosis of joints, 102, 136; coins term *tumor albus,* 102; on tonsil surgery, 172–73

Withering, William: clinical observations on scarlet fever, 32–33; on occupational influences in tuberculosis, 104; on tuberculosis as infectious disease, 104

Wollaston, William Hyde, demonstrates sodium urate in tophi: 129

THE HISTORY AND CONQUEST OF

common diseases

has been composed on the Linotype machine in
Granjon, a type which has enjoyed wide popularity for some thirty years because of its unobtrusive
clarity, and has been printed directly from type.
The paper is fifty-pound antique wove.

UNIVERSITY OF OKLAHOMA PRESS

NORMAN